Oxford Textbook of

Infectious Disease Control

Start using the online version today at www.oxfordmedicine.com

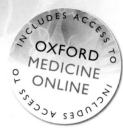

Thank you for purchasing this work from Oxford University Press. The purchase price includes twelve months' access to the online version. To get started, register your access token, which you'll find bound into the front of this book, at

https://subscriberservices.sams.oup.com/token

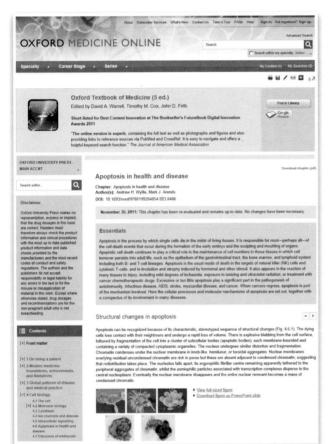

THE ONLINE VERSION ENABLES YOU TO:

- Find exactly what you're looking for, using the 'quick search' and advanced search functions

- Navigate around the content quickly and easily

- Share content with colleagues using integrated tools including social bookmarking, email and citation export

- Return to frequently-used content by saving searches and favourite chapters

- Enlarge images and charts, or download them to PDF or PowerPoint

- Access the content wherever you are, from your desktop, mobile device or tablet

Once your twelve months' access has expired, you can extend your online access by taking out a subscription, and take advantage of our renewal discounts for book purchasers.

Start using your online access today.

Visit https://subscriberservices.sams.oup.com/token and register your access code

(Inclusive online access is only available to individuals.)

And why not recommend Oxford Medicine Online to your librarian?

Free trials are available for institutions, simply visit www.oup.com/online/freetrials/

Oxford Textbook of
Infectious
Disease Control

A Geographical Analysis from Medieval Quarantine to Global Eradication

Andrew Cliff

Matthew Smallman-Raynor

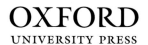

OXFORD
UNIVERSITY PRESS

OXFORD
UNIVERSITY PRESS

Great Clarendon Street, Oxford, OX2 6DP,
United Kingdom

Oxford University Press is a department of the University of Oxford.
It furthers the University's objective of excellence in research, scholarship,
and education by publishing worldwide. Oxford is a registered trade mark of
Oxford University Press in the UK and in certain other countries

British Library Cataloguing in Publication Data
Data available

Library of Congress Cataloguing in Publication Data
Data available

ISBN 978–0–19–959661–4

Printed in China through
Asia Pacific Offset

Oxford University Press makes no representation, express or implied, that
the drug dosages in this book are correct. Readers must therefore always check
the product information and clinical procedures with the most up-to-date
published product information and data sheets provided by the manufacturers
and the most recent codes of conduct and safety regulations. The authors and
the publishers do not accept responsibility or legal liability for any errors in the
text or for the misuse or misapplication of material in this work. Except where
otherwise stated, drug dosages and recommendations are for the non-pregnant
adult who is not breast-feeding.

Contents

Acknowledgements

The authors and publisher are grateful for permission to reproduce the following material:

World Health Organization (Figures 1.5, 2.1 lower, 2.24, 2.25 group photograph, 2.30, 2.32, 2.39, 2.40, 3.18 lower, 3.32 cottage, 4.8, 5.4, 5.5, 5.12, 5.13, 5.19, 6.17, 6.36)

Wellcome Library, London (Figures 1.1, 1.4 upper and lower centre, 2.8A, 2.13A, 3.1, 3.13, 3.16, 3.17, 3.19, 3.23, 3.24 upper, 3.31 upper, 4.2 left and centre, 6.1)

Wellcome Photo Library, London (Figure 3.18 upper)

Pan American Health Organization/World Health Organization (Figures 4.9, 5.8, 5.22, 5.23)

UNICEF (Figure 2.25 Rajchman)

WHO Regional Office for South East Asia (SEARO) (Figures 2.36, 2.37)

National Academy of Sciences, USA, copyright 2006, Figure 3 (Figure 5.25)

© Corbis Images (Figure 3.31 lower)

© Mary Evans Picture Library (Figure 3.32 newspaper)

Office of the New York County Clerk (Figure 3.32 index card)

Dixson Gallery, State Library of New South Wales, call number DGD 3/7 (Figure 3.15 inset)

Local Population Studies (Figure 3.21)

English Heritage (Figure 3.25)

Western Pacific Region/World Health Organization (Figure 3.46)

John Wiley and Sons/RightsLink® (Figure 4.7)

Australian War Memorial (Figure 6.6 upper right)

John Oxley Library, State Library of Queensland Neg: 44398 (Figure 6.6 lower left)

Oxford Journals/Oxford University Press RightsLink® (Figure 6.7)

Although every effort has been made to trace and contact copyright holders, this has not always been successful. We apologise for any apparent negligence.

Preface

This book begins seven centuries ago among the lazarettos of Venice and ends among the saints of Palermo. Both lazarettos and saints in different ways – the first by quarantine and isolation and the second by alleged cure – attempted to control the geographical spread of communicable diseases. Although modern readers will show askance at the notion of saints against disease, saints for and against almost anything were deeply embedded in the life and culture of medieval Europe. And it was in medieval Europe that the first significant attempts at controlling the spread of communicable diseases began. Religion was central and scientific knowledge scant. Against what we now know to be communicable diseases, saints like Rosalia of Palermo (1130–70), who was alleged to have halted the spread of the Plague of Palermo in 1624, were and still are commonly appealed to. There are six cities in Latin America alone named after her. In the twenty-first century, like Rosalia, the world is still working at disease control, eradication and elimination. As this book is being written, in an initiative dubbed the *London Declaration on Neglected Tropical Diseases*, a coalition of 13 global drugs companies brought together by the Bill and Melinda Gates Foundation aims to provide 1.4 billion treatments annually to eradicate five neglected tropical diseases and to bring a further five under control in the developing world. The World Health Organization's roadmap to elimination in support of the London Declaration appears in the **Preface table**.

The geographical control of human communicable diseases is touched on in many books but this is the first systematic monograph devoted to the topic. In six chapters it tackles surveillance, quarantine, vaccination, and forecasting for disease control. In the twenty-first century, with an armoury of early warning and vaccination methods at our disposal, it is easy to forget that, by the middle of the seventeenth century, the states of Italy had already developed a sophisticated spatial system to try to control the spread of plague, a system which involved surveillance, border controls, medical passports for goods and people, quarantine and forecasting. As noted in Cipolla (1976, pp. 65–6), the concept of health organisation as developed in the renaissance Italian states eventually found systematic expression and elaboration in the late 1770s in the *System einer vollständigen Medizinischen Polizey* by Johann Peter Frank (1745–1821), volumes 1–4 of which were first published in Mannheim in 1779–88. Volume 5 appeared in Tübingen in 1813, and volume 6 in Vienna in two parts in 1817–19. But the philosophical mood of the times by the end of the eighteenth century favoured the individual, and the state was seen as a centralised oppressor. Plague also disappeared, and with its disappearance, opposition to health controls and regulations became progressively more vociferous. *Laissez faire* prevailed and when cholera struck *The Times* observed people "would rather take the risk of cholera and the rest than to be bullied into health", Italian ideas on control were regarded as obsolete and abandoned until the modern period. Then it took the vision and energy of people like Benjamin Disraeli and Sir John Simon once again to develop the concept and to set up a system of Public Health. There was rediscovery rather than continuity on methods of disease control and this time the British and the French led the way, uncovering once more many of the Italian ideas now used in current disease control systems. And so in Chapter 1 we begin our story of the geographical control of human communicable diseases by describing the elements of the Italian system and their operation as a backcloth to our substantive treatment of infectious disease control in the five chapters which follow.

Infectious diseases spread from person to person and so from place to place. Thus the control of spread has a strong geographical component which, given our own interests and a lifetime working as professional geographers, is central to our consideration of the control problem. We explore the geographical dynamics of control through our selection of diseases and themes which can either be analysed statistically over substantial historical time spans or which can be mapped in specific geographical settings. In each chapter, we have tried to assemble representative maps to illustrate the ideas we explore.

As we have noted elsewhere, for the authors, this book is part of a much larger canvas on which we have been painting for more than a generation. There has been a series of epidemic disease monographs which focus on specific infectious diseases (notably measles, influenza and poliomyelitis), on specific epidemiological sources (the United States consular records of disease), and on specific themes (such as island epidemiology and the role of conflict in epidemic generation), and there have been atlases – on AIDS, disease mapping and epidemics in Britain. As on previous occasions, we have been particularly blessed by the resources made available to us by Tomas Allen at the library and archives of the World Health Organization. These resources were placed at our disposal to complement the great collections on epidemic history in our own university libraries and medical schools. We record with gratitude the contributions of all the skilled staff in these places who have helped us.

Preface table Elimination and eradication of neglected tropical diseases. Target milestones by 2020

Disease	2015					2020			
		Elimination					Elimination		
	Eradication	Global	Regional	Country	Eradication	Global	Regional	Country
Rabies			Latin America					South-East Asia and Western Pacific regions	
Blinding trachoma							Yes		
Yaws					Yes				
Leprosy							Yes		
Chagas			Transmission by blood transfusion interrupted					Intra-domiciliary transmission interrupted in Americas	
Human African trypanosomiasis				In 80% of foci		Yes		
Visceral leishmaniasis								Indian subcontinent	
Guinea worm	Yes								
Lymphatic filariasis							Yes		
Onchocerciasis			Latin America	Yemen					Selected African countries
Schistosomiasis			Eastern Mediterranean, Caribbean, Indonesia, Mekong river basin					Americas and Western Pacific regions	Selected African countries

Source: World Health Organization (2012, Table 1a, p. 4).

We have also received financial help and generous support in kind. One of us (AC) was fortunate in retirement to be awarded a Leverhulme Trust Emeritus Fellowship which made the Geneva work possible, while the Department of Geography at the University of Cambridge has provided office space and, crucially, cartographic help. Philip Stickler, Head of the Cartographic Unit in the Department, has sustained the authors with his superb maps, graphs and diagrams for several books now, the last five of which have been published by Oxford University Press. At the Press, Nicola Wilson as medical commissioning editor and Viki Mortimer as production editor oversaw the complex task of integrating a large number of illustrations with a brief text. The design team must have wept on more than one occasion with the high image to text ratio.

Manuscript preparation is always an individual affair, and the authors have had a base for several years now at the Bull and Swan in Stamford where we meet regularly to exchange material – generally monthly which, for a time, was as frequently as the inn changed hands! Happily, stability has now returned. Those closest to us have inevitably borne the brunt of our obsession with research, with its periods of pre-occupation from other tasks. We let these pages stand as a token of our thanks to them.

ANDREW CLIFF
MATTHEW SMALLMAN-RAYNOR
Bull and Swan, Stamford
Feast of Santa Rosalia di Palermo, 2012

Front cover figure description: Painted panel, southern Italy (Kingdom of the Two Sicilies) c.1800. This scene shows the main elements of the context in which Italian states developed defences against the plague from the middle of the fourteenth century. The town with watch-towers on the hillside for surveillance, defensive walls penetrated by gates at which travellers and goods arriving would have had to show passports to gain entry, the estuary essential for trade and communication, and the harbour wall in the foreground. The system developed in Italy is described in detail in Chapter 1.

Rear cover figure description: The global eradication of smallpox. Statue erected outside the entrance to the main World Health Organization (WHO) building in Geneva, Switzerland. The bronze and stone statue was unveiled on 17 May 2010 by Dr Margaret Chan, Director-General of the WHO, to commemorate the thirtieth anniversary of the WHO's declaration of the global eradication of smallpox. The statue depicts four persons, one of whom is a girl who is about to be vaccinated by a health worker with a bifurcated needle. The bifurcated needle was designed to hold freeze dried smallpox vaccine between two prongs, with the vaccine administered by a technique (multiple puncture vaccination) that involved up to 15 insertions delivered in rapid succession in a circle of about 5 mm in diameter. The base of the statue shows the continents, while the plaques surrounding the statue (written in the six official languages of the WHO) state that the eradication of smallpox was made possible through the collaboration of nations.

CHAPTER 1

Containing the Spread of Epidemics

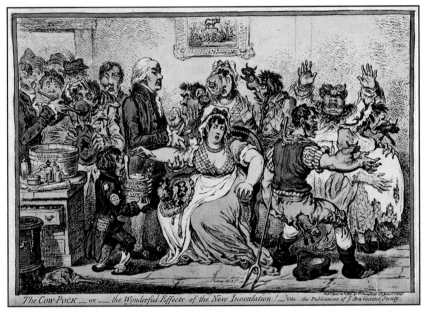

The COW-POCK __ or __ the Wonderful Effects of the New Inoculation!

Figure 1.1 Vaccination. Edward Jenner (1749–1823), whose general practice was located in Berkeley, Gloucestershire, is generally credited with the discovery in 1796 of cowpox vaccination to provide protection against smallpox. But it was in fact a Dorset farmer, Benjamin Jesty, who was the first person recorded as having inoculated a person with cowpox matter in order to protect against smallpox – the procedure subsequently known as vaccination. He carried out this procedure on his wife and sons in 1774, some twenty years before Edward Jenner independently performed the same operation in Gloucestershire. It was, however, certainly Jenner who made the procedure public and widely available to the population of his local area at the Temple of Vaccinia in Berkeley. The method was initially regarded with scepticism in many quarters as James Gillray's (1802) cartoon makes clear. It shows Jenner among patients at the Smallpox and Inoculation Hospital, St Pancras, London, vaccination point in hand, and a tin of cowpox held for him by a young ruffian. Recipients of the brew could expect to grow bits of cows. Notice also the use of "OPENING MIXTURE" on those queuing for vaccination to make it more efficacious! *Source*: Wellcome Library, London.

1.1 Introduction

From the time humans first lived in groups and communicable diseases of humans began to emerge, fear of the spread of infection from one person to another, from one community to another, from one country to another, and from one continent to another grew. And means were sought to contain such spread. The fear of pestilential spread found its way into early writing – for example, the biblical Pharonic plagues of Moses which selectively killed the firstborn of Egypt (Exodus, 12, 13); being spared of pestilence (1 Chronicles 22; Mark 5, 34); and the pale horse of Revelation 6 with dominion over a quarter of the earth and the power to kill *inter alia* by pestilence.

In medieval times, mystical writing about pestilence (one of the "wages of sin") was allied with practical methods to control the geographical diffusion of communicable disease. This reached a first zenith in Italy during the five plague centuries beginning with the Black Death of 1346–52. In the modern era, medical progress led to a second zenith by enabling the physical controls on disease spread used from early times, such as quarantine and barriers to movement, to be complemented by prophylactic methods and education. The first generally successful vaccinations were employed by Edward Jenner at the end of the eighteenth century to control the spread of smallpox (**Figure 1.1**). The medical developments of the twentieth century ushered in an apparently golden era of communicable disease prevention by vaccination against the great epidemic killing diseases of history. To smallpox, control was added for infections like diphtheria, whooping cough, scarlet fever, measles, mumps, rubella and poliomyelitis so that, by the last quarter of the twentieth century, the geographical spread of epidemic communicable diseases appeared largely to have been achieved. But it proved a false dawn as epidemics of new infections like HIV (human immunodeficiency virus) and SARS (severe acute respiratory syndrome) emerged alongside the growing drug resistance of others like tuberculosis to refocus the debate on how to control the geographical spread of communicable or infectious diseases.

It is this topic – controlling the spatial or geographical diffusion of infectious diseases – which forms the subject of this book. Many are capable of causing epidemics with widespread public health, demographic, social and economic consequences. As we shall see, there is a large literature on aspects of epidemic control, but very little of it is geographical. And yet control is an inherently geographical problem with surveillance at its core. In England, the importance of the spatial dimension and the need for surveillance was incisively summarised at the end of the nineteenth century by Tatham (1888, p. 403):

> Again and again we have had to complain of the importation of infection into Salford [England] from non-notification outside districts immediately contiguous to our boundaries…[E]ven between towns which possess powers for the compulsory notification of infectious disease, there exists at present no organization by which one sanitary authority may receive timely warning of the presence of infectious disease in the district of a neighbouring authority.

If epidemic diseases did not spread from person to person, and infected individuals move from area to area, containment would be relatively straightforward. But diseases and people do move. In the twenty-first century, mass airline travel has ensured that all inhabited points of the globe are within a day's flying time – within the incubation period of all communicable diseases of public health importance – and so, as W.H. Auden's 1938 poem, *Gare du Midi*,

succinctly summarises, it is possible for the seeds of an epidemic silently to arrive in a new geographical location unwitnessed until the damage is done. To this element of spread we can add the increasing tropicalisation of the human population as global warming increases the spatial extent of many diseases and grows the geographical range of "tropics" north and south from 23.5° North and South, potentially exposing populations in previously temperate zones to a spectrum of new infections.

Contemporary geographical disease control systems employ several elements: surveillance, isolation or quarantine, vaccination, and forecasting models of spread to inform intervention strategies. This book devotes a single chapter to each of these elements. Many of the concepts underpinning these themes were developed into an interlocking system by the states and cities of Italy from the thirteenth century in an attempt to control the spread of bubonic plague to and within Italy. In this chapter, the development of the Italian system is described. Then the system which was developed is cast into a theoretical framework to underpin the individual chapters on surveillance, quarantine, vaccination and forecasting which comprise the remainder of the book.

1.2 Disease Control in Italy: The Plague Centuries, 1342–1851

After the great pandemic of Black Death which affected Europe for some seven years from 1346, plague became endemic in Europe (Hirsch, 1883; Simpson, 1905; Pollitzer, 1954). Italy was entrained in 1347–8, with epidemics continuing there over the next four and a half centuries (**Figures 1.2** and **1.3**). The epidemic history of Italy in this period is reviewed in detail by Corradi (1865–94), while summary overviews of the major outbreaks of plague and plague-like disease are provided by Biraben (1975–76) and Scott and Duncan (2001). To these general surveys can be added many local investigations of plague mortality (Carmichael, 1986, p. 174). Illustrative are the studies of Carmichael (1991) and Zanetti (1976) on fifteenth- and sixteenth-century Milan, Morrison, *et al.* (1985) and Carmichael (1986) on fifteenth-century Florence, Ell (1989) on seventeenth-century Venice and Cipolla (1981a) on seventeenth-

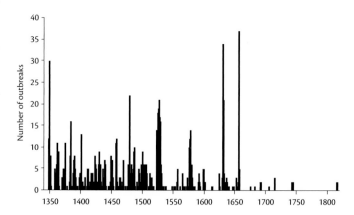

Figure 1.2 Plague outbreaks in Italy, 1347–1816. Annual time series of number of localities reporting plague. The generalised epidemics of 1348, 1383, 1457, 1478, 1522–28, 1577, 1630 and 1656 stand out from the annual background of 4–5 outbreaks which occurred in one place or another throughout the period. *Source*: data in Biraben (1975–76, Annexes III and IV, pp. 363–74, 394–400).

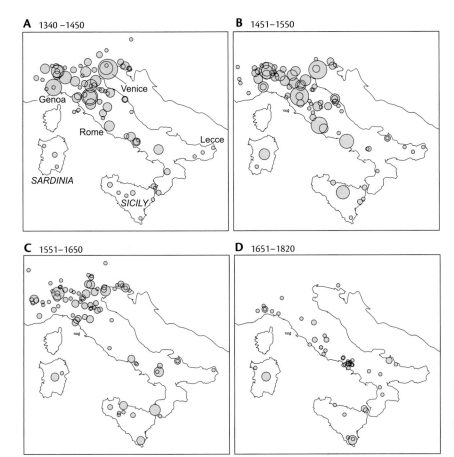

Figure 1.3 Geographical distribution of number of recorded plague outbreaks in Italy, 1340–1820. (A) 1340–1450. (B) 1451–1550. (C) 1551–1650. (D) 1651–1820. Outbreaks declined in number and became more widely dispersed spatially over the period. *Source*: data in Biraben (1975–76, Annexe IV, pp. 394–400).

century Pistoia. As described in these and similar works, the repeated outbreaks of plague deeply affected culture, society and economy at all levels. In response to the threat posed by plague visitations, three main groupings of states emerged (Scott and Duncan, 2001, p. 303): (i) the city states of the north (particularly Venice, Milan and Genoa), wealthy and jealous of each other; (ii) the Santa Sede (Holy See/Papal States); and (iii) in the south two very different and poor regions, the Kingdoms of Naples and Sicily (eventually the Kingdom of the Two Sicilies).

It was the northern group of states which led the fight against the disease. Despite its (then) unknown aetiology, these states gradually evolved a system of public health which, by the middle of the seventeenth century, had reached a high degree of sophistication. The northern Italian focus of this evolution was driven by the position of Italy at the interface of Europe and Asia, its location on arms of the Silk Road, and the dependence of the great republics like Venice and Genoa upon trade with Asia for their prosperity, factors which combined to ensure that importation of the plague, especially by ships returning from the Levant, was an ever-present threat. Similar developments to those in northern Italy took place north of the Alps but remained at a much more primitive level – as they did in Italy south of the Dukedom of Tuscany (Cipolla, 1981a, pp. 4–5).

The system which evolved was based upon special Magistracies which, while they combined legislative, judicial and executive powers in all matters pertaining to the public health, had as their prime focus prevention of the plague. By the middle of the

sixteenth century, all major cities of northern Italy had permanent Magistracies, reinforced in times of emergency by health boards set up in minor towns and rural areas. All boards were subordinate to and directly answerable to the central Health Magistracies of their respective capital cities (Cipolla, 1981a, p. 4). The Magistracies stressed prevention rather than cure, and out of their organisational genius came the ideas of surveillance and quarantine that have persisted to the present day. The nature and operation of Italian plague defences has attracted a specialised literature (see Carmichael, 1986, p. 175). In the English language, the volumes by Cipolla (1973, 1981a, b) are well known, while Italian-language studies and reports in relation to such cities as Florence (Ciofi, 1984), Milan (Beltrami, 1882; Decio, 1900; Bottero, 1942) and Venice (Preto, 1978; del Fiumi, 1981) are illustrative of local investigations. A recent study by Konstantinidou, *et al.* (2009) adds further context for the discussion which follows.

Surveillance

Underpinning the system was surveillance and inter-state communication. During the sixteenth and seventeenth centuries, the Health Magistracies of the capital cities of the republics and principalities of Italy north of the Santa Sede established the custom of regularly informing each other of all news they gathered on health conditions prevailing in various parts of Italy, the rest of Europe, North Africa, and the Middle East. For example, Florence 'corresponded' regularly with Genoa, Venice, Verona, Milan, Mantua, Parma, Modena, Ferrara, Bologna, Ancona and Lucca. The frequency of the correspondence with each of these places ranged from one let-ter every two weeks in periods of calm to several letters a week in times of emergency (Cipolla, 1981a, p. 21).

Spies and later official observers were also present in the major cities who reported back to their employers on the state of health in the various republics and principalities. But it was the great plague epidemic of 1652 which ultimately led to agreed, coordinated and enforced action among the north Italian states in a *Capitolazione* (Convention) between Florence, Genoa and the Santa Sede. The Convention bound the three powers to common practices and health measures in the principal ports of Genoa, Leghorn (Livorno) and Civitavecchia. Each state agreed to allow the other two to station one representative of their respective health boards in the main harbour – a forerunner of "international controls and the voluntary relinquishment of discretionary powers by fully sov-ereign states in the matter of public health" (Cipolla, 1981a, p. 34). The *concerto* between Tuscany and Genoa came rapidly to pass, but attempts to bring in the state groupings (ii) and (iii) mentioned earlier (the Santa Sede and Naples) proved meagre. Even the *con-certo* between Tuscany and Genoa collapsed a few years later, but it was a remarkable early attempt at international health collabo-ration not repeated for 200 years until the international control of the great nineteenth-century cholera pandemics became para-mount (Huber, 2006).

When contagious disease was uncovered anywhere by a par-ticular Magistracy, a proclamation of *ban* (when the presence of communicable disease was positively ascertained) or *suspension* (precaution because there was legitimate suspicion of disease) was issued. Bans were long term, suspensions short term. Bans and suspensions were used to denote the interruption of regular trade and communication. With banishment and suspension, no person, boat, merchandise or letter could enter the state issuing the order except at a few well-specified ports or places of entrance where quarantine stations were set up. At the stations, incoming people, boats and merchandise were subject to quarantine and disinfection even if they carried health certificates issued at the point of depar-ture (**Figure 1.4**). The health certificates were the seventeenth- and eighteenth-century equivalents of the twentieth-century interna-tional vaccination certificates, certifying that travellers and boats were free of disease. The authorities also reserved the right to refuse access to anything or anybody from banished areas – even, if nec-essary, to the quarantine stations. People attempting to violate the ban or enter the territory of the banishing state were commonly executed (**Figure 1.5**).

Cordon Sanitaire

The regular attacks by Turks, Barbary Coast and Corsican pirates from the Middle Ages onwards upon the coastlines of the states and towns of Italy meant that there existed an extensive system of coastal defensive towers, castles and forts which formed the basis of a maritime *cordon sanitaire* in time of plague. The sanitary observation posts encircled the entire Italian coastline. Some of the maps, generally fugitively catalogued and largely unknown, show-ing the locations of these posts have survived (**Figure 1.6**). They are described in Cliff, Smallman-Raynor and Stevens (2009) upon which this subsection is based. In Figure 1.6, the strings of posts are denoted by the solid lines. The identity numbers correspond with the numbered list of sources given in Appendix 1.1.

The cordon comprised two elements: (i) in both the Adriatic and the Mediterranean, armed sailing boats (*feluccas, trabaccoli, baragozzi*) to prevent illegal landings; and (ii) coastal observation towers and sentry boxes manned by armed infantry who stopped and recorded people and merchandise passing through the post. In addition, so-called "flying corps" of cavalry were deployed in some locations in the rear of the observation posts. The role of the flying corps was to act as a rapid response force, mopping up sources of infection which penetrated the outer rings of boats and observation posts. Finally, within the overall ring, individual defensive quaran-tine rings were constructed from time to time along land borders and around individual towns as necessary to keep out local disease threats.

The observation posts were constructed within sighting dis-tance of each other; communication between posts was primarily by sephamore (daylight) and beacon (night) signals. The reporting system was hierarchical: *local observation posts ⇒ district central command post ⇒ regional reporting centre*. Some of the maps give an indication of the manning – around 2–5 soldiers per observa-tion post, with periodic forts of around 30–50 men. Observation posts not only recorded the traffic passing, but also tried to prevent illegal passage so that ships, goods and travellers were routed into fixed quarantine stations.

The Northern States

Venice

Because of its maritime supremacy and trading connections, the Venetian Republic was visited by plague at regular intervals over nearly five centuries. Accordingly, the Republic established an extensive ring of sanitary guard or signal posts around its borders from an early date. **Figure 1.7** illustrates an extract from one of the surviving maps around Monfalcone. The individual posts appear as tents (see added enlarged inset in bottom left corner), while the 76 *casselli* (signal posts) are named in the entablature. **Figure 1.8** illustrates the frontier ring erected along the borders of the terri-tory of Friuli in 1713 at times of epidemics. This print shows the guard posts for the infantry (*appostamenti di infanteria*) in the fore-ground, as well as men at arms and supporting cavalry. The guard posts were designed primarily to prevent the arrival of plague over-land. The Ottoman Dominions were regarded as the main threat. On arrival, persons and goods suspected of carrying disease were confined in one of the city's two lazarettos for a statutory quaran-tine period of 40 days (see 'Quarantine and Isolation').

Genoa

The defensive quarantine ring, as well as the location of other infrastructure used to protect the public health of the Republic of Genoa, was mapped in a remarkable atlas by Matteo Vinzoni in 1758 (Appendix 1.1 (13)). In the first half of the eighteenth century, Liguria was divided into 36 health districts, each over-seen by a Commissioner for Health. Using one plate per district, Vinzoni charted the locations of the hospitals, lazarettos and san-itary (health) observation posts serving each district. The man-ning information recorded by Vinzoni varied by health district and is of three types: (i) the complement by day and night at each of the guard posts; (ii) post complement plus information on the military support in the district; (iii) simple lists of the post names.

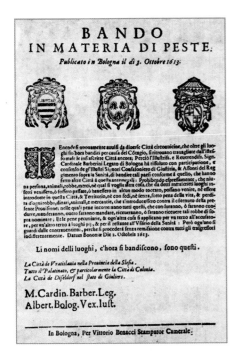
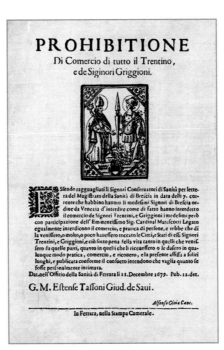
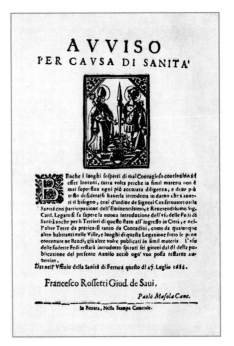
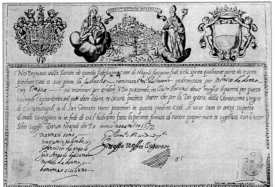
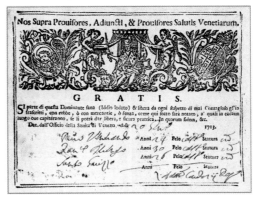
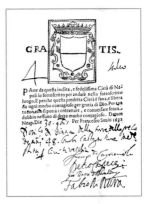

Figure 1.4 Certificates issued at times of plague. (*Upper, left to right*) Bologna, 1613, poster proclaiming no contact, on pain of death, with people or animals from Cologne, Düsseldorf or Vratislavia where there was plague; Ferrara, 1679, poster proclaiming restrictions on trade to help combat the transmission of plague; Ferrara, 1682, poster stating health passes to be introduced in six days. (*Lower, left to right*) travel documents issued by Naples and Venice. Left and centre are two health passports. The document on the left, dated 1632 and measuring 35 × 25 cm, is embossed with coats of arms and a panorama of Naples. It was issued to the captain of the fellucha (a type of boat) named *Santa Maria del Rosario*, which was sailing from Naples to Civitavecchia, the port of Rome, with five sailors on board. Their names are listed at the end of the certificate. It declares Naples to be free of all infectious disease, and asks for unrestricted and secure *pratique* (*prattica*: a licence to deal with a port after quarantine or on producing a clean bill of health). Nearly a hundred years later (1713) and the health passport for Venice (centre) appears essentially the same as that for Naples. The document on the right, measuring 16 × 12 cm and embossed with the arms of the city of Naples, was given in plague periods to each traveller from the port of Naples at embarkation. It declares the city to be healthy and free of all morbid contagions. It also declares that it is safe to trade and negotiate with the bearer without fear of infection. The almost illegible handwriting gives the date (30 June or July 1632), the name and a description of the bearer, his destination, and the signatures of the four representatives of the city authorities. The anonymous source author (p. 32), interprets the script as Giovanni Angelo Baucano, of the Greek Tower (*de la Torre dello Greco* barely recognisable at the end of line 1), age 48 (de anni 48, line 2), with a dark chestnut moustache (*castagno*, middle of line 2) and a mole on the upper left cheek, travelling to Civitavecchia (line 3). The signatories are: Francesco Caracciolo, Delio Capece, Giov. Battista d'Alessandro, and Fabio di Ruvo. Such certificates were issued to try to guarantee free passage and continuance of travel in the face of bans and suspensions. *Sources*: (*Lower, left and right*) Ministero dell'Interno, Direzione Generale Della Sanità Pubblica, Napoli (1910, Plates II and III following p. 32). Remainder: Wellcome Library, London.

Archival documents indicate how the system operated. Regular armed soldiers were assigned to the posts, supported by men from the local area on a rotation basis. Some posts were manned day and night while others were manned only at night. Nocturnal manning was more intensive because inter-post communication and observation was restricted by darkness. Logs were kept at each post of the visitors passing through the post.

Figure 1.9 illustrates the map for the health district of San Pier d'Arena which comprised the subdistricts of Cornigliano and Sampierdarena [*sic*]. The plate shows that 10 smaller observation posts (*guardia*) were supported by a castle (*castello*) (site 9). Some of the accompanying text details the night patrols. The two for San Pier have been added to Figure 1.9. The guard posts of the two subdistricts were visited by three patrols nightly. Each patrol

A

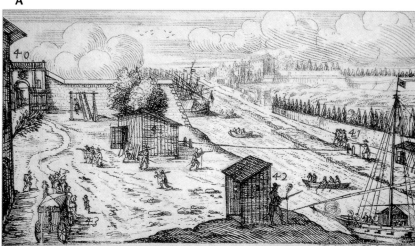

40. Porta Portese. 41. Corpo di Guardia al Canapo che trauerſa Fiume a Ripa, perche non e'ntrino barche ſenza notitia 42. Sentinella. 43. Carrozza de gli Ecc.^{mi}

B

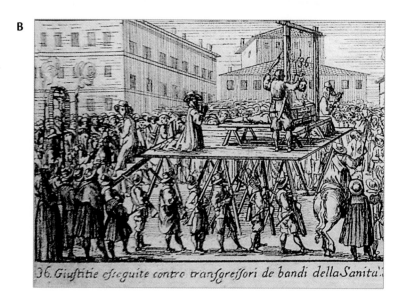

36. Giuſtitie eſeguite contro tranſgreſſori de bandi della Sanita'.

Figure 1.5 The plague in Rome, 1656. Extracts from G.G. de Rossi's 1657 three-part etching of episodes of the 1656 outbreak of the plague in Rome. (A) Guarded river crossing point (41) to ensure boats did not land illegally with a sentry (42) at his post. (B) Execution of persons who broke the quarantine rules. *Source*: World Health Organization Library, Geneva.

consisted of two men from the castle who had been collected by a patrol leader from each subdistrict. The first patrol ran between 0100–0500 hours, the second between 0500–0900 hours and the third from 0900–1300 hours. At the conclusion of each patrol, the guard was returned to the castle by the patrol leader. This intensity was judged sufficient for the number of visitors to San Pier (90 per day) (source: Appendix 1.1 (13, p. 12)).

The Santa Sede (Holy See/Papal States)

Two maps exist showing the *cordon sanitaire* for the Santa Sede, one for the Mediterranean coast, and one for the Adriatic coast including the land border with the Kingdom of Naples.

Mediterranean coast (Appendix 1.1 (14))

This map (**Figure 1.10**) plots and tabulates the sanitary, military and customs posts along the 226 km Mediterranean coast

of the Santa Sede from the border with the Grand Duchy of Tuscany to Graticciare on the border with the Kingdom of Naples. Operationally, the coast was divided into four Divisions, Civitavecchia (12 observation posts), Fiumicino (5 posts), Porto d'Anzio (7 posts) and Terracina (10 posts), at average spacing of 6.6 km.

Adriatic coast, Ravenna to Ascoli (Appendix 1.1 (15))

The map of this 80 km section of coast was divided into four geographical Divisions, each under the command of an army captain and his adjutant. The extract in **Figure 1.11** (figure located in the colour plate section) shows the First Division from Ancona to Ascoli, and the Fourth Division (the land border with the Kingdom of Naples). The Divisions were divided into Sections (for example, 10 in the case of the First Division). Within each Section, lookout posts (serially numbered 1,

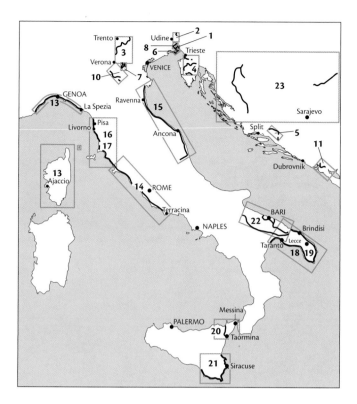

Figure 1.6 *Cordon sanitaire* **and containment of the plague in Italy by the eighteenth century.** Geographical locations of surviving maps showing observation posts which comprised the defensive isolation ring maintained around Italy against the plague. Map extents are shown by boxes, and strings of posts by heavy lines. The identity numbers correspond with the sources listed in Appendix 1.1. *Source*: Cliff, Smallman-Raynor and Stevens (2009, Figure 5, p. 207).

2, ... within each Division) were established at regular intervals, approximately 0.33 km apart. Nearly all Sections had their own sanitary officer (location marked with an asterisk). There was a reporting hierarchy; Section lookout posts reported to a central lookout post occupied by the Commander of the Section and the Sanitary Superintendent. In their turn, the central lookout posts returned their data to Divisional reporting lookout posts which were responsible for transmitting the information to the Commander-in-Chief of the *cordon sanitaire* (Captain Guiseppe Vaselli), whose seal appears in the lower right corner of Figure 1.11.

The map also gives the military complement of each post (italic script on the seaward side of each bar). In addition to the infantry, flying corps (cavalry; cf. Figure 1.8 for Venice) were based in Ascoli to support the lookout posts in maintaining the *cordon* along the land border with the Kingdom of Naples. The flying corps operated an offensive containment policy. The map includes a summary table of the manning of the *cordon* – for the four Divisions, nearly 1,900 men. Armed sailing boats (*trabaccoli*) cruised the Adriatic and completed the protection ring (one appears in Figure 1.11). The area around Ravenna (Section 5 of the Third Division) must have been especially vulnerable, adjacent as it was to the great trading city of Venice, and with many inland rivers. Here the quarantine defences were reinforced by squadrons of 4–6 small sailing boats (*baragozzi*). Thus consistent with the system around Venice, the surveillance ring was three layers deep; an outer ring of armed boats in the Adriatic, a middle ring of coastal observation posts manned by infantry, and an inner ring of what in modern terms would be called a rapid response force of cavalry providing additional offensive cover – here at the land frontier with the Kingdom of Naples.

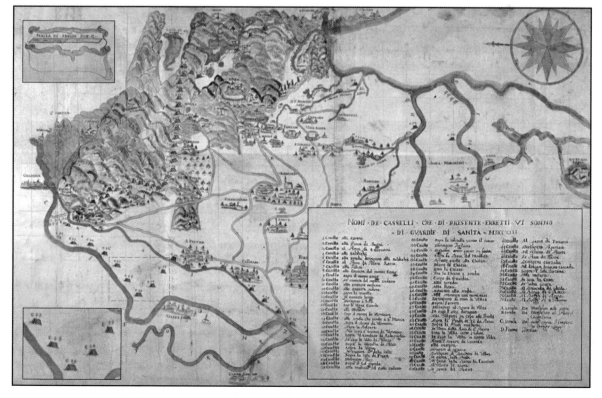

Figure 1.7 Sanitary guard posts of Monfalcone. Map of the territory of Monfalcone between the lake of Pietra Rossa and the River Isonzo, showing the towns, posts and sanitary guard huts at the border with the Granducale (Tuscany). *Source*: Appendix 1.1 (8).

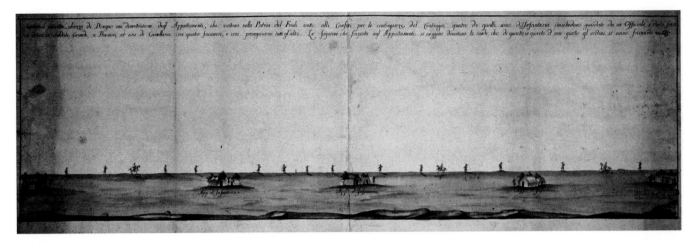

Figure 1.8 Sanitary guard lines in Friuli. Acquatint drawing of the infantry and cavalry posts erected along the borders of the territory of Friuli in times of epidemics. *Source*: Appendix 1.1 (9).

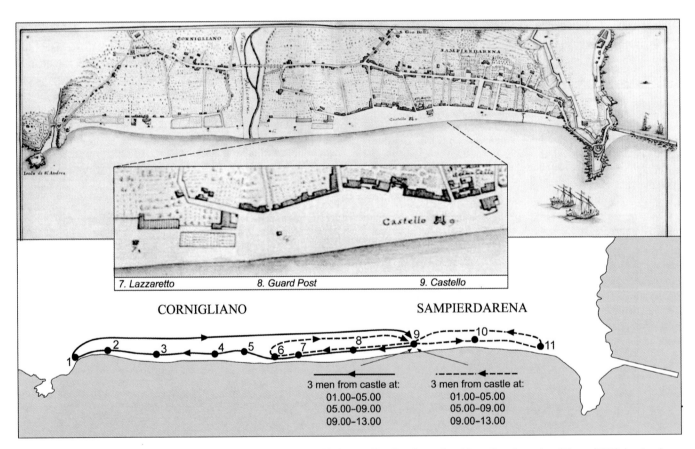

Figure 1.9 Sanitary guard posts of Genoa. Extract from the map of the health district of San Pier d'Arena from Vinzoni's sanitary atlas of Genoa (1758) showing the guard posts (*guardia*) along the coast, along with the routes followed by the night patrols (added). The enlargement shows that Vinzoni numbered the posts serially on his maps, and this was linked to an account of the manning and nature of each guard post in his Atlas. See text for examples. *Source*: Appendix 1.1 (13, 1758, pp. 8–9).

Quarantine and Isolation

Once plague entered an area, quarantine and isolation were deployed to limit spread. The first rudimentary steps in the eastern Mediterranean area were taken in 1377 when the Republic of Ragusa, a former Venetian colony on the Dalmatian Coast, instituted a legal system for the quarantining of visitors from plague-affected areas (Stuard, 1973; Kiple, 1993, p. 14; Frati, 2000; Sehdev, 2002). The Republic was also the location of the first permanent health office. As described in Frati (2000) and Palmer (1978, p. 208), the Ragusean approach was a compromise between the (potentially)

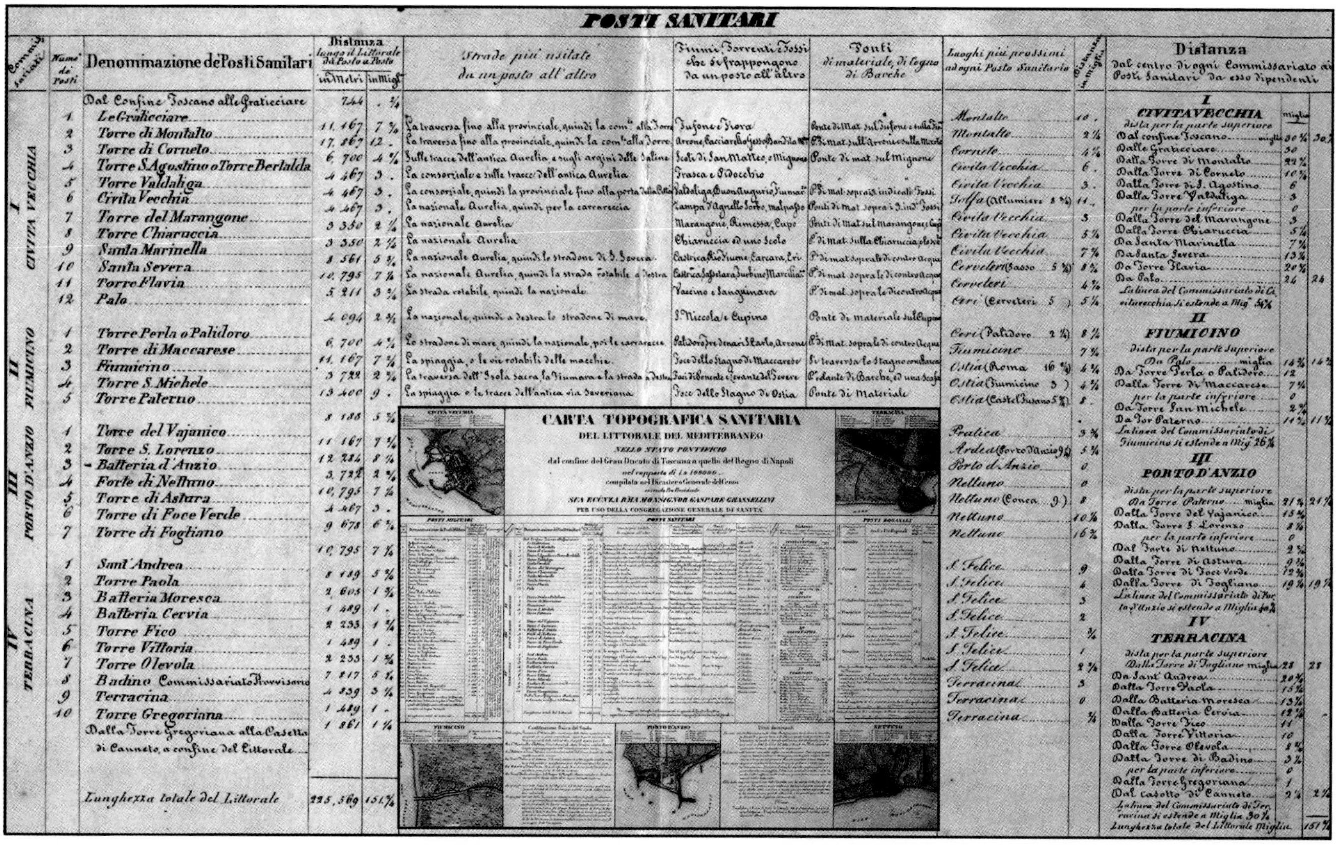

Figure 1.10 Sanitary guard posts of the Mediterranean coast of the Papal States. The whole map appears as the inset. The enlarged extract details the location of each sanitary post, inter-post distances, condition of the route, rivers and bridges between each post, and the distances from posts to reporting centres, all geared to produce rapid surveillance and reporting of infringements. *Source*: Appendix 1.1 (14).

complete blockade of human and commercial intercourse generally practised in western Europe in plague periods and the complete absence of intervention in the Ottoman east. The Ragusean system of regulation aimed to protect business in Ragusa, one of the great medieval maritime trading republics in the region.

As regards the Italian states, maritime quarantine was pioneered by the Venetian administration with the establishment of a lazaretto on the island of Santa Maria di Nazareth in 1403 (Simpson, 1905; Hirst, 1953; Gensini, *et al.*, 2004). Trying to prevent plague arriving by sea is described in a mid-eighteenth-century booklet by Venice's *Magistrato della sanità* (1752):

> Experience has shewn [sic], that in the *Ottoman* Dominions, the Plague is never utterly extinct: Hence it is an immutable Law with the Magistrate of the Office of Health, to consider the whole Extent of the *Ottoman* Dominions and every State dependent on it, as always to be suspected to be in an infected Condition, to such a Degree, as not to receive, in any Part of the Dominions of the Republick [Venice], either confining to or commercing with them, any Persons, Merchandizes, Animals, or any other Thing coming from thence, without the necessary Inspection of the Office of Health, and the previous purifications (*Magistrato della sanità*, 1752, p. 4).

Although the Ottoman Dominions were perceived as the prime risk, the same procedures were followed for "every Vessel, coming from any Part of the World, that is either infected, or suspected to be so" (*Magistrato della sanità*, 1752, p. 4). Vessels were normally expected to stop at Istria to take on board a pilot, or were towed up to Venice. Spies were maintained on the high tower of San Marco to watch for approaching vessels. The Magistrate sent one of his 60 Guardians to meet the ship which was moored in distant canals up to 25 km from the city according to the level of perceived risk. Ships were guarded throughout the quarantine period. They were unloaded of goods and passengers and both were dispatched to one of the city's two lazarettos. Generally, unless they were afflicted with full-blown plague, new arrivals were confined in the *Nuovo Lazzaretto* (New Lazaretto). The unfortunate creatures suffering from full plague either on arrival or during quarantine were dispatched to *Lazzaretto Vecchio* (the Old Lazaretto); see **Figure 1.12** for locations and descriptions. Only when the ship had been fully unloaded did the statutory 40 day quarantine period begin.

The Old and New Lazarettos were isolation hospitals on islands (Figure 1.12). The Old was 525 feet by 425 feet, the New 560 feet by 460 feet. Each was capable of holding 6,730 bales of merchandise. The Old could properly house about 300 passengers, the New 200 (Palmer, 1978, pp. 183–210; 29). The lazarettos were not only externally isolated but constructed to provide internal isolation of goods and passengers to the individual level. Conditions were frequently appalling. It was not uncommon for people to die at the rate of 500 per day in *Lazzaretto Vecchio* during plague outbreaks in the sixteenth century, while *Lazzaretto Nuovo* was recorded as

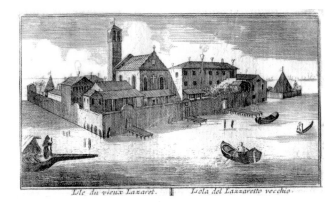

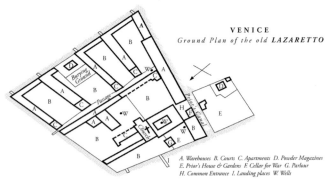

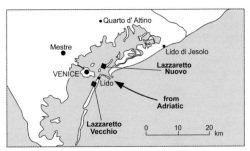

Figure 1.12 Lazarettos of Venice. Location map of the Old (*Lazzaretto Vecchio*) and New (*Lazzaretto Nuovo*) Lazarettos of Venice. The engravings show the ground floor plan of *Lazzaretto Vecchio* and a prospect of the lazaretto from the northwest corner. *Lazzaretto Vecchio* was established in 1403 about 2 km from Venice on a small island then known as Santa Maria di Nazareth, close to modern Lido. *Lazzaretto Nuovo* was established in 1468 on the island then known as Vigna Murada, separated by a navigable channel from the southern tip of the island of Sant' Erasmo, about 3 km from Venice. It occupied a strategic location at the entrance to the Venetian lagoon from the Adriatic and, when visited by John Howard in 1786, was used primarily to quarantine Turks, soldiers and crews of plague-infected ships (Howard, 1791, p. 11). By decree, ships, passengers and goods were isolated for a limited period to allow for the manifestation of any disease and to dissipate imported infection. Originally the period was 30 days, *trentina*, but this was later extended to 40 days, *quarantina*. The choice of this period is said to be based on the period that Christ and Moses spent in isolation in the desert. *Source*: ground floor plan of *Lazzaretto Vecchio* from Howard (1791, Plate 12); prospect is a mid-eighteenth-century copper engraving by the Venetian artist, Giuseppe Filosi. The ground floor plan has been distorted to conform with the prospect.

holding 8,000 inmates on one occasion, far beyond the capacities of either lazaretto to do anything worthwhile (Palmer, 1978, p. 195 for example).

The captain of the vessel was taken ashore by a guarded way to a point of examination. The examination turned upon whence the vessel had come, duration of the journey, places visited and their health, visits ashore, contact with other vessels at sea, the health of the ship's crew and passengers, and the nature of the cargo. Account had to be rendered of any crew or passengers who had died on board or who had left the ship en route "and particularly the Condition of that Person who is wanting" (*Magistrato della sanità*, 1752, p. 8). If the examining officer was satisfied "if the Vessel really come from a place that is free, it [the vessel] is declared free; if from a suspected one [place], the ship was placed in quarantine."

The principles of quarantine for goods were frequent handling, airing and smoke fumigation with aromatic herbs. Cloth and untreated animal hides were regarded as especially risky. Although the procedure varied in detail by product, bales were generally opened, aired, rummaged and cleaned up to twice a day, and moved from one location to another once a week. For people, social interaction was prevented, and each individual had his/her own cell, garden plot and cooking facilities. Individuals who died in quarantine were checked for plague marks before being buried in lime in holes at least 12 feet deep. In the event that any disease broke out during a quarantine period, the process was repeated so that second and third quarantines were not unheard of for individual ships.

These examples are important for illustrating certain repeating features of quarantine systems down the ages, namely: separation of suspected goods/animals and travellers from the populous for a period long enough to reduce the risk of transmission of infection to the public at large; the idea of a ring system of health check posts around an area; isolation hospitals in which suspected individuals and chattels were housed until cleared; and identification of parts of the world where infection was likely to be found.

Other Lazarettos

Lazarettos came in all shapes and sizes, and **Figure 1.13** illustrates two others – the large and complex merchandise lazaretto at Fortezza Santa Maria near Portovenere, Genoa, and, for the people of Rome, the modest hospital on Isola Tiberina in the middle of the River Tiber. Santa Maria served the entire Ligurian coast and was constructed in 1723 especially to receive suspected and contaminated imported goods for cleaning or burning (cf. Venice's New Lazaretto); see items 8, 9, 11, 12, 13 and 18 for example, in the key. Howard (1791) gives a full account of the principal lazarettos of Europe, along with views and plans. Island locations like those of Venice and Rome were, for obvious reasons, preferred locations, but pseudo-islands like Santa Maria were chosen where islands were not available. Conditions in all were appalling.

Foreward Planning and Control

In 1700, the eminent Bolognese naturalist and geographer, Luigi Ferdinando Marsili (1658–1730) produced the remarkable map shown in **Figure 1.14** (figure located in the colour plate section), 15 months after the Treaty of Karlowitz (1699) which concluded the Austro-Ottoman War of 1683–97. The map was either prepared for or by Marsili who was serving the Habsburg Emperor Leopold I in a Danubian campaign against the Ottoman Empire at the time. Marginal map notes describe Marsili's map as a "copy", and hint that it may have been copied from a [Habsburg?] original. It appears to have been one of two maps in a series, the second of which is missing (Jarcho, 1983, p. 11 and Appendix 1.1 (23)). Turkey was one of the principal conduits of plague into Europe, and the Habsburgs were

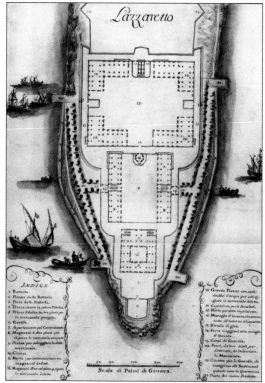

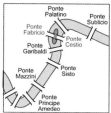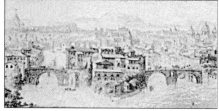

Figure 1.13 Lazarettos of Italy. (*Upper*) Portovenere. (*Lower*) Rome. The quarantine island for Rome in the middle of the Tiber at Ponte Fabricio is seen in this seventeenth-century view. *Sources:* (*Upper*) Appendix 1.1 (13, 1773, map 40). (*Lower*) Etching by Jacob Baptist, seventeenth century.

constructing a *cordon sanitaire* against plague in this area from the latter years of the seventeenth century (Rothenberg, 1973) which, by 1770 extended along more than 1,000 miles of frontier between Austria and the Ottoman Empire (Rothenberg, 1973, p. 16).

The map is entitled *Mappa geographica qua preacautio contra pestem post factam locorum, iuxta Pacis Instrumenta, Evacuationem ac Demolitionem in Confinibus istis Cis-Danubialibus instituenda ostenditur* (*A Geographical map in which are shown the precautions that are to be taken against the plague within these Cis-Danubial regions after the evacuation and demolition of places in accordance with the peace treaties*). The map is at a scale of roughly 1:200,000 and was drawn with south at the top. It shows the eastern coast of the Adriatic from Sebenico (now Šibenik) to Fiume (now Rijeka), a distance of approximately 220 km, and the territories of Croatia, Bosnia, "Sclavonia" and Sirmium as far inland as Belgrade.

The map shows provincial boundaries, two plague cordons (solid black lines and dots) determined by mountain tops, and several lazarettos. A linear scale of hours (travel times) appears in the lower left and a detailed explanation in the upper left. To control the spread of plague if it visited the region, the map proposes that

the residents of the region lying south of the yellow line have to be assumed to be susceptible to the disease, and should be detained in the lazar houses which appear at road intersections, to serve their quarantine. Merchants could continue to follow the roads shown by the double pecked lines but all other roads were to be closed to prevent spread of infection. The defence against the plague was not limited to isolation by cordon and lazaretto since the descriptive note states that the system was to be instituted after depopulation of the area by evacuation and demolition of houses. The combined preservation of commercial routes, cordons, lazarettos and checkpoints amounts to "an almost complete depiction of the way in which plague was resisted" (Jarcho, 1983, p. 11).

1.3 **Prato, 1630**

How did the various elements of the Italian system mesh together in a single location? One of the best illustrations is provided by the response of the city of Prato, 21 km northwest of Florence in Tuscany, in the face of the great plague of 1630 (Figures 1.2 and 1.3C). This was the second largest outbreak to hit Italy during the plague centuries. It devastated the northern states over a period of a year from the autumn of 1630. A qualitative account of its course is given in Cipolla (1973, pp. 16–75). Here we map the sequence of events in Tuscany and Prato to illustrate the highly integrated nature of the control system as surveillance, bans and quarantine were ratcheted up over some four months to try to counter the ever-increasing disease threat.

Figure 1.15 shows Prato was a typical walled Italian town. Originally walled for defence, five main gates penetrated the walls which, in times of plague, could be readily controlled or closed. Communications between Prato and other towns followed the main valleys – along the valley of the River Arno west to Pisa and east to Florence, or northwards towards Bologna (**Figure 1.16**). Prato fell under the Magistracy of Florence.

The opening moves of the epidemic began in the autumn of 1629 when plague was carried by French armies from the northwest and German armies from the north via Lake Como who entered Italy as part of the Thirty Years' War, 1618–48 (**Figure 1.16A**). By the end of 1629, the Milan Health Board had quarantined Savoy, other areas of Piedmont, and Turin. Guards had been placed at all the gates of Milan, the laws governing the use of health passports for goods and people throughout the state of Milan had been reinforced, and communities with fifty or more families were required to enclose inhabited areas and barricade gates. All was in vain and, by the end of 1629, the states of Milan, Savoy, and Piedmont had been banned by surrounding states as far south as Rome to try to prevent spread south into Tuscany and beyond, and east into the Venetian Republic. At the end of October, the health officers in the Magistracy of Florence instructed their opposite numbers in Prato to implement two defence lines – one at the borders of the Grand Duchy to check travel north/south through the mountain passes and fords (Figure 1.16B), and the second around the city itself by placing guards at all the gates.

Spread of the plague was checked over winter, but flowered in full vigour in the spring of 1630 (Figure 1.16B). Plague reached Bologna in mid May, so that Florence required health passes (cf. Figure 1.4) for all travellers into the Grand Duchy. Prato appointed an issuing officer for the purpose. On 12 June Florence reinforced the northern border of the Duchy with more troops and a guard post every three miles (cf. Figure 1.8), banned Bologna on 13th,

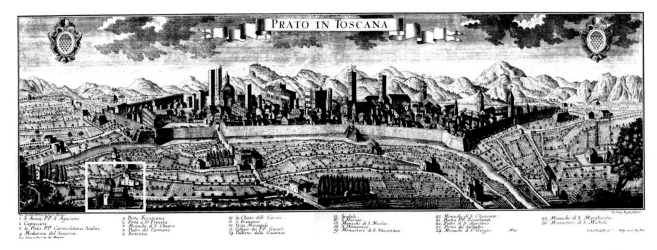

Figure 1.15 Prato in Tuscany, c. 1700. Piere Giovanni Fabbroni/Jon. Georg Ringle, 80 × 27 cm. Prospect of Prato from the east showing the walled city with few entry points through the walls. The Convent of St Anne ultimately became the plague hospital. Located well outside the city walls, it appears in the lower left foreground (white box). At this period around 7,000 lived within the walls and 11,000 outside.

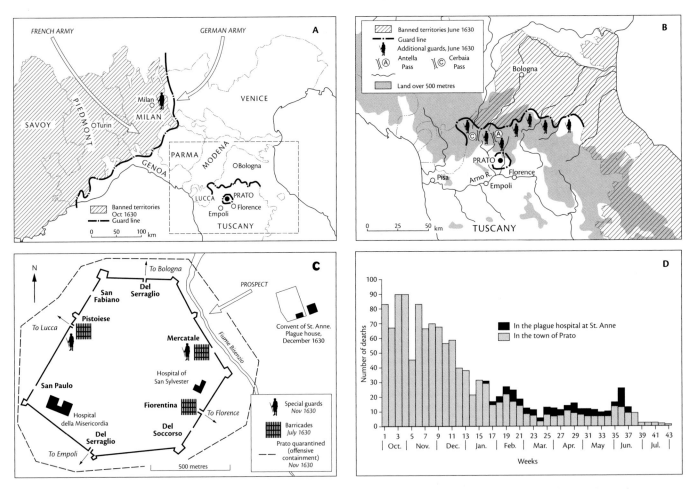

Figure 1.16 Controlling the plague in Prato, 1630–31. Sequence of steps taken in Prato in an attempt to defend itself from the great plague epidemic of 1630. (A) 1629. (B) 1630. (C) Prato, 1630. (D) Epidemic curve, Prato, October 1630–July 1631. *Source*: based on written account in Cipolla (1973, pp. 15–69).

and raised a general alert to health officers in all walled towns and villages to exercise extreme care when issuing health passes.

On July 1, the grand Duke seconded part of his personal guard further to reinforce border controls in Tuscany. On July 6, movements of friars were stopped. In Prato on July 10th the three most frequently used gates (Mercatale, Fiorentina and Pistoiese) were reinforced with barricades, and the number of health officers increased from four to eight (Figure 1.16C). Despite all this, plague arrived in the city in late September. By 14 November all the city's gates had been permanently closed except the Mercatale and Pistoiese which had special guards put in place. By the year end, all communications with Prato had been severed; the city was isolated. A plague house for victims was in operation by 31 December. Given the land-locked location of Prato and after much wrangling among vested interests, it was eventually settled to be the Convent of St Anne, outside the city walls. It was to be many more months before the epidemic finally subsided in Prato and the city began to return to normal.

1.4 Models of Control

At the heart of all modern control systems for communicable diseases lies an understanding of how each disease is transmitted from person to person. While this is a medical problem in the first instance, this knowledge is commonly taken forward mathematically both to devise control models and to assess their effectiveness and cost. Such models have attracted mathematical interest from Bernoulli onwards: the classic accounts are given by Bailey (1975) in his *Mathematical Theory of Infectious Diseases* and by Anderson and May (1991) in their *Infectious Diseases of Humans: Dynamics and Control*. To give a flavour of their approach to which we return in detail in Chapter 6, a very simplified diagram of the spread of an infectious disease through a human population, which does not involve an intermediate vector like mosquitos in malaria and dengue, is illustrated in **Figure 1.17**. The population is divided into three sub-populations – those at risk (susceptibles, S), those with the disease (infectives, I), and those who have recovered (recovereds, R). Propagation of an epidemic occurs by homogeneous mixing (mass action) between the S and I populations at a rate β. This generates new cases by the transition $S \Rightarrow I$. Infectives recover or die at a rate μ, while the susceptible population is renewed for future epidemics by births at the rate γ. Population stocks are updated by simple accounting equations. That for I is shown in Figure 1.17 – i.e. the number of new infectives at $t + 1$ is given by the number at t, plus new infectives generated by the transition $S \Rightarrow I$, minus those infectives at t who recover or die by $t + 1$. If an epidemic is to be sustained, a continuous chain of infectives must be maintained. Such a chain will continue as long as transmission of infection from infectives to susceptibles can occur.

Spatial Mass Action Models

Using the communicable disease of measles, a number of early writers, notably Bartlett (1957) and Black (1966), developed the *SIR* model into a geographical setting by studying the mixing process between susceptibles and infectives in populations distributed in systems of towns of different sizes. Under these conditions, the parameter β cannot be assumed to be constant in different geographical locations, even for the same disease. Neither can the homogeneous mixing assumption within geographical areas be regarded as reasonable. The upshot of their work was to establish a direct relationship between the population size of a town and the frequency of epidemic waves. They divided waves into three types found in towns of successively smaller population size: *Type I* waves (large towns), where chains of infection remained continuous and major epidemics flared up at regular intervals; *Type II* waves (medium-sized towns), in which regular epidemics occurred but where the disease disappeared completely between epidemics; and *Type III* waves (small towns) in which epidemics occurred irregularly and infrequently, separated by long inter-epidemic periods of unpredictable duration when no cases of the disease were reported. The population threshold crossed when towns cease to display Type II waves and experience Type I waves is called the *critical community size*; it defines the transition from epidemic to endemic behaviour (**Figure 1.18A** and **B**).

A large literature has developed around the *SIR* model in which refinements have been added to the model to allow (for example) for: inhomogeneous mixing among the population subgroups, especially spatially; vaccination; the latent period of the disease; carrier states; and population recycling from $R \Rightarrow S$ (see, for example, Keeling and Grenfell, 1997). The model has often given profound insights into the spread of epidemics, but it is complex to fit to space–time data without heroic assumptions about the stationarity of model parameters and isotropisms of the underlying processes. The longer the time series and the greater the geographical area being studied, the less likely are such assumptions to be tenable, not least because the sensitivity and specificity of disease reporting is unlikely to have remained constant over time.

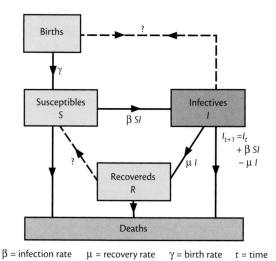

β = infection rate μ = recovery rate γ = birth rate t = time

Figure 1.17 Simplified model of an infection process. The mass action model is based upon person to person contact between infectives, *I*, and susceptibles, *S*, at a rate β which generates new cases of the disease. Infected individuals recover or die at a rate μ and enter the recovered (removed) population, *R*. *Source*: Cliff, *et al.* (1993, Figure 16.1 upper, p. 414).

Barriers to Spread

Thus the spatial dimension to checking communicable disease spread becomes superficially simple to state. It consists of breaking chains of infection by preventing a disease moving from endemic

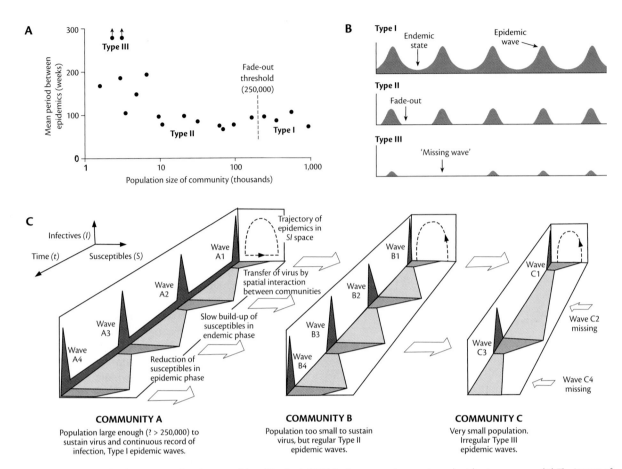

Figure 1.18 Measles propagation in a system of settlements. (*Upper*) Bartlett's (1957) findings on settlement size and epidemic recurrence. (A) The impact of population size on the spacing of measles epidemics for 19 English towns. (B) Characteristic epidemic profiles for the three types indicated in (A). In the Type I settlements, which have populations ≥ 250,000, measles is continuously present and there are regularly spaced large epidemics. In Type II settlements (< 250,000) which are still large, there are regular epidemics but there are also gaps between the epidemics when no cases are reported. In the very small Type III settlements (< 10,000 population), there are gaps between epidemics and settlements may miss an entire epidemic. (*Lower*) (C) Spatial version of the Bartlett model. Conceptual view of the spread of a communicable disease (measles) in communities of different population sizes. Stages in spread correspond to the Bartlett model. Settlements like A, in which measles is permanently present, provide the reservoir of infection which sparks a major epidemic when the population at risk (susceptibles, S) builds up to a critical level (see Figure 1.17). When an epidemic happens, the S population is diminished and the stock of infectives, I, increases as individuals are transferred by infection from the S to the I population. This generates the characteristic 'D'-shaped relationship over time between the sizes of the S and I populations shown on the end plane of the block diagram. If the total population of a community falls below the quarter of a million size threshold, as in settlements B and C, measles epidemics can only arise when the virus is introduced into it by the influx of infected individuals (so-called *index cases*) from reservoir areas. These movements are shown by the broad arrows. In such smaller communities, the S population is insufficient to maintain a continuous record of infection. The disease dies out and the S population grows in the absence of infection. Eventually the S population becomes big enough to sustain an epidemic when an index case arrives. Given that the total population of the community is insufficient to renew by births the S population as rapidly as it is diminished by infection, the epidemic will eventually die out. It is the repetition of this basic process which generates the successive epidemic waves experienced in most communities. *Source*: Cliff, *et al.* (1981, Figure 3.2, p. 40) and Cliff and Haggett (1988, Figure 5.5A, p. 246).

reservoirs to seed infection in smaller communities where the population size is insufficient to sustain the disease on a permanent basis. As shown in **Figure 1.19**, spatial protection against the spread of infection can be undertaken at two points. The first method, (i), is to interrupt the mixing of infectives and susceptibles with protective spatial barriers. This may take the form of isolating an individual or a community, or of restricting the geographical movements of infected individuals by quarantine. Potential spatial strategies which achieve these goals are illustrated schematically in **Figure 1.20**. In the two maps, infected areas have been shaded, while disease-free areas have been left blank. In Figure 1.20A, the disease-free areas need to be protected by isolation. Such *defensive isolation* entails the building of a spatial barrier (a *cordon sanitaire*)

around the perimeter of the disease-free areas, the aim being to prevent infectious cases in any diseased area beyond the pale from gaining access to susceptibles inside the pale. *Offensive containment* (Figure 1.20B) is the flip side of this, where a containment barrier is interposed between known diseased and disease-free areas to prevent spread from the former to the latter. The diseased area is then cleared of infection by some means or another.

The second method of interrupting the chains of infection, (ii) in Figure 1.19, is to short-circuit the route from susceptible to removed states by creating population immunity through immunisation. Although immunisation in the present era of mass vaccination usually results in generalised population immunity in developed economies, this is not true for many diseases in developing economies

Alternative intervention strategies

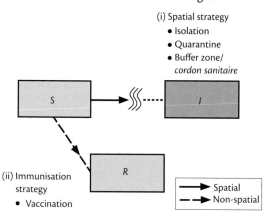

(i) Spatial strategy
- Isolation
- Quarantine
- Buffer zone/ *cordon sanitaire*

(ii) Immunisation strategy
- Vaccination

→ Spatial
⇢ Non-spatial

Figure 1.19 Interrupting chains of infection. Alternative intervention strategies based on (i) a *spatial strategy*, blocking links by isolation and quarantine between susceptibles and infectives and (ii) a generally *aspatial strategy*, opening of new direct pathways from susceptible to recovered status through immunisation. This outflanks the infectives (*I*) box. *Source*: Cliff, *et al.* (1993, Figure 16.1, p. 414).

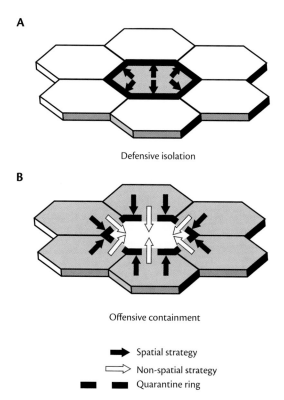

A

Defensive isolation

B

Offensive containment

➡ Spatial strategy
⇨ Non-spatial strategy
▬ Quarantine ring

Figure 1.20 Spatial control strategies. Schematic diagram of two spatial control strategies to prevent epidemic spread. (A) Defensive isolation. (B) Offensive containment. Infected areas are shaded; disease-free areas are left blank. Geographical areas are shown arbitrarily as hexagons. *Source*: Cliff, *et al.* (1993, Figure 16.9, p. 423).

or where, for one reason or another, so-called *herd immunity* has failed or not been achieved (e.g. war zones, refugee camps). Then immunisation takes on a geographical component of where to vaccinate to achieve the best disease control results. These issues form the subject matter of Chapter 4.

A final method of population protection is to relocate susceptible populations into supposedly safe areas (cf. Marsili's approach in Figure 1.14). Although this may be possible in some instances for animal populations, it is not generally a realistic strategy today for human populations.

Sicily, 1743: The Plague of Messina

Defensive isolation and offensive containment were used in the heel of Italy (Puglia) and in Sicily in 1743 successfully to thwart generalised spread of what turned out to be the last major outbreak of plague in Europe – the Plague of Messina. The regulations under which plague control operated in the Kingdom of the Two Sicilies is best summarised in the *Regolamento generale di servizio sanitario marittimo, sanzionato da S.M. il 1 gennajo 1820, in esecuzione dell'articolo 20 legge de' 20 ottobre 1819* (5). *Inter alia*, paragraphs 219–235 of the general service regulations specify the geographical structure of a defensive isolation *cordon sanitaire* to be applied around coastlines, its manning, operation and reporting system. **Table 1.1** lists the critical elements, while **Figure 1.21** converts these into a schematic diagram; (A) shows the implied arrangement of guard posts along the coast and (B) illustrates the hierarchical reporting system. Many of the features of (A) and (B) – for example, the siting of posts within viewing distance of each other, the complement of three soldiers per post, and the reporting structure – have been noted earlier as the practice for the coastlines of the Republic of Genoa and the Santa Sede.

Figure 1.22 (located in the colour plate section) illustrates a practical articulation of these arrangements in the *cordon sanitaire* for the province of Lecce, across the Ionian Sea from Sicily and Messina. Consistent with the legislative framework summarised in Table 1.1 and Figure 1.21, the figure shows the division of the coastline into sections (pecked lines), with the regular and dense network of masonry towers (*torre*, housing the local sanitary official and section commander; large red circles on Figure 1.22) and guard huts (*barracca*, each housing three guards or *uomini di guardia*; black lozenges on Figure 1.22). Armed patrol boats (*feluccas*) appear offshore (Article 235 in Table 1.1). The entablature gives the manning details for this *cordon*: 494 guard huts, 79 towers, 2,319 *uomini* and 160 *cavallari* (horsemen) along c. 400 km of coast.

Messina had been free from plague since 1624, and the Sicilians prided themselves on the rigour of their quarantine laws which they thought had preserved them. A protective *cordon sanitaire* of observation posts existed around Sicily as part of this enforcement (**Figure 1.23**, located in the colour plate section). In May 1743 a Genoese vessel arrived in Messina (**Figure 1.24**, located in the colour plate section) from Morea (near Patras in the Little Dardanelles), on board of which had occurred some suspicious deaths (plague was present in the Levant at this time). The ship and cargo were burnt but, soon after, cases of a suspicious form of disease were observed in the hospital and in the poorest parts of the town. *The Supremo Magistrato di Commercio* preferred commercial expediency to rigorous enforcement of the sanitary laws and a major epidemic of plague developed which killed an estimated 40,000–50,000 persons. It was this plague which led to the establishment of the island-wide permanent sanitary magistracy with jurisdiction over the pre-existing local health deputations which had existed for decades to control the importation of infectious diseases.

Table 1.1 Kingdom of the Two Sicilies: geographical structure of the *cordon sanitaire* specified in the general service regulations of 1820

Paragraph	Regulation	Cordon structure
Geographical features		
221	La distanza tra un posto e l'altro dev' esser tale, che l'uno sia sempre a vista dell' altro	Each guard post to be within sighting distance of its neighbours
222	Quando in una provincia o valle vi sieno delle coste inaccessibili, per le quali vi ha bisogno di poca o niuna custodia, l'Intendente deve impiegare questo risparmio di forze de cordone per assicurare le spiagge aperte, ed i siti più esposti a degli sbarchi furtive	Any economies in manpower from not having to patrol inaccessible coastal sections to be used to guard open beaches and places most available for clandestine landings
Manning		
223	In ogni posto devono montar di guardia tre individui ed un basse uffiziale, che farà le funzioni di capo posto. Quando le spiagge sieno aperte ed esposte in modo che non bastion a custodirle in quattro individui destinati per ciascun posto, può allora aumentarsene il numero a seconda del bisogno e delle circostanze	Normally three guards per post with a low-level official as head of post; four on open beaches difficult to guard, augmented if necessary to suit the conditions
224	La guardia dee recarsi al suo posto la mattina, ed esserne rilevata il domane alla stess'ora, durante il qual tempo è vietato agl'individui che la compongono, il potersi appartar dal posto sotto qualunque pretesto. Il capo-posto dee rimaner fisso per un'inera settimana, ad oggetto di conoscer bene le consegne e trasmetterle, e di conoscere i segnali e le pratiche da osservarsi. Egli ha l'obbligo particolare d'invigilar sulla condotta de'suoi subalterni	Guards must be on station from daylight and relieved the following morning. The head guard has a one-week tour of duty; he has recording, reporting and supervisory duties
225	Per ogni sei posti vi sarà un'Uffizial comandante, che dee rimaner distaccato per un"intera settimana, e tener presso di se una o più persone a cavallo per la sollecita diramazione degli ordini. La posizione da assegnarsi al suddetto Comandante sarà, per quanto è possibile, la centrale. Egli avrà specialmente l'incarico d'invigilare all'adempimento degli obligi ingiunti a(i)l capi-posti	A sanitary official every six posts, centrally located, on a weekly tour of duty. The official is responsible for distributing orders rapidly using horsemen
226	Per ogni tre distaccamenti di sei posti l'uno, vi sarà un sottoispettore, che anche deve avere una situazione centrale. Il suo incarico è quello d'invigilare alla regolarità del servisio de'tre distaccameni che compongono la sua sotto-ispezione	Three detachments per six posts under the supervision of an under-inspector in a central position
Reporting system		
228	Tra tutt' i capi del cordone vi deve essere una corrispondenza giornaliera ed esatta, onde si rilevi il modo con cui si attende al servizio, e le novità che possono aversi luogo. Affinchè la corrispondenza suddetta proceda colla massima regolarità, e nel modo più celere, i capi-posti devono corrispondere coi rispettivi Comandanti di distaccamento, questi col sotto-ispettore, il sotto-ispettore col' Ispettore, l'Ispettore contemporaneamente coll' Intendente, e col Comandante militare della provincia o valle. Da siffatta regola sono eccettuati i casi di seria considerazione ne' quali, oltre del rapporto regolare da passarsi col cennato metodo, i Comandanti di distaccamento sono autorizzati di far rapporto straordinario, e spedirlo con espresso all' Intendente ed al Comandante della provincia o valle	Cordon commanding officers must communicate daily with each other. The normal upwards reporting system is from local guard post heads via intermediate officers to the provincial military commander and the sanitary superintendent (Figure 1.21B); the intermediate officers can be by-passed in an emergency
Integrity of the cordon		
229	Gli obblighi di tutti gl'individui destinati a formare il cordone, si riducono generalmente ad impedir nelle spiagge l'approdo di qualsivoglia legno, qualunque ne sia la provenienza, obbligandolo a dirigersi ne'punti più vicini, ove risiede una deputazione de salute	All individuals in the cordon must act to prevent, through a general reduction of manpower, unauthorised beach landings by boat by funnelling those concerned towards the nearest points manned by sanitary officers
230	Ne' casi di burrasca, i legni amici o nemici possono, quando il naufragio è quasi sicuro, farsi approdare nelle spiagge, impiegando all' uopo tutte le cautele di custodia, ed un rigoroso cordone *parziale*, sino a che non accorrano i deputati di salute corrispondenti per applicarvi l'analogo trattamento sanitaria	Shipwrecks to be quarantined by a local *cordon sanitaire* until sanitary officers can attend
231	Se qualche posto fosse minacciato da gente, che volesse sbarcare a viva forza, ed alla quale non potesse resistere, il capo posto deve innalzare un bandiera di convenzione, ed a questo segnale deve accorrere subito la forza de' posti limitrofi. Avvenendo questo caso in tempo di notte, il segnale per aver soccorso sarà di due fuochi consecutive	Post heads must signal for support from neighbouring posts if a forced landing is threatened. Two consecutive fire signals used at night

Table 1.1 (*Continued*)

Paragraph	Regulation	Cordon structure
232	In ogni posto devono farsi, durante la notte, de'fuochi convenuti di corrispondenza, a fin di assicurarsi della vigilanza de'posti limitrofi.	Fire signals to be agreed between adjacent posts for night communication
233	Nei tempi di cordone l'esercizio della pesca non è più libero. Le barche pescarecce possono uscire dal levare al tra montar del sole; ed in questo periodo è anche proibito loro di allontanarsi dal lido oltre le quattro miglia. I padroni di queste barche devono essere allora muniti di una *bolletta*, che i deputati di salute corrispondenti devono loro vistare giorno per giorno	A charge is made for fishing during times of cordon, collected daily by the sanitary inspectors from the boat captain. Fishing is permitted only during daylight hours and not more than four miles from the beach.
235	I cordone sanitari marittimi possono anche stabilirsi per mezzo di altrettante crociere di barche armate, applicandosi a queste, sotto certe tali necessarie modificazioni, le norme di sopra indicate per la distribuzione, il servigio e la dipendenza de' posti situati a terra su i littorali	Armed boats (*felucca*) patrol the coastline

Source: based on Petitti (1852, pp. 318–55).

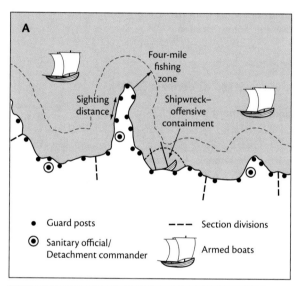

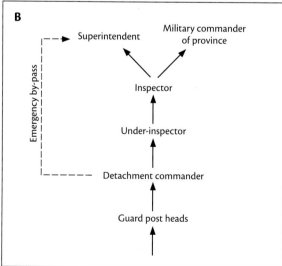

Figure 1.21 Kingdom of the Two Sicilies: Maritime *cordon sanitaire*. (A) Arrangement of guard posts along the coastline recommended in the general service regulations of 1819–20 (Table 1.1). (B) Reporting system for the *cordon*.

Defensive Isolation: Sicily

To prevent spread within Sicily, three internal *cordon* lines were established in August 1743 by the health officials in Palermo, stretching across the neck of land from Milazzo on the north coast to Taormina on the south (Figure 1.24, located in the colour plate section). From east to west, the *cordon* lines were: (east) 26 miles (42 km) long, number of posts and men unrecorded; 23 miles (37 km), 152 posts, 700 men; 21 miles (34 km), 130 posts, 633 men (west). This defensive isolation appears to have worked for there is no surviving evidence that plague spread to other parts of the island.

Offensive Containment: Lecce

As noted in Figure 1.20B, an alternative approach to defensive isolation is *offensive containment* to prevent disease propagation into disease-free areas. During the Plague of Messina, a Turkish ship was unfortunate enough to be shipwrecked off the port of Lecce. Following Article 230 of the General Regulations in Table 1.1, a local cordon was established around the wreck, the boat and contents burned, and the sailors quarantined (**Figure 1.25**).

1.5. Conclusion

This book considers how the geographical spread of communicable diseases from one area to another may be prevented or at least controlled. Using largely unknown maps in Italian state archives, this chapter has shown how, from the establishment of the first quarantine station by the Republic of Ragusa (modern-day Dubrovnik) in 1377, the states and principalities of Italy developed a sophisticated system of control to try to protect themselves from the ravages of plague. A *cordon sanitaire* existed around the Italian coast for five centuries, consisting of three elements: (i) an outer defensive ring of armed sailing boats in the Mediterranean and the Adriatic, (ii) a middle coastal ring of forts and observation towers, and (iii) an inner defensive ring of land-based cavalry. Health passports, and restrictions on travel and trade during plague epidemics were added to the surveillance system based on spies and the *cordon sanitaire*.

The procedures developed were largely unsuccessful in their primary aim of preventing the spread of plague, a disease whose aetiology was then unknown. And yet it is clear that, apart from vaccination, unavailable at the time, the elements developed in

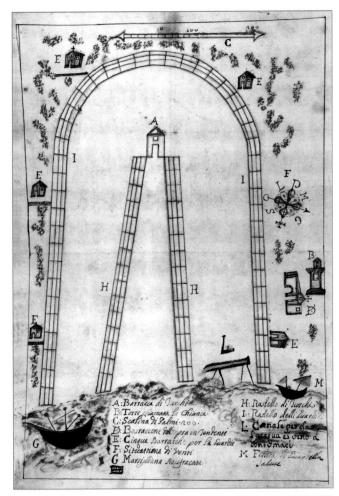

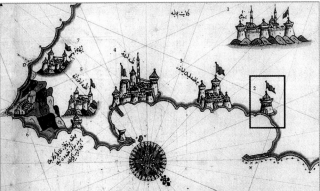

Figure 1.25 City of Lecce, tower of Chianca, 1743: local *cordon sanitaire*. At the time of the Plague of Messina, a Turkish boat was unfortunate enough to be shipwrecked near the tower of Chianca, Lecce harbour. The upper map illustrates the local containment *cordon sanitaire* erected around the wreck to prevent any risk of plague being carried by the sailors into Lecce. It shows the hut for the Turks (A), Chianca tower (B), the five sanitary guard huts (E), the stockades used to separate the Turkish compound from the guards (H, I), an armed patrol boat (*felucca*, G) and the *felucca* with the public health officers on board (M). The lower map of the heel of Italy is an extract from a sixteenth-century Ottoman map of the area. The town of Lecce (1) is a few miles inland from the port (3) with its disembarkation point (2, boxed) where the wreck occurred. Other towns marked are Roca Vecchia (4), Otranto (5) and Tricasi (7). (6) is Capo Santa Maria di Leuca. The towns are all walled. *Source*: (main map) Appendix 1.1 (19); (inset map) Salierno (2010, p. 41).

northern Italy during the plague centuries form the nucleus of contemporary control systems for communicable diseases – surveillance, isolation, barriers to spread such as health passports, bans on travel, quarantine and forward planning. The system was largely forgotten when plague ceased to be a problem. It was reinvented north of the Alps from the middle of the nineteenth century when cholera pandemics swept the globe; then countries like England, Germany and France led the way, rather than Italy.

With the Italian ideas as historical context, we now move in the remainder of the book to bring the disease control problem into a modern framework with chapters on surveillance (Chapter 2), quarantine (Chapter 3), vaccination (Chapter 4), eradication of infectious diseases (Chapter 5), and planning for control in the twenty-first century (Chapter 6).

Appendix 1.1: Map Sources

This Appendix gives the sources of the maps used in this chapter. The item numbers correspond with the key map shown in Figure 1.6. All plates with sources cross-referenced to this Appendix have been reproduced by kind permission of the Directors of the State Archives and Libraries cited.

Venice

Archivio di Stato di Venezia (ASV)

1. Giancomo Binard

Mappa del territorio del basso Friuli compreso tra Palma la linea formata dal- l'Iudri, il Torre e l'Isonzo e Cervignano, con l'indicazione delle postazioni sanitarie. 4 marzo in Udine; scala di miglia 3 = mm 30; dim mm 940 × 650. Disegno a mano, su carta, con colorazioni ad acquarello. ASV. Provveditori alla Sanità, Disegni, B2N8.

2. Iacopo Spinelli

Mappa con parte del corso del fiume Natisone e tracciate le postazioni di guardia al confine tra il Friuli e la Schiavonia veneta in caso di epidemie. 1714; scala di miglia = mm 90; dim mm 1,025 × 720. Disegno a mano, su carta, con colorazioni ad acquarello. ASV. Provveditori alla Sanità, Disegni, B3N12.

3. Tommaso Pedrinelli

Mappa comprendente parte del territorio Vicentino dei Settecommni e Bassanese al cinfine con il Trentino e con l'indicazione dei posti e guardie sanitarie. 28 febbraio 1739, Bassano; scala di miglia italiane 5 = mm 155; dim mm 1,140 × 975. Disegno a mano, su carta, con colorazioni ad acquarello. ASV. Provveditori alla Sanità, Disegni, B3N16.

4. P. Guiseppe Di San Francesco

Mappa con la linea di confine tra l'Istria veneta ed il territorio austriaco e gli appostamenti sanitari posti da Zaule, territorio di Muia e Fiauona, territorio d'Albona. 1712; scala di miglia italiane 5 = mm 162; dim mm 1,230 × 1,305. Disegno a mano, su carta, con colorazioni ad acquarello. ASV. Provveditori alla Sanità, Disegni, B1N16.

5. Pietro Soranzo

Mappa del territorio di Imoschi (Dalmazia veneta) confine con l'Impero Ottomano, con il territorio Sign, di Duare e di Vergoraz ed i caselli ed appostamenti sanitari. 18 novembre 1783; scala passi veneti 2400 = mm 130; dim mm 1,570 × 765. Disegno a mano, su carta, con colorazioni ad acquarello. ASV. Provveditori alla Sanità, Disegni, B4N21.

6. Giancomo Pellegrini

Mappa con il litorale di Monfalcone da Porto Anfora al castello di Duino e con l'indicazioni dei posti di guardia sanitari al confine con gli arciducali. 13 novembre 1713, Monfalcone; scala miglia Quattro = mm 140; dim mm 1,430 × 675. Disegno a mano, su carta di più pezzi uniti insieme e riforzati con tela, con colorazioni ad acquerello. ASV. Provveditori alla Sanità, Disegni, B1N3.

7. (Unknown)
Colognese (Territorio)

Mappa del territorio colognese, al confine con le province di Padova e Vicenza, con i castelli e le separazioni stabilite dal Provv. Gen. in T.F. in occasione di una epidemia bovina. 10 guigno 1747; dim mm 420 × 340. Disegno a mano, su carta, con colorazioni ad acquerello. ASV. Provveditori alla Sanità, Disegni, B4N19.

8. Gio. Giancomo Pelligrini
Monfalcone (Territorio)

Mappa del territorio di Monfalcone compreso tra il lago di Pietra Rossa e il corso del fiume Isonzo con l'indicazione delle ville, posti e caselli di guardia sanitari al confine con il granducale. 1713; di miglia due = mm 123; dim mm 1,400 × 700. Disegno a mano, su carta, di due pezzi uniti insieme rinforzati con tela, con colorazioni ad acquerello. ASV. Provveditori alla Sanità, Disegni, B5N26.

9. Bartolo Riviera
Friuli

Disegni con raffigurati gli appostamenti di cavalleria e di fanteria creati ai confini del Friuli in occasione di epidemie. (Att. Linea di confine per contaggio dei Bovini fatta nel Friuli – 87). Sec. 18; dim mm 1,040 × 395. Disegno a mano, su carta di due pezzi uniti insieme, con colorazioni ad acquerello. ASV. Provveditori alla Sanità, Disegni, B5N27.

10. Gio Batta Cavalcaselle
Veronese (Territorio)

Mappa con parte del territorio veronese al confine con il mantovano e il ferrarese e con la descrizione di vari caselli sanitari. Sec 18; scala di miglia di circa = mm 125; mm 958 × 730. Disegno a mano, su carta rinforzata su tela con colorazioni ad acquerello. ASV. Provveditori alla Sanità, Disegni, B5N29.

11. Unknown
Budua (Territorio Di)

Mappa comprendente un tratto di mare tra Porto Rose e Castel di Lastva ed i territori di Cattaro Zupa, Budua, Maini e Pastroviech con l'indicazione dei posti di confine. Sec 18; dim mm 785 × 580. Disegno a mano, su carta di due pezzi uniti insieme e rinforzata con tela, con colorazioni ad acquerello. ASV. Provveditori alla Sanità, Disegni, B6N34.

12. Vicenzo Bernardi
Adige (Fiume)

Parte del corso del fiume Adige all'altezza di Ossevigo in territorio veronese, con l'indicazione degli appostamenti al confine, lungo la strada postale. Sec 18; scala pertiche veronesi 100 = mm 180; dim mm 1,260 × 720. Disegno a mano, su carta di più pezzi uniti insieme, con colorazioni ad acquerello. ASV. Provveditori alla Sanità, Disegni, B7N43.

Genoa
Biblioteca Civica Berio

13. Matteo Vinzoni

Piante delle due Riviere della Serenissima Repubblica di Genova. Divise Ne. Commissariati di Sanita. Cavate Dal M. Col. Ing. Matteo Vinzoni. Per Ordine Dell' Ill Mag. di Sanita. 1758; mm 528 × 355; cc. 119 complessive, num nel sec XVIII per pagg 230 (escluso il foglio di guardia ant. e il front.). Mostra di manoscritti e libri rari della Biblioteca Civica di Berio di Genova.

Il Dominio della Serenissima Republica de Genov in Terrafirma. 1773. Facsimile edition; mm 340 × 240; Mostra di manoscritti e libri rari della Biblioteca Civica di Berio di Genova. Genova: Compagnia Imprese Elettriche Liguri, 1955.

Santa Sede (Holy See)
Archivio di Stato di Roma (ASR)

14. Gaspare Grassellini

Carta topografica sanitaria del littorale del Mediterraneo nello Stato Pontificio dal confine del Gran Ducato di Toscana quello del Regno di Napoli nel rapporto di 1 a 1000000. Compilata nel Dicastero Generale del Censo essendo Pro Presidente sua eccnza RMA Monsignor Gaspare Grassellini per uso della Congregazione Generale di Sanità. 9 decembre 1843. Scala 1:100,000; dim mm 2,790 × 415; disegno a penna su carta, colorato. ASR. Disegni, Coll I cart 106f, 215.

15. Guiseppe Vaselli

Topografica del Littorale Pontificio, nell' Adriatico, e del confine terrestre col Regno di Napoli portante l'armamento del cordone sanitario, ripartito in quattro Divisioni (Stato generale della forza impiegata dell' Adriatico, e confine col Regno di Napoli). Ancona, marzo 1816; dim mm 550 × 1,580; disegno a penna su carta, colorato. ASR. Disegni, Coll I cart 106f, 218.

Tuscany
Archivio di Stato di Firenze (ASF)

16. Unknown
Livorno (Torri Costiere)

Piano specificazione e stato delle Torri e Posti che sono situati sul Lido del Mare da Livorno fino a Torre Nuova, aumentati in occasione della contumacia della Città di Messina dell'anno MDCC XLIII (1743). 1743. Scala di miglia italiane 10 = mm 215; dim mm 435 × 1,385; disegno a penna su carta, colorato. ASF. Miscellanea di piante 5/20, 38.

17. P. Giovanni Fabbroni
Toscana (Torri Costiere)

Pianta della costa del Mare Toscano guarnita con tutte le sue Torri e Casotti fatta in occasione della Peste di Messina l'anno MDCCXXXXIII principiando dalla Torre del Cinquale fino alla Torre di Cala del Forno che confina con lo Stato di Orbetello. 1754. Scala di miglia 6 = mm 76; dim mm 770 × 2,110; disegno à penna su carta telata, colorato. ASF. Disegni, Miscellanea di piante 5/20, 258.

Naples
Archivio di Stato di Napoli (ASN)

18. Augustin De Bargas Machuco
Lecce

Piano dimostrativo della marina di Lecce e del suo cordone marittimo. 1743. Scala di miglia quindici italiane pari a mm 95; dim mm 355 × 485 (350 × 480); disegno a inchiostro acquerellato. Segreteria di Stato d'Azienda, fs. 253, fascic. 20.

19. Soprintendenza Generale Della Salute
Lecce, Chianca Di

Pianta delle baracche e rastelli fatti costruire per la custodia dei Turchi naufragati nella marina della torre della Chianca di Lecce. 1743. Scala di palmi 200 pari a mm 110; dim mm 415 × 285 (385 × 265); disegno a inchiostro acquerellato. Segreteria di Stato d'Azienda, fs. 252, fascic. 38.

20. Vicari Generali (General Vicars)

MESSINA, 1743. *Relazione topografica dell' intèro cordone, commandato dalli 3: Vica^i Gener^i il quale hà li suoi termini nelli due mari di Milazzo, e Taormina che per linea retta saria miglia so mà per tortuosa come al pres ritrouasi si estende a miglia.* Dim mm 910 × 920; disegno a inchiostro acquerellato. Piante e disegni, busta XXXIII, 8.

Palermo
Archivio di Stato di Palermo (ASP)

21. Alì Innocenzo: Ministero E Real Segreteria Di Stato Presso IL Luotenente Generale in Sicilia, Ripartiment Lavori Pubblica

Pianta topografica del littorale della valle di Siracusa distinto nei littorali rispettivi di ogni comune e con l'indicazione dei posti di cordone sanitario terrestre. Siracusa 30 April 1837. Miglia siciliani; dim mm 920 × 1,310; disegno a penna su carta, colorato.

Bari
Wellcome Trust Medical Photographic Library, London

22. F. De Arrieta

Ragualio historico del contaggio occorso nella provincial di Bari negli anni 1690, 1691, e 1692. (Naples, Parrino and Mucii, 1694.) 324 × 180 mm. Scale ≈ 1:500,000. The map is on p. 183.

University of Bologna
Library of the University of Bologna

23. L. F. Marsili

Mappa geographica, qua praecautio contra pestem post factam locorum, juxta pacis instrumentum, evacuationem ac demolitonem in confinibusistis Cis Danubialibus instituenda ostenditur. See Frati, L. (1928). *Catalogo dei Manoscritti di Luigi Ferinando Marsili Conservati nella Biblioteca Universitaria di Bologna,* p. 213, entry 25 (Firenze: Olschki). A manuscript map prepared by or for Marsili and dated April, 1700. Dimensions: mm 224 × 130. Scale ≈ 1:500,000.

CHAPTER 2

The Surveillance of Communicable Diseases

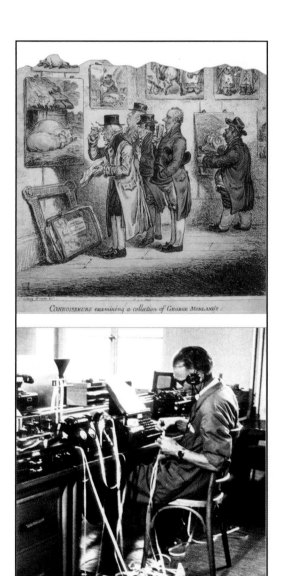

Figure 2.1 Two views of surveillance. James Gillray's (1807) send up of connoisseurs inspecting some of George Morland's (1763–1804) sentimental rural scenes recognises that early surveillance was primarily observational, with little data recording. In contrast the lower image shows epidemiological information being received at Geneva post office via paper tape when machine-generated tables of surveillance data first began to be published by the World Health Organization in the mid-1950s. *Source:* (*Lower*) Fee, *et al.* (2008, Image 1, p. 630), reproduced courtesy of the World Health Organization.

2.1 Introduction

If we are to control the spread of a communicable disease, knowledge by surveillance of the existence – where, when and how much – of a disease is a necessary prerequisite (**Figure 2.1**). Although the idea of using morbidity and mortality data as a basis for public action to inhibit the spread of infection can be traced back to medieval times (Chapter 1), the modern concept of 'disease surveillance' as a scientific basis for such action rests with the establishment of the US Communicable Disease Center in 1946. Beginning with the national malaria control programme, the mandate of the Center was to initiate the investigation of health events through the systematic collection and analysis of morbidity and mortality data. In 1955, the term 'disease surveillance' was applied to these activities by Alexander D. Langmuir, chief epidemiologist (**Figure 2.2**), who defined disease surveillance activities as:

> the continued watchfulness over the distribution and trends of incidence through the systematic collection, consolidation and evaluation of morbidity and mortality reports and other relevant data. Intrinsic in the concept is the regular dissemination of the basic data and interpretations to all who have contributed and to all others who need to know (Langmuir, 1963, pp. 182–3).

At the global level, Langmuir (1976) observes that the term 'surveillance' was given expanded meaning in the course of the World Health Organization's Malaria Eradication Programme (Section 5.4) and was extended to embrace active measures of control such as the administration of chemotherapy and the use of insecticides. In the Smallpox Eradication Programme (Section 5.2), the term became synonymous with containment, including the delivery of vaccines. Subsequently, the US Centers for Disease Control and Prevention (CDC), successor to the Communicable Disease Center, has defined disease surveillance as the:

> Ongoing systematic collection, analysis and interpretation of health data in the process of describing and monitoring a health event. This information is used for planning, implementing, and evaluating public health interventions and programs (Centers for Disease Control, 1988, p. 1).

An understanding of the purposes and methods of data compilation under the aegis of disease surveillance is a necessary prerequisite to effect analysis of the resulting data. Disease surveillance systems vary in method, orientation and scope depending upon the nature of the health event being observed, and they thus vary in their simplicity, acceptability, sensitivity, representativity and timeliness (Centers for Disease Control, 1988).

Layout of Chapter

In this chapter, we focus upon the role of surveillance in informing control strategies for communicable diseases. We begin in Section 2.2 by examining how morbidity and mortality are recorded and classified to form the basis of surveillance systems. In Sections 2.3–2.8, we examine the business of gathering surveillance data over time and space, beginning with the earliest systematic data recording, the bills of mortality for London and other cities in Europe and North America (Section 2.3). Geographically, the bills are local-scale. In Section 2.4, we move up the geographical scale to national surveillance systems, as well as forward in time, and study the evolution of surveillance systems in the United States from colonial days to the present. Sections 2.5–2.7 shift up the geographical scale yet again to the world regional and global levels by examining international disease surveillance articulated through

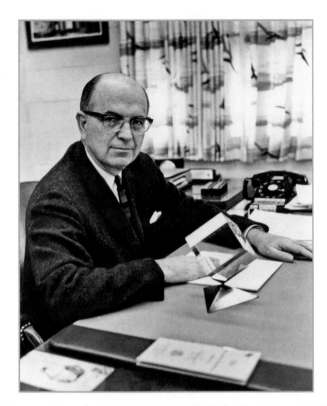

Figure 2.2 Alexander D. Langmuir (1910–93). Chief epidemiologist at the US Communicable Disease Center (forerunner of the Centers for Disease Control and Prevention), 1949–70, and founder of the Disease Investigations branch of the US Epidemic Intelligence Service. He is credited with the modern development of the concept of surveillance in relation to public health. *Source*: CDC (Public Health Image Library ID #8148).

such historical bodies as the Office International d'Hygiène Publique and the League of Nations Health Organisation and, today, through the World Health Organization. Over time, collection strategies have evolved in response to changing technologies, from pen and paper, through the electric telegraph, paper tape and punch cards, to the worldwide reach and instantaneity of the Internet. The Internet-age has spawned a number of 'informal' real-time disease surveillance mechanisms, while enhancing the opportunities for multiple-source disease tracking tools. At the same time, the global range of diseases and the global population have mushroomed, so that the blanket surveillance of former times is now evolving into sampling procedures by time, disease and geographical location. These developments form the basis of the chapter's final substantive section, Section 2.8.

2.2 Disease Classification and Recording: General Considerations

Disease Classifications

Early attempts to devise a systematic classification of diseases include the works *Nosologia Methodica* by François Bossier de Lacroix (1706–77) in 1763, *Genera Morborum* by Linnaeus (1708–78) in 1759, and *Synopsis Nosologiae Methodicae* by William Cullen (1710–90) in 1785. Major advances in disease classification, however, awaited the mid-nineteenth century and the First International Statistical Congress, held in Brussels in 1853 – the first in a series of nine meetings with the underpinning aim of achieving uniformity in national statistics. The Congress requested that both William Farr of London and Marc d'Espine of Geneva should prepare uniform classifications of causes of death that were internationally applicable. A compromise list of 138 rubrics was agreed at the next Congress in 1855. Much revised at subsequent meetings, the Farr–d'Espine list formed a basis for the present *International Classification of Diseases* (*ICD*) which began formally in Chicago in 1893 with the adoption by the International Statistical Institute of Bertillon's International List of Causes of Death. In 1898, the American Public Health Association recommended the adoption of the Bertillon classification by the civil registrars of Canada, Mexico and the United States, adding that the classification should be revised every 10 years. The first revision of the Bertillon classification appeared in 1903 (**Figure 2.3**). Since that time, the classification now known as the *ICD* has gone through a total of 10 revisions

and runs to several weighty volumes (World Health Organization, 2011a).

The *ICD* is the international standard diagnostic classification for all general epidemiological and many health management purposes. It is used to classify diseases and other health problems recorded on health and vital records including death certificates and hospital records. The idea of such a classification is to ensure comparability of data recording over space and time, thus facilitating the storage and retrieval of diagnostic information for clinical and epidemiological purposes. These records also provide the basis for the compilation of national mortality and morbidity statistics by country-level surveillance organisations. The latest (tenth) classification (*ICD*-10) came into use in WHO Member States from 1994; see www.who.int/classifications/icd/en for a history.

Figure 2.4A shows the time series of the number of infectious diseases appearing in the *ICD* since its inception. The diseases

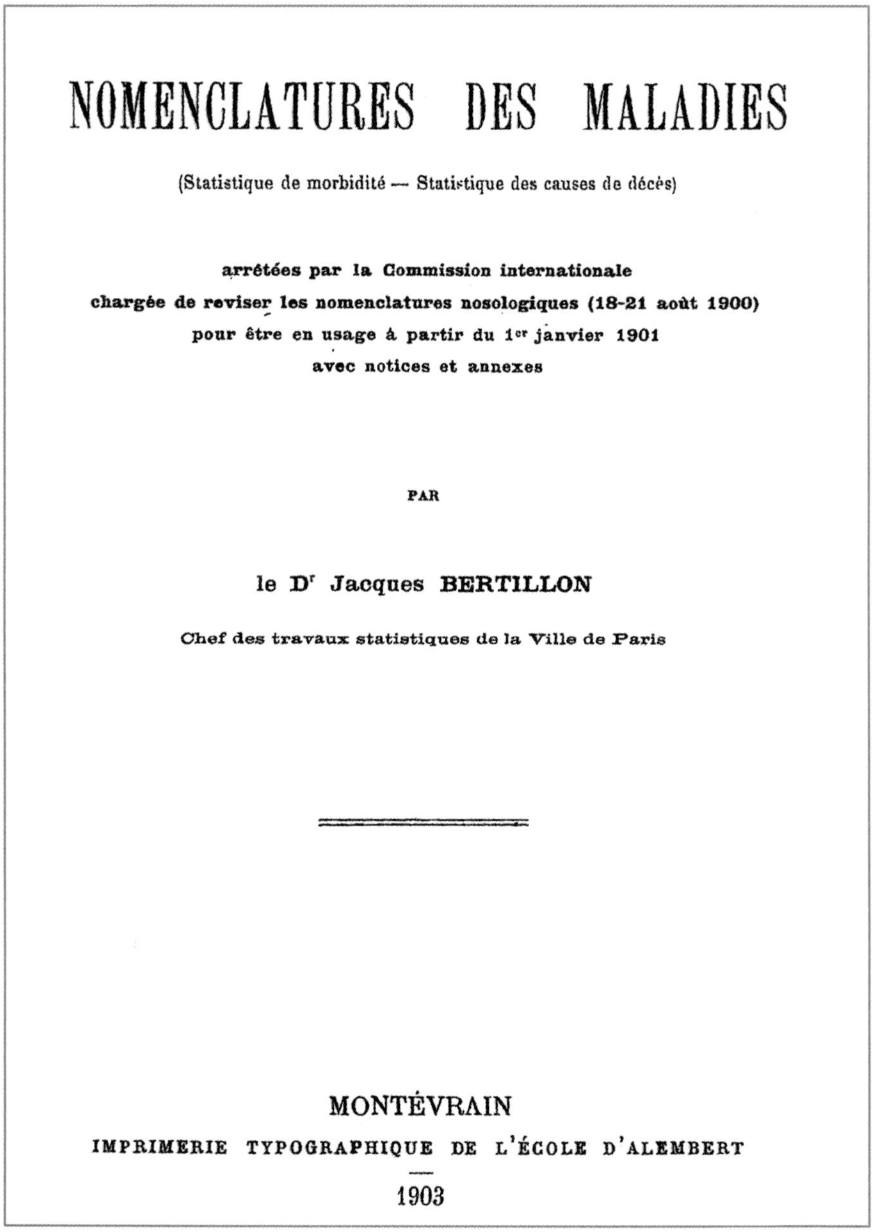

NOMENCLATURES DES MALADIES

(Statistique de morbidité — Statistique des causes de décès)

arrêtées par la Commission internationale
chargée de reviser les nomenclatures nosologiques (18-21 août 1900)
pour être en usage à partir du 1er janvier 1901
avec notices et annexes

PAR

le Dr Jacques BERTILLON

Chef des travaux statistiques de la Ville de Paris

———

MONTÉVRAIN

IMPRIMERIE TYPOGRAPHIQUE DE L'ÉCOLE D'ALEMBERT
——
1903

Figure 2.3 Bertillon's *Nomenclatures des Maladies (Statistique de Morbidité – Statistique des Causes de Décès)*, better known as the *International List of Causes of Death*. Title page to the first revision of the List, published in 1903, and providing a detailed classification of causes of death into 179 groups.

included are those in the so-called A and B lists. The number of diseases listed remained at around 100 for the first 65 years of *ICD*'s existence. In the ninth and tenth revisions, however, the number rose sharply from around 350 (*ICD*-9) to over 1,000 (*ICD*-10). Figure 2.4B gives, on the same decennial basis, the dates of discovery of the main disease agents which have shaped this curve. The switch from bacterial to viral agents identified over the course of the twentieth century is evident.

Disease Collecting Systems

Primary Surveillance Networks

The various routes by which a case of a particular disease may enter the statistical record at the primary (local) level are shown schematically in **Figure 2.5**. The left-hand path describes a *reactive* process in which an individual may experience symptoms of a disease but may or may not be able (or inclined) to visit a medical practitioner. Such a consultation may or may not result in a correct diagnosis and the physician may or may not have to pass the record up the reporting chain. Primary data collection by general practitioners, consultants, hospital clinics and others may or may not become part of a country's official disease records. Only diseases of major public health importance are subject to statutory notification (that is, notifiable by law) and the quality of the data record will depend on many factors: the complexity of the disease and associated complications; the diagnostic skill of the physician; the case load of other clinical work, and so on. The routine reporting of some diseases is supplemented by the right-hand path in Figure 2.5. This path describes a *proactive* process in which screening or surveys of 'healthy' or 'at risk' populations may reveal evidence of infection or disease (for example, HIV/AIDS or tuberculosis) either unrecognised by the individual or for which medical advice had not been sought in the first instance.

Secondary Surveillance Networks

Figure 2.6 shows the reporting routes whereby disease-related information finds its way from the primary level, via secondary reporting routes of varying complexity, to national (e.g. the Health Protection Agency in the United Kingdom and the Centers for Disease Control and Prevention in the USA) and to international recording agencies like the World Health Organization.

Time Span of Disease Records

The availability of disease data varies greatly over time. As we shall see in Section 2.3, a written record of the incidence of some diseases goes back to the sixteenth century for a few great cities. Before this, historical and even prehistoric archaeological records can cast a dim and fitful light on the presence or absence of a few specific diseases. With improvements in DNA testing on palaeopathological specimens, there is hope for some extension. But, as **Figure 2.7** shows, there is little consistent archival material until the second half of the nineteenth century. At this time, legislation was passed in the United States, Scandinavia and Great Britain which ensured disease records were kept for afflictions considered to be of public health importance to national populations. As described earlier, internationally-endorsed classifications of causes of death (and, later, causes of morbidity) which could be used by international agencies for the compilation of disease statistics became available in the early twentieth century. From that time, international agencies such as the Pan American Sanitary Bureau, the League of Nations Health Organisation and the World Health Organization have served as sources of international data on health and disease.

In interpreting Figure 2.7 it is important not to assume that disease recording over time has become ever more accurate. In recent decades, the recording of some common diseases has been downgraded as their incidence and perceived threat have fallen. In some countries, disease recording has moved from statutory reporting of all recognised cases to one of sampling and surveillance using devices such as 'sentinel' medical practices.

Sources of Disease Data

Over the centuries, many sources of disease-related data have developed. These include: mortality registration; morbidity case reporting; epidemic reporting; laboratory reporting; individual case reports; epidemic field investigations; surveys; animal reservoir and vector distribution studies; and demographic and environmental data (Declich and Carter, 1994). To these can be added: hospital and medical care statistics; general practitioner records; public health laboratory reports; disease registries; drug and biologics utilisation and sales data; absenteeism data; health and general population surveys; and media reports. Different data sources present their own advantages and disadvantages. Their availability varies from country to country and they differ in their level of sophistication, quality, utility and extent.

2.3 Early Surveillance Systems: Local Bills of Mortality

The early history of bills of mortality, which were printed or written abstracts from parish registers of the number of people who had died in a given place and time (**Figure 2.8**), is reviewed by Walford (1878). Ancient Rome had bills in the form of *Rationes Libitinæ*, maintained in the Temple of Libitina, the Goddess of Funerals. The Temple of Libitina, in which the last rites were transacted, served as a registration office, and an account (*ratio ephemeris*) was kept of those who died (Walford, 1878). In modern form, bills of mortality date to the sixteenth and seventeenth centuries. The London *Bills of Mortality* (Figure 2.8A) represent one of the earliest examples of a disease surveillance system in that they involved data collection and analysis, interpretation and dissemination of information for action in the context of the repeated plague epidemics in the late sixteenth and seventeenth centuries (Declich and Carter, 1994), and the London *Bills* form our point of departure in this section.

The London *Bills of Mortality*

The history of the London *Bills of Mortality* is reviewed by Marshall (1832) and Walford (1878) and we draw on their accounts here. The *Bills* originated in the sixteenth century as a device for providing the Royal Court with warning when plague was abroad in the city. Responsibility for the preparation of the *Bills* rested with the Parish Clerks of London, with the first known *Bills* issued in the plague year of 1532 and then irregularly throughout the remainder of the sixteenth century as and when plague appeared in the city. Regularity was established early in the seventeenth century, with the first of the uninterrupted series of weekly *Bills* appearing in December 1603 and the first of the annual *Bills* from 1606. In 1625, the Worshipful Company of Parish Clerks obtained a decree under

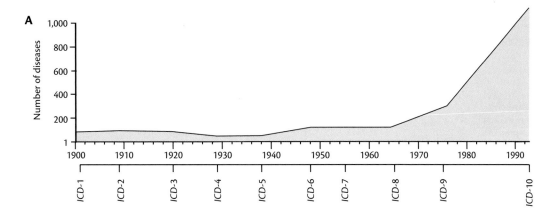

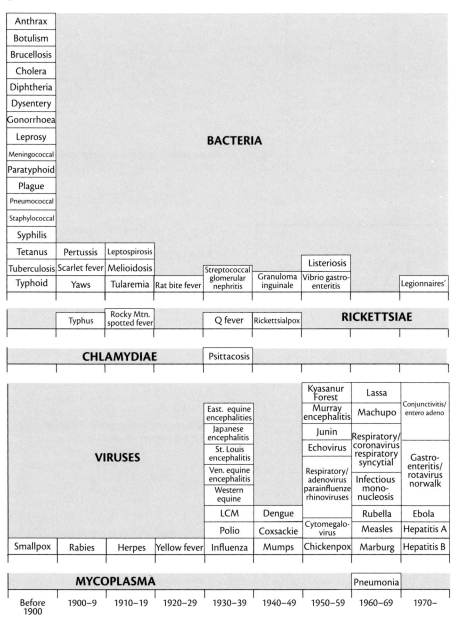

Figure 2.4 *International Classification of Diseases (ICD) 1900–1994.* (A) Number of infectious diseases of humans recorded in *ICD*-1 to *ICD*-10. (B) Decade of discovery of principal infectious disease agents by taxonomic division of agents. *Source:* redrawn from Cliff, Smallman-Raynor, Haggett, *et al.* (2009, Figure 1.8, p. 34).

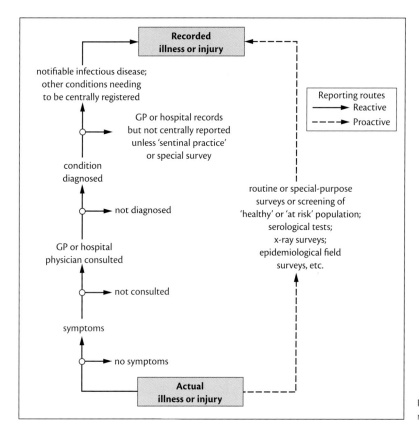

Figure 2.5 Disease recording at the primary level. *Source*: redrawn from Cliff, *et al.* (1993, Figure 2.16, p. 39).

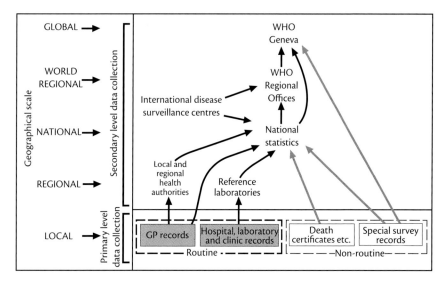

Figure 2.6 Secondary level systems of disease reporting. Schematic representation of the sequence of events whereby a disease event at the primary level is eventually recorded in official statistics up to the global level. *Source*: Cliff, *et al.* (2004, Figure 1.5, p. 4).

the seal of the High Commission Court (Star Chamber) to establish a printing press in their hall and, for this purpose, a printer was assigned by the Archbishop of Canterbury. The quantity of information included in the *Bills* expanded from thereon, with the number of burials in each parish included from 1625, specific causes of death (other than plague) from 1629 and, somewhat later, age at death from 1728. Publication of the *Bills* continued until the mid-1830s, when they were superseded by the *Returns* of the Registrar General.

Surveillance Operations, Geographical Reach and Data Quality

For the purpose of data collection, the Parish Clerks appointed two female 'searchers' in each parish. A contemporary account of the duties of the searchers is provided by John Graunt:

> When any one dies … The Searchers hereupon (who are ancient Matrons, sworn to their office) repair to the place, where the dead Corps lies, and by view of the same, and by other inquiries, they examine by what *Disease* or *Casualty* the Corps died. Hereupon they make their Report to the *Parish-Clerk*, and he, every *Tuesday* night,

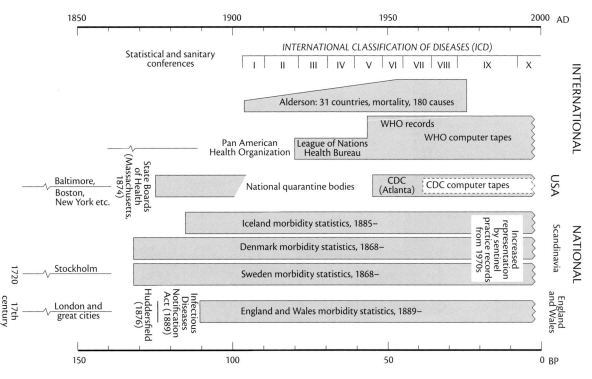

Figure 2.7 Time span of the disease record. The diagram provides a schematic representation of the length of archival records for sample countries and international health organisations, 1850–2000. The sequence of revisions of the *International Classification of Diseases* (*ICD*) is shown towards the top of the diagram. The period encompassed by Alderson's (1981) systematic compilation of standardised mortality data for 31 countries, 1901–75, is also indicated. *Source*: Cliff, *et al.* (1998, Figure 1.7, p. 34).

carries in an Accompt of the *Burials*, and christenings, happening that Week, to the *Clerk* of the *Hall*. On Wednesday the general Accompt is made up, and Printed, and on Thursdays published, and dispersed to the several Families, who will pay four shillings *per Annum* for them (Graunt, 1662, p. 11).

The progressive expansion of the area encompassed by these surveillance operations is mapped to the mid-eighteenth century in **Figure 2.9**. When regular reporting began in 1603, the activities of the searchers were limited to an area of approximately 1,853 acres, encompassing 96 parishes within the walls of the city and several out-parishes. The inclusion of the City of Westminster and several out-parishes in Middlesex and Surrey contributed to a threefold increase in the area under surveillance by the late 1620s, while the incorporation of the parishes of Hackney, Islington, Lambeth, Newington, Rotherhithe, Stepney, Poplar and Bethnal Green brought the total area covered by the *Bills* to over 22,500 acres by the mid-1600s. The geographical reach of the *Bills* was further extended as the city grew over the following century (Walford, 1878) (Figure 2.9).

Contemporary views on the quality of the information included in the London *Bills* are provided by Graunt (1662) and, towards the end of their compilation, Marshall (1832); Landers (1993, pp. 91–3, 193–4) and Boulton and Schwarz (2010) provide more recent perspectives. Suffice it to note here that, officially, the *Bills* only include information relating to burials within Anglican grounds. Even then, it seems doubtful that the records are entirely accurate and both systematic and random elements impinge on the confidence that can be placed in the available data; see Cliff, Smallman-Raynor, Haggett, *et al.* (2009, p. 94).

The Investigations of John Graunt

Although many contemporary physicians held the *Bills* in contempt, not least because "they were based on the diagnoses of ignorant women" (Gale, 1959, p. 21), a mid-seventeenth-century analysis of their content by John Graunt (1620–74), a haberdasher by trade, allowed him to establish some of the fundamental principles of public health surveillance. Graunt's observations were published in *Natural and Political Observations Made upon the Bills of Mortality* in 1662 (**Figure 2.10**), where the motivation for his investigations was laid out:

> Having been born, and bred in the City of *London*, and having always observed, that most of them who constantly took in the weekly Bills of *Mortality*, made little … use of them … I casting mine Eye upon so many of the General *Bills*, as next came to hand, I found encouragement from them, to look out all the *Bills* I could … which, when I had reduced into Tables … I did then begin, not onely to examine the Conceits, Opinions, and Conjectures, which upon view of a few scattered *Bills* I had taken up; but did also admit new ones, as I found reason, and occasion from my *Tables* (Graunt, 1662, pp. 1–2).

Through his tables, Graunt developed the fundamental principles of disease-specific death counts and death rates; he attempted to define the basic laws of natality and mortality; and he is generally credited as the first to estimate the population of the City of London (Declich and Carter, 1994; Thacker, 2010).

Historical Mortality Patterns

The *Bills of Mortality* have informed a substantial literature on the historical demography and mortality of London since Graunt's time, including the major studies and overviews of Creighton (1891–94),

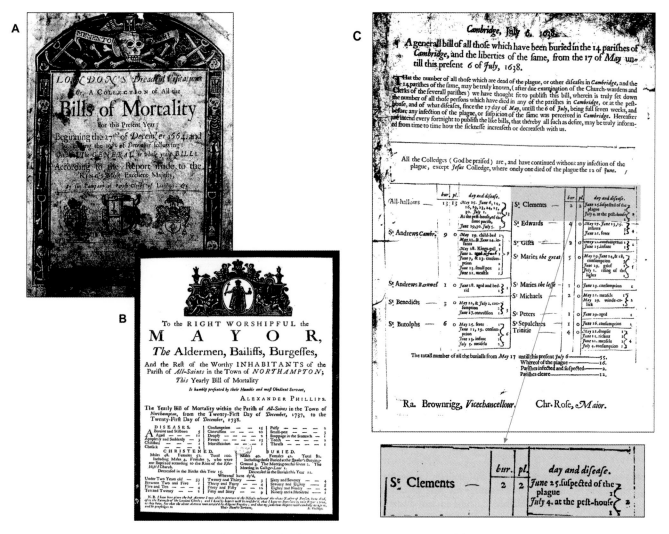

Figure 2.8 Seventeenth- and eighteenth-century bills of mortality for sample English towns and cities. (A) London: cover of the annual collection of weekly *Bills of Mortality* for the infamous plague year of 1665, a year in which 68,596 Londoners are recorded as having died from plague. (B) Northampton: bill for 25 December 1737–21 December 1738, showing the cause of death and age category of the 82 people buried in the period. (C) Cambridge: bill for 17 May–6 July 1638, giving deaths by day and cause in the colleges and parishes of Cambridge. A total of 55 burials were recorded in the period, of which 16 (including a solitary death at Jesus College) were associated with plague. *Source*: (A) Wellcome Library, London.

Finlay (1981), Matossian (1985) and Landers (1993). Because the data in the *Bills* are temporally and spatially coded, both longitudinal and spatial analyses are possible as the following examples show.

Temporal series

The graphs in **Figure 2.11** plot the estimated annual burial rate per 1,000 population in London for all causes (graph A) and seven sample communicable diseases (graphs B–H), 1603–1829. Consistent with the early stages of Omran's epidemiological transition model (Omran, 1971), graph A shows a high background level of burials (30–50 burials per 1,000), punctuated by a series of plague-related 'mortality crises' in 1603, 1625, 1636 and 1665. From the mid-eighteenth century, overall burial rates began a secular decline that continued until the end of the series.

In addition to the sample communicable diseases shown in Figures 2.11B–H, many others were long-present in London but were not formally recorded in the *Bills* as separate disease categories until relatively recent times – an indicator of growing medical

awareness of the conditions. Influenza, for example, emerged from the 'epidemic agues' as a distinct clinical entity in the *Bills* at the end of the eighteenth century, while scarlet fever was formally differentiated from fevers, measles and other causes of death in the 1830s, "long after it had become an important factor in … mortality" (Creighton, 1891–94, Vol. II, p. 719).

Spatial cross-sections: plague

As we have noted, the original purpose of the *Bills* was to provide warning when plague was abroad in London so that its great citizens could retire to the relative epidemiological security of the countryside. Up to 1665, the city was subjected to repeated plague epidemics (Figure 2.11D). Some impression of the spatial manifestation of a sample of these events (1593, 1625, 1636 and 1665) can be gained from **Figure 2.12**. Here, circles plot the total number of burials from all causes in aggregations of parishes; shaded segments indicate the proportion of burials that were plague-related. The Great Plague of London in the year 1665 stands out as a particularly dramatic event (Figures 2.8A, 2.11D and 2.12D). This epidemic is

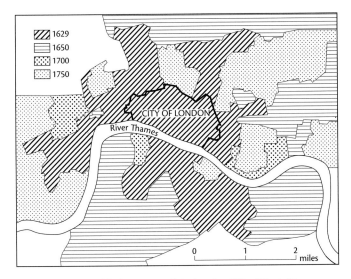

Figure 2.9 Geographical coverage of the London *Bills of Mortality*. The map shows the area covered by the *Bills* in 1629, with an approximate delimitation of additional parishes included by 1650, 1700 and 1750. The city walls are delineated by the black line. *Source*: drawn from information in Marshall (1832).

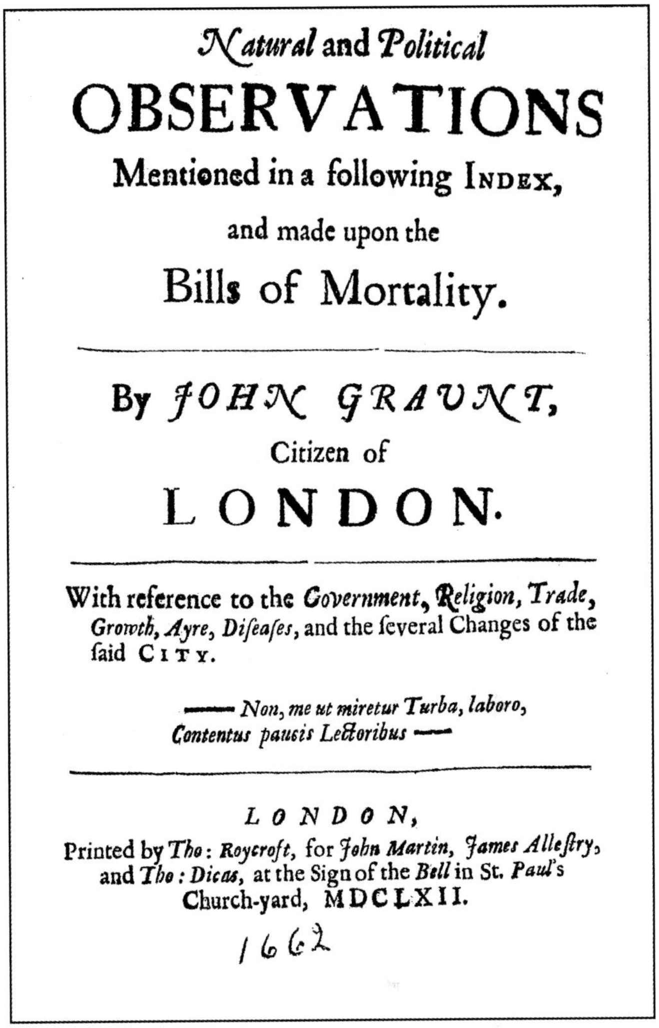

reputed to have begun in the slums of St Giles, in the Fields (then a London out-parish) to the west of the city, spreading thereafter to the east and south and resulting in 68,596 recorded deaths by the end of the year (Creighton, 1891–94, Vol. I, pp. 646–92).

Bills for Other Cities: Continental Europe and North America

Continental Europe

Early Italian 'bills': Books of the Deceased

Cipolla (1978) reports that 'bills of mortality' for some cities of northern Italy become available from the late fourteenth century: Florence (1385), Milan (1452), Bologna (1456), Mantua (1496) and Venice (1504). The bills for these cities were not published at the time but were compiled in unpublished Books of the Deceased and held in city archives. With the exception of Bologna, the registration of deaths on which the bills were based were independent of vital registration at the parish level, and the motivation for their collation ranged from demographic accounting to epidemic intelligence. In Florence, for example, two series of Books of the Deceased were compiled: (1) a 20-volume series, 1385–1778, compiled by the Board of the *Grascia* and concerned with provisioning for the city; and (2) a 23-volume series, 1450–1808, compiled by the Guild of Physicians and Apothecaries. Both series were compiled from information supplied by the town's gravediggers, although the material contained in the two series does not always agree. More generally, deaths in hospitals were omitted from the records of both series, while deaths of children were only erratically and incompletely recorded – the latter, probably, because these were viewed as a normal fact of life (Cipolla, 1978).

Other European countries

Bills of mortality had come into general usage in many parts of Europe by the second quarter of the eighteenth century, as revealed by Sir Conrad Sprengell's extracts of bills for 'considerable towns' in Austria (Lobau, Vienna), Denmark (Copenhagen), Germany (Berlin,

Natural and *Political*

OBSERVATIONS

Mentioned in a following INDEX,

and made upon the

Bills of Mortality.

By *JOHN GRAUNT*,

Citizen of

LONDON.

With reference to the *Government*, *Religion*, *Trade*, *Growth*, *Ayre*, *Diseases*, and the several Changes of the said CITY.

——— *Non, me ut miretur Turba, laboro,* *Contentus paucis Lectoribus* ———

LONDON,

Printed by *Tho: Roycroft*, for *John Martin*, *James Alleſtry*, and *Tho: Dicas*, at the Sign of the *Bell* in St. *Paul's* Church-yard, MDCLXII.

1662

Figure 2.10 Title page of *Natural and Political Observations Made upon the Bills of Mortality* (first edition) by John Graunt, published in 1662. The book went through five editions in 15 years and served to engender an interest in the demographic and epidemiological worth of the London *Bills*.

Dresden, Erfurt, Freiberg, Leipzig, Nurenberg, Weimar), Netherlands (Amsterdam) and Poland (Breslau, Danzig) (Sprengell, 1727). Of these, the bills for Breslau are of particular historical significance as they formed the basis for the first modern life table, constructed by Edmund Halley and published in the *Philosophical Transactions* of the Royal Society in 1693 (Halley, 1693; Bellhouse, 2011) (**Figure 2.13**).

North America

Books of births, marriages and deaths for the city of Boston, Massachusetts, can be traced back to the 1630s. Between 1701 and 1774, the keepers of burial grounds in Boston were required to submit weekly reports of the number of deaths in the city and an annual statement of deaths was compiled and published on the basis of these returns. A new system of registration was established in Boston in the early nineteenth century. In October 1810, the Board of Health divided the city into three districts, within each of which the age, sex, cause of death and other details of all burials was recorded. The information so garnered was printed annually from 1811 in *A General Abstract of the Bill of Mortality*. The *Bills* continued to be

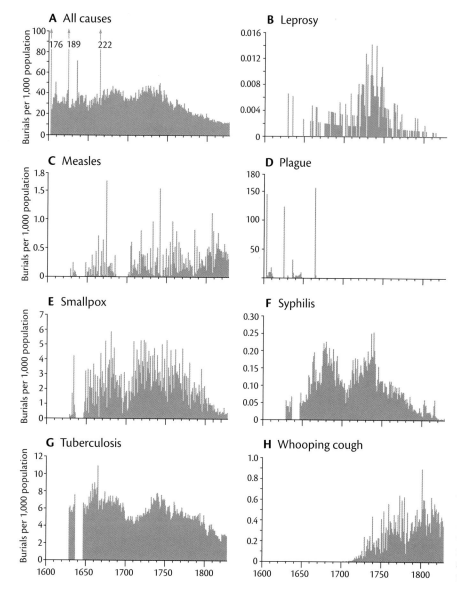

Figure 2.11 Estimated annual burial rates per 1,000 population, London, 1603–1829. (A) All causes. (B) Leprosy. (C) Measles. (D) Plague. (E) Smallpox. (F) Syphilis. (G) Tuberculosis (pulmonary). (H) Whooping cough. Note that, with the exception of plague (D), no cause-specific data are available for the periods 1603–29 and 1637–46. While the 1670s marked the final extinction of plague in the city, other diseases were in the ascendancy. Smallpox, which is said to have begun to attain significance as a cause of death in the reign of James I (1603–25), had achieved the status of an "alarming disease" in London by the mid-seventeenth century (Creighton, 1891–94, Vol. II, p. 436) – a situation that was gradually quelled by inoculation, among other factors, from the late eighteenth century (Hardy, 1983). As smallpox retreated, mortality due to two other long-term incumbents of the city (measles and whooping cough) was increasing, with the great measles epidemic of 1807–8 marked out as "the first of a series of epidemics in which the disease established not only its equality with smallpox as a cause of infantile deaths but even its supremacy over the latter" (Creighton, 1891–94, Vol. II, p. 650). Shortly thereafter, cholera exploded onto the epidemiological scene in the 1830s and 1840s. The remaining graphs chart the rise and fall of leprosy, syphilis and tuberculosis at various times during the seventeenth to nineteenth centuries.

published until 1849, when the Registrar's Department was established in the city (Registry Department, Boston, 1893).

2.4 National Surveillance: The United States

Over a quarter of a millennium, local and national disease surveillance in the advanced economies has developed from the comparatively primitive bills of mortality into a highly sophisticated, real-time data gathering machine. This is particularly so in the United States, and so in this section, we examine as a case study the evolution of surveillance systems for communicable diseases in this country.

Background

Thacker and Berkelman (1988) trace the basic elements of disease surveillance in the American colonies back to the mid-eighteenth century. In 1741, the colony of Rhode Island passed an act that required tavern keepers to report the occurrence of contagious diseases among their patrons. Within a few years, the colony passed a law requiring the statutory reporting of smallpox and yellow fever. National monitoring of disease in the United States began in 1850 when mortality statistics, based on the decennial census, were first published for the entire country. By the start of the twentieth century, laws were in place for the notification of selected communicable diseases to local authorities and, in 1914, Public Health Service personnel were appointed to state health departments to telegraph weekly summaries of notifications to the Public Health Service. By the mid-1920s, all states were engaged in national morbidity reporting. The US Communicable Disease Center was established in Atlanta, Georgia, in July 1946. Initially concerned with diseases such as malaria, murine typhus and smallpox, the new institution expanded its interests to include all communicable diseases in the United States. In 1970, the Communicable Disease Center became the Center for Disease Control and, subsequently, the Centers for Disease Control and Prevention (CDC) (Etheridge, 1992).

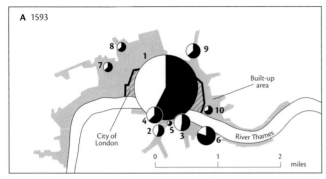

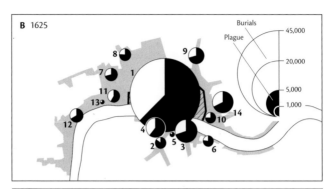

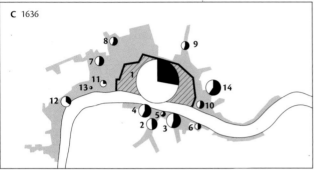

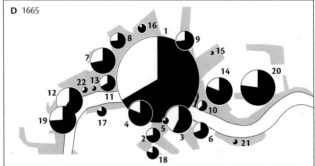

Figure 2.12 Plague in London. Plague assumed epidemic proportions in London in 1593, 1625, 1636 and 1665. The maps are based on information included in the London *Bills of Mortality* and plot, as circles, the total number of burials from all causes in the various divisions of London; shaded segments indicate the proportion of burials attributed to plague. 1 = City parishes, north of the River Thames; 2 = St George, Southwark; 3 = St Olaves, Southwark; 4 = St Saviours, Southwark; 5 = St Thomas, Southwark; 6 = St Mary Magdelen, Bermondsey; 7 = St Giles, in the Fields; 8 = St James, Clerkenwell; 9 = St Leonard, Shoreditch; 10 = St Katherine, by the Tower; 11 = St Clement Danes; 12 = St Martin, in the Fields; 13 = St Mary Savoy Precinct; 14 = St Mary, Whitechapel; 15 = St John, Hackney; 16 St Mary, Islington; 17 = St Mary, Lambeth; 18 = St Mary, Newington; 19 = St Margaret, Westminster; 20 = St Dunstan, Stepney; 21 = St Mary, Rotherhithe; 22 = St Paul, Covent Garden. *Source*: drawn from data in Marshall (1832, p. 68).

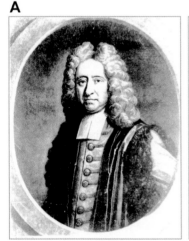

Figure 2.13 Edmund Halley (1656–1742).
English scientist and author of the first known modern life table. The life table was based on the bills of mortality for the city of Breslau (in present-day Poland), 1687–91, and published in *Philosophical Transactions* in 1693. (A) Mezzotint of Halley, 1722. (B) Title page to Halley's 1693 contribution to *Philosophical Transactions*. (C) Halley's population table for Breslau. (D) Halley's worked example of the likelihood of a 30-year-old living to the age of 57–58 years. *Sources*: (A) Wellcome Library, London.

Morbidity and Mortality Weekly Report (MMWR), 1952–2005

In this subsection, we examine the contents of the principal surveillance publication of CDC, and one of the most familiar journals in the epidemiological world: *Morbidity and Mortality Weekly Report*. Universally abbreviated as *MMWR*, it has landed on thousands of desks each week since 1952 – first in paper format and now electronically via the Internet. Published since 1961 by CDC in Atlanta, *MMWR* contains a mix of current information on the distribution of outbreaks and epidemics around the world, reports on vaccines, protective devices, disease definitions and other developments of epidemiological importance, as well as statistical tables of notifiable diseases in the states and territories of the United States. *MMWR* is valued for its timeliness and immediacy. Somewhat akin to the headlines of a newspaper, the mixture of reports, notices and summaries contained within *MMWR* provides a means of tracking headline trends in the contemporary occurrence of communicable diseases of national and international importance.

The MMWR Weekly Data Set

Volume 1, Number 1, of the weekly series of *MMWR* appeared on Friday 11 January 1952 (**Figure 2.14**). In the 60 years since that first edition, around 3,100 issues have been published. Cliff, Smallman-Raynor, Haggett, *et al.* (2009, pp. 133–59) have carried out a content analysis of the first 54 years, 1952–2005 (Vols. 1–54), and the results presented in this subsection are based upon that work. Volumes 1–54 comprise 2,798 issues of *MMWR Weekly*. In addition to the standard tables of notifiable disease counts in the states and other administrative divisions, these issues contain some 16,300 separate reports, articles, notices, updates and related items that appear under a variety of section headings, including 'Current Trends', 'Brief Reports', 'Epidemiologic Notes and Reports', 'International Notes', 'Special Reports', 'Surveillance Summaries' and 'Updates'. The topics covered in this class of item, which we refer to for convenience as 'entries' in the remainder of the present section, range from ciguatera fish poisoning to diabetic retinopathy, iron deficiency to foetal alcohol syndrome, and dental health to childhood pedestrian deaths during Halloween. And scattered among these entries are the early notices and groundbreaking reports of a half-century-long series of newly emerging infectious diseases. Summary details of these entries are given in **Table 2.1**. Geographically, the majority were related to domestic US issues (85 percent) and the Americas Region (87 percent) more generally. Epidemiologically, just under two-thirds of all contributions were associated with sample categories of communicable disease that were drawn primarily from Chapter I ('Certain Infectious and Parasitic Diseases', A00–B99) of the *ICD*-10 list (64 percent), with viral and bacterial agents and their associated diseases accounting for almost 60 percent of the entries.

Global trends

Figure 2.15A plots the annual count of entries in *MMWR Weekly* for all topics (upper line trace) and sample categories of communicable disease encompassed by *ICD*-10 codes A00–B99 (lower line trace). In the first three decades, the annual count of entries for all topics waned gradually, from an early peak of > 400 per annum to a low of < 150 per annum in the early 1980s. The number of entries then rose again, reaching > 300 per annum from the late 1990s. The curve for communicable diseases tracks the overall pattern – albeit at a lower level – until the early 1980s. Thereafter, the divergence of the two curves reflects both (i) the establishment of new publications (*Recommendations and Reports* and *Surveillance Summaries*) as outlets for communicable-disease related information in the *MMWR* series and (ii) the widening scope of *MMWR Weekly* as CDC's activities expanded beyond communicable diseases; see Etheridge (1992) and Centers for Disease Control and Prevention (1996).

New communicable disease categories

One of the interesting features of the data set is the way in which it picks up newly-emerging diseases over time. The main graphs in **Figure 2.16** show a progressive shift in the pattern of publishing activity, with disease categories first included in the 1950s (graph A) and 1960s (graph B) displaying a pronounced reduction in levels of coverage in the pages of *MMWR Weekly* from the late 1970s. With the retreat of these longer-recognised diseases, the episodic spikes of activity associated with the graphs for the 1970s (graph C) and 1980s–2000s (graph D) flag the early reports of such diseases as Legionnaires' disease (1976–78), human immunodeficiency virus (HIV) (1985), hantavirus pulmonary syndrome (HPS) (1993) and severe acute respiratory syndrome (SARS) (2003). To these developments can be added the trans-Atlantic extension of West Nile fever, evidenced by the early twenty-first-century resurgence of the curve in Figure 2.16B.

Primary Data Generation

MMWR represents, as we have noted, the principal published face of surveillance for communicable diseases in the United States. It is based on primary data which arrives at CDC in two main ways: (i) from individual physicians and state health departments that undertake real-time reporting of data to CDC; and (ii) reactive field investigations by CDC staff from the Epidemic Intelligence Service (EIS). We consider sources (i) and (ii) in turn. Full accounts appear on the CDC website (www.cdc.gov).

Physician and State Epidemiological Recording

The structure of public health case reporting in the United States is summarised in **Figure 2.17**. The origins of modern-day reporting through the National Notifiable Diseases Surveillance System (NNDSS) can be traced to 1878 when Congress authorised the US Marine Hospital Service (the forerunner of the Public Health Service) to collect reports on the occurrence of certain communicable diseases from US consuls overseas. As described in Section 3.2, this information was to be used for the implementation of quarantine measures to prevent the introduction of the diseases into the United States. In 1893, Congress expanded the authority for the collection and publication of these overseas reports to include domestic data from states and municipal authorities. Uniformity of disease reporting was subsequently aided by a law, enacted by Congress in 1902, which required the provision of forms for the purposes of data collection, compilation and publication at the national level. A decade later, in 1912, state and territorial health authorities recommended that five diseases should be subject to immediate telegraphic reporting, while an additional 10 diseases should be reported on a monthly basis by letter. The list of notifiable diseases expanded in the following decades such that, by 1928, all states (including the District of Columbia), Hawaii and Puerto Rico were engaged in the national reporting of 29 diseases. The CDC assumed responsibility for the collection and dissemination of nationally notifiable disease data in 1961. Today, the Council of State and Territorial Epidemiologists (CSTE), in conjunction with

Morbidity and Mortality Weekly Report

FEDERAL SECURITY AGENCY Public Health Service
NATIONAL OFFICE OF VITAL STATISTICS

Vol. 1, No. 1   Washington 25, D. C.   January 11, 1952

Provisional Statistics for Specified Notifiable Diseases in the United States for Week Ended January 5, 1952

For the current week there was a total of 9,284 cases of measles reported which was 14 percent higher than for the previous week and nearly 70 percent greater than the number reported for the same week of 1951. The disease is being reported in increasingly large numbers in several of the South Atlantic States. Incidence still remains high in the northeastern part of the country.

The revised list of diseases recommended for weekly reporting by States to the Public Health Service formed the basis for the current week. The diseases being reported for the first time are brucellosis, dengue, infectious hepatitis, trichiniasis, endemic typhus fever, and rabies in man. Cases of dengue and rabies in man will be shown only in footnotes when they occur.

Of the diseases reported for the first time on a regular weekly basis, there were few cases of brucellosis. A considerable number of cases of infectious hepatitis (157) were reported. States reporting the largest numbers were: Georgia with 48, Tennessee with 20, and Kentucky with 16. Only 2 cases of trichiniasis, and 3 of endemic typhus were reported.

In addition to the above changes all cases of scarlet fever and streptococcal sore throat will be combined in one figure. Paratyphoid fever has been ommitted, but typhoid fever cases will be reported. Influenza and pneumonia will no longer be included in morbidity tabulations.

EPIDEMIOLOGICAL REPORTS

Infectious Hepatitis

Dr. J. P. Ward, Arizona Director of Public Health, has reported an extensive outbreak (approximately 275 to 300 cases) of infectious hepatitis in a boarding school for Indians in Tuba City. Preliminary reports indicate that scattered cases occurred in October, but since that time increasing numbers have occurred. Staff members are also reported to be ill. A second nearby community consisting of 600 Indians has had frequent contact with the school, and it appears that some members of this group may be involved in the outbreak. Drs. L. A. Byers, and C. M. Clark, Jr., of the Indian Medical Service, and State health department officials in cooperation with other Federal officials are conducting an intensive investigation. Gamma globulin is being used in an attempt to prevent infection in those not yet ill.

Rabies in Man

Dr. C. R. Freeble, Ohio Department of Health, has reported a case of rabies in a man who died less than 24 hours after seeking medical advice. He had not been feeling well for several days, however. Profuse salivation and violence were noted a few hours before death. Microscopic examination of the brain demonstrated the presence of Negri bodies,

which was confirmed by another laboratory. No animal inoculations were done. Three weeks prior to the patient's illness he shot a fox while hunting in an area where rabies was known to have occurred in these animals. However, no history of a bite was established. The family's hunting dogs had been well and had had antirabies vaccine.

Gastro-enteritis

Dr. Dean Fisher, Maine Director of Health, has reported an outbreak of food poisoning among 8 adults following a meal at which cooked chicken was eaten. Two chickens were cooked, and all 8 cases resulted from eating one of them. Persons eating the other were not ill.

Influenza

Dr. Morris Schaeffer, Public Health Service Communicable Disease Center, has reported through the Influenza Information Center, National Institutes of Health, that a set of paired serum specimens taken from a patient in Indiana showed a significant rise in titer to type A influenza virus. The pair of specimens was received from the Indiana State Board of Health on December 27, 1951. No date of onset was given nor was clinical information furnished.

Botulism

Dr. M. H. Merrill, California Department of Health, has reported 2 fatal cases of botulism which occurred in Fresno County. The onset of these cases was December 29 and both died on December 31. No other persons were present at the meal when infection took place. Laboratory examinations of food collected from the home have not been completed.

Primary Atypical Pneumonia

Dr. G. D. Carlyle Thompson, Executive Officer, Montana Board of Health, has supplied preliminary information on several cases of primary atypical pneumonia which occurred during the latter half of December at the Montana State Training School at Boulder, Montana. Considerable concern developed over this situation as the first 2 cases were severe, and the institution houses 550 individuals. Onset of the disease was sudden with slight sore throat, slight cough, chest pain, and temperatures ranging from 101° to 104°. Penicillin had little or no effect, but aureomycin promptly relieved all symptoms. However, as evidenced by X-ray, the pulmonary infiltration process continued after the administration of aureomycin. A total of 25 cases was hospitalized during a 3-week period. Ten of these gave findings significant of such an infection. Cold-hemagglutinin tests were performed on these 25 cases. Pharyngeal and nasal washings have been submitted to the Public Health Service Rocky Mountain Laboratory in order to isolate a specific virus, if possible.

Figure 2.14 The inaugural issue of *Morbidity and Mortality Weekly Report* (MMWR). Volume 1, Number 1, published by the US Public Health Service on Friday 11 January 1952. Responsibility for the publication of *MMWR* passed to CDC in 1961.

CDC, makes annual recommendations for diseases to be reported through the NNDSS (Centers for Disease Control and Prevention, 2012d). The list of notifiable diseases for 2012 is given in **Table 2.2**.

National Electronic Disease Surveillance System (NEDSS)

The route by which nationally notifiable disease data arrives at CDC today is via NEDSS, a web-based infrastructure for public health surveillance data exchange between CDC and the 50 states (Centers for Disease Control and Prevention, 2011c). The NEDSS project was launched in 2001 to integrate and replace existing CDC surveillance systems, including the National Electronic Telecommunications System for Surveillance (NETSS, adopted in all states by 1985), HIV/AIDS reporting systems, vaccination programmes and tracking systems for other communicable diseases. NEDSS has been designed, *inter alia*, partly to feed other CDC data systems, including the following:

WONDER (Wide-ranging OnLine Data for Epidemiologic Research). This is an Internet system that makes CDC information resources available to public health professionals and the public at large. It provides access to a wide array of public health information. Its purposes are (1) to promote information-driven decision making by placing timely, useful facts in the hands of public health practitioners and researchers, and (2) to provide the general public with access to specific and detailed information from CDC (Centers for Disease Control and Prevention, 2012a).

Epi-X (Epidemic Information Exchange). Launched in December 2000, Epi-X is a web-based communications system that facilitates the access and sharing of preliminary health surveillance information by CDC officials, state and local health departments and other public health professionals. Epi-X also has the facility to notify users of the occurrence of health events in real-time. Since inception, the system has been used to post reports on a range of topics, including SARS, West Nile virus and foodborne outbreaks and multi-state food recalls (Centers for Disease Control and Prevention, 2012b).

Epi Info™ and Epi Map™. *Epi Info™* is a public domain software package designed to facilitate public health education, disease surveillance and analysis and to encourage collaboration between

Table 2.1 Summary details of entries in *MMWR Weekly*, 1952–2005

Category[1]	Number of entries
All entries	16,297
Domestic/international	
Domestic (U.S.) only	13,838
International (non-U.S.) only	1,650
Combined (domestic & international)/no geographical reference	809
WHO world region	
Africa	291
Americas	14,211
Eastern Mediterranean	184
Europe	514
South-East Asia	80
Western Pacific	208
Multiple region/other[1]	809
Sample communicable disease groups (*ICD*-10 code)	
Intestinal infectious diseases (A00–A09)	2,014
Tuberculosis (A15–A19)	244
Certain zoonotic bacterial diseases (A20–A28)	551
Other bacterial diseases (A30–A49)	889
Infections with a predominantly sexual mode of transmission (A50–A64)	394
Other spirochaetal diseases (A65–A69)	44
Other diseases caused by chlamydiae (A70–A74)	262
Rickettsioses (A75–A79)	112
Viral diseases of the central nervous system (A80–A89)	1,282
Arthropod-borne viral fevers and viral haemorrhagic fevers (A90–A99)	505
Viral infections characterised by skin and mucous membrane lesions (B00–B09)	1,284
Viral hepatitis (B15–B19)	495
HIV disease (B20–B24)	397
Other viral diseases (B25–B34)	76
Mycoses (B35–B49)	89
Protozoal diseases (B50–B64)	302
Helminthiases (B65–B83)	188
Influenza and pneumonia (J09–J18)	1,334
Severe acute respiratory syndrome (U04)	28
Infectious disease agents	
Bacteria	4,000
Helminths	188
Protozoa	345
Rickettsiae	111
Viruses	5,392
Multiple/other	156

Notes: [1] Includes entries with no primary geographical reference.
Source: Cliff, Smallman-Raynor, Haggett, *et al.* (2009, Table 3.5, p. 138).

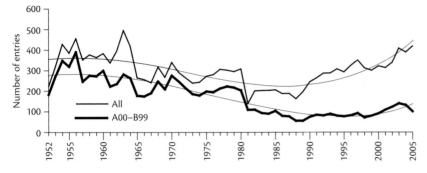

Figure 2.15 Publishing trends in *MMWR Weekly*, 1952–2005. The graph plots the annual count of entries on all topics (upper line trace) and sample categories of communicable disease encompassed by *ICD*-10 codes A00–B99 (lower line trace). Trends are shown by polynomial regression lines. *Source*: redrawn from Cliff, Smallman-Raynor, Haggett, *et al.* (2009, Figure 3.8, p. 139).

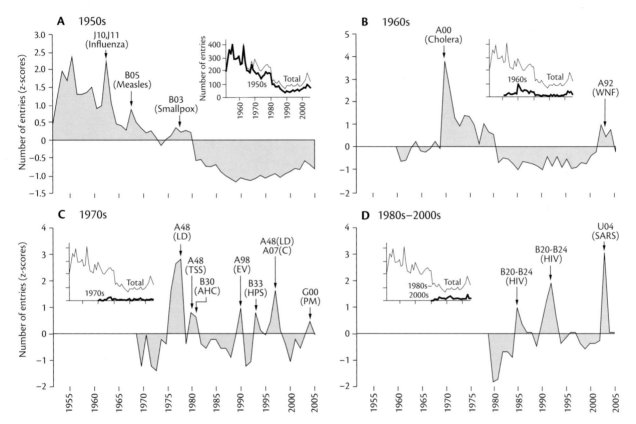

Figure 2.16 Publishing trends for sample communicable diseases by decade of first inclusion in *MMWR Weekly*, 1952–2005. The graphs are based on a sample set of 126 categories of communicable disease and plot the annual count of entries associated with the subset of categories first included in *MMWR Weekly* in the (A) 1950s, (B) 1960s, (C) 1970s and (D) 1980s–2000s. Annual counts are plotted as standard Normal scores (z-scores) (main graphs) and as absolute counts (inset graphs, heavy line traces), with the latter also giving the annual count of entries for all 126 disease categories. Specific diseases (with their three-character *ICD*-10 codes) associated with periods of increased coverage in *MMWR Weekly* are indicated. AHC = acute haemorrhagic conjunctivitis. C = cyclosporiasis. EV = Ebola virus. HIV = human immunodeficiency virus. HPS = hantavirus pulmonary syndrome. LD = Legionnaires' disease. PM = pneumococcal meningitis. SARS = severe acute respiratory syndrome. TSS = toxic shock syndrome. WNF = West Nile fever. *Source*: redrawn from Cliff, Smallman-Raynor, Haggett, *et al.* (2009, Figure 3.9, p. 140).

local, national and international partners, state and territorial epidemiologists, national centres, institutes and government offices, foreign ministries of health and the WHO. It provides questionnaire and database construction, data entry and analysis with epidemiological statistics, graphs and geographical information system (GIS) mapping capability via *Epi Map*™ (Centers for Disease Control and Prevention, 2012c).

Field Investigations: The US Epidemic Intelligence Service (EIS), 1946–2005

Since inception in the early 1950s, the Epidemic Intelligence Service (EIS) of the CDC has been called on by state, federal, national and international health authorities to assist in the field investigation of thousands of disease outbreaks and other events of public health importance. The history and operations of the EIS are reviewed by Langmuir (1980), Goodman, *et al.* (1990), Koplan and Thacker (2001) and Thacker, *et al.* (2001). The EIS Program was established in July 1951 to provide capacity to respond to threats of bioterrorism. Underpinning the initiative, however, was a broader vision to provide a trained cohort of field epidemiologists that would be available at all times for the surveillance and control of diseases in outbreak situations. Since then, some 3,000 EIS Officers have participated in more than 4,000 epidemic assistance investigations in the United States and worldwide (**Figure 2.18**). In

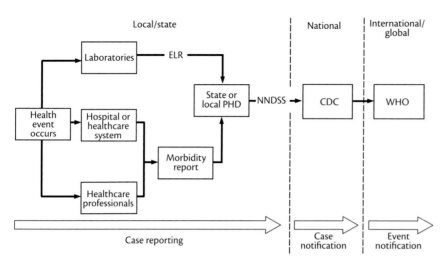

Figure 2.17 Public health case reporting in the United States. Schematic diagram of the process of disease reporting to the Centers for Disease Control and Prevention (CDC) and the World Health Organization (WHO). ELR = Electronic Laboratory Report. NNDSS = National Notifiable Diseases Surveillance System. PHD = Public Health Department. *Source*: courtesy of S.B. Thacker.

Table 2.2 Nationally notifiable diseases in the United States, 2012

Anthrax	Plague
Arboviral neuroinvasive and non-neuroinvasive diseases	Poliomyelitis, paralytic
Babesiosis	Poliovirus infection, nonparalytic
Botulism	Psittacosis
Brucellosis	Q fever
Campylobacteriosis	Rabies, animal and man
Chancroid	Rubella (German measles)
Chlamydia trachomatis infection	Rubella, congenital syndrome
Cholera	Salmonellosis
Coccidioidomycosis	SARS-CoV disease
Cryptosporidiosis	Shiga toxin-producing *Escherichia coli* (STEC)
Cyclosporiasis	Shigellosis
Dengue	Smallpox
Diphtheria	Spotted fever rickettsiosis
Ehrlichiosis/Anaplasmosis	Streptococcal toxic shock syndrome
Free-living amoebae, infections caused by	*Streptococcus pneumoniae*, invasive disease
Giardiasis	Syphilis
Gonorrhoea	Tetanus
Haemophilus influenzae, invasive disease	Toxic shock syndrome (other than streptococcal)
Hansen disease (leprosy)	Trichinellosis (trichinosis)
Hantavirus pulmonary syndrome	Tuberculosis
Hemolytic uremic syndrome, post-diarrheal	Tularemia
Hepatitis A, B and C	Typhoid fever
HIV infection	Vancomycin-intermediate *Staphylococcus aureus* (VISA)
Influenza-associated hospitalizations	Vancomycin-resistant *Staphylococcus aureus* (VRSA)
Influenza-associated paediatric mortality	Varicella (morbidity)
Legionellosis	Varicella (deaths only)
Listeriosis	Vibriosis
Lyme disease	Viral hemorrhagic fevers, due to:
Malaria	Ebola virus
Measles	Marburg virus
Melioidosis	Crimean–Congo haemorrhagic fever virus
Meningococcal disease	Lassa virus
Mumps	Lujo virus
Novel influenza A virus infections	New World arenaviruses
Pertussis	Yellow fever

Source: Centers for Disease Control and Prevention (2012d).

line with the original remit of CDC, the early investigations were largely concerned with outbreaks of communicable diseases. As the responsibilities of CDC have broadened, however, the public health problems addressed by EIS Officers have expanded to include chronic diseases, injuries, drug/vaccine reactions and reproductive, environmental and occupational health issues (Goodman, *et al.*, 1990; Thacker, *et al.*, 2001).

Within the framework of EIS operations, an epidemic assistance investigation (Epi-Aid) is a specific form of investigation that is undertaken by CDC in response to external requests for assistance by states, federal agencies, international organisations and other countries. A request for assistance follows a prescribed administrative mechanism which, if granted, results in the preparation of an initial memorandum ('Epi-1') and, following the investigation, a full report on the work undertaken ('Epi-2') (**Figure 2.19**). Although the Epi-1 and Epi-2 documents are for administrative use and have limited circulation, descriptions of investigations of special interest are frequently published in *MMWR Weekly* and elsewhere in the scientific literature.

The first 60 years of EIS investigations, 1946–2005, are reviewed by Thacker and colleagues (Stroup and Thacker, 2007; Thacker and Stroup, 2007a, b, 2008; Thacker, *et al.*, 2011). A total of 4,484 EIS investigations were initiated in the period and, while the vast majority of these investigations were based in the United States, EIS activities had a global reach (Figure 2.18). Almost 75 percent of all investigations were associated with infectious diseases, but with chronic diseases, environmental/injury and other/unknown categories accounting for an important share of all requests for assistance since the mid-1960s (**Figure 2.20A**). Of the communicable disease investigations, viruses and bacteria accounted for the overwhelming majority (82 percent) of causative agents, but with a pronounced growth in investigations concerned with other agents

(including mycobacteria, parasites and fungi) over the observation period (Figure 2.20B). The communiable disease investigations are noteworthy for including a number of emerging disease events, including Legionnaires' disease, Ebola haemorrhagic fever and HIV/AIDS in the period 1976–85, the first occurrence of meat as a vehicle for *Listeria monocytogenes*, the first documented outbreak caused by *Escherichia coli* O104:H2 and the identification of apple cider as a vehicle for *E. coli* O157:H7 in the period 1986–95, and West Nile virus and SARS in the period 1996–2005 (Thacker, *et al.*, 2011).

2.5 International Health Cooperation: Before the League of Nations

Proto-Systems: Regional Health Bodies in the Nineteenth Century

By the mid-nineteenth century, a number of maritime powers in the Mediterranean area recognised that the control of epidemic diseases extended beyond quarantine in home ports. Effective measures of disease control required international cooperation and, as described by Goodman (1952, pp. 234–42) and the World Health Organization (1958, pp. 32–4), this formed the basis of regional health bodies in Constantinople, Alexandria, Tangier and Tehran.

Constantinople. The Conseil Supérieur de Santé de Constantinople was formed as an agreement between the Ottoman Empire and European powers in 1839 with a view to regulating the sanitary control of foreign shipping in Ottoman ports. The Conseil oversaw local health offices, distributed throughout the Ottoman Empire, which were responsible for reporting on the health of their areas, the supervision of hygienic measures and the implementation of sanitary regulations received from the Conseil. The Conseil

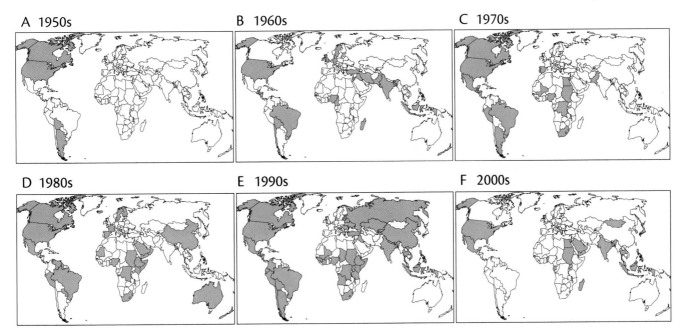

Figure 2.18 Sites of EIS epidemic assistance investigations (Epi-Aids). Countries in which investigations were undertaken in a given time period are shaded. (A) 1950s. (B) 1960s. (C) 1970s. (D) 1980s. (E) 1990s. (F) 2000s. *Source:* redrawn from Cliff, Smallman-Raynor, Haggett, *et al.* (2009, Figure 3.16, p. 160), originally from Centers for Disease Control and Prevention (2005).

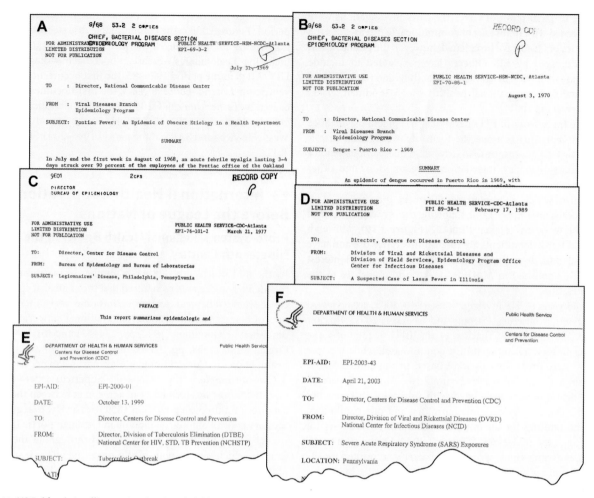

Figure 2.19 US Epidemic Intelligence Service. Sample field investigation memoranda (Epi-1) and reports (Epi-2) for selected outbreaks of communicable diseases. (A) Outbreak of Pontiac fever, Oakland County, Michigan, 1968. (B) Outbreak of dengue fever, Puerto Rico, 1969. (C) Outbreak of Legionnaires' disease, Philadelphia, 1976. (D) Suspected case of Lassa fever, Illinois, 1989. (E) Outbreak of tuberculosis, Columbia, South Carolina, 1999. (F) Hospital-based exposure to a probable SARS case in Pennsylvania, 2003. *Source*: Cliff, Smallman-Raynor, Haggett, *et al.* (2009, Plate 3.4, p. 163).

was finally abolished in 1914 with the outbreak of the First World War.

Alexandria. The Conseil Sanitaire Maritime et Quarentenaire d'Egypte, later to become known as the Egyptian Quarantine Board, was established in Egypt in 1843. International regulation of the Board was instituted following the International Sanitary Conference at Venice in 1892 when it was entrusted with the sanitary regime of the Suez Canal. The work of the Board included the port health administration of Alexandria, Suez, Port Said and the Suez Canal, along with the sanitary control of pilgrims returning from Mecca. For the purposes of epidemic intelligence, it was recognised as a regional epidemiological bureau of the Office International d'Hygiène Publique under the International Sanitary Convention of 1926. Although the Board was abolished in 1938, the Egyptian authorities continued to support a Regional Epidemiological Intelligence Bureau in Alexandria, with its functions transferred to the WHO Regional Office for the Eastern Mediterranean in 1949.

Tangier and Teheran. The Conseil Sanitaire de Tangier was established in the 1840s with the intention of limiting the spread of plague, cholera and other epidemic diseases in the Empire of Morocco by pilgrims, although it failed to operate as an effective instrument of international quarantine. The Conseil Sanitaire de

Téhéran, established in 1867, was similarly limited in its effectiveness and came to an end with the outbreak of war in 1914 (World Health Organization, 1958).

The Office International d'Hygiène Publique (1907–46)
The International Sanitary Conferences and Conventions

The mid-nineteenth century and the first of the International Sanitary Conferences marked the beginning of a new phase in international health cooperation (**Table 2.3**), forming a broad platform for the development of international health offices and legislative responses to infectious diseases in the next century (**Figure 2.21**). The primary objective of the First International Sanitary Conference, opened in Paris in 1851, was for the 12 participating states (all European) to reach agreement on the minimum quarantine requirements for cholera, plague and yellow fever, with a view to facilitating trade and safeguarding public health. Although an international sanitary convention and associated sanitary regulations were formulated, some participants were slow to ratify the convention and it had become inoperative by 1865. Part of this failure lay in the state of medical knowledge regarding cholera and the contradictory views of the delegates regarding the role of quarantine in its control (World Health Organization, 1958).

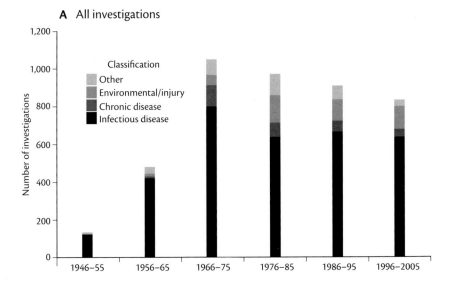

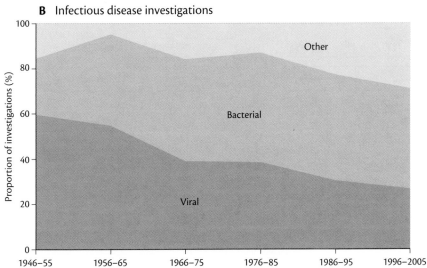

Figure 2.20 EIS epidemic assistance investigations (Epi-Aids), 1946–2005. (A) Count of investigations by 10-year period. (B) Percentage proportion of communicable disease investigations associated with viral, bacterial and other agents in each 10-year period. *Source*: drawn from data in Thacker, *et al.* (2011, Table 1, p. S6).

Further International Sanitary Conferences were held in the second half of the nineteenth century, each centred on the containment of cholera, plague and yellow fever and with their agendas dictated by epidemics of whichever disease was considered to be the most pressing at the time (Table 2.3). The first of the effective International Sanitary Conventions, concerned with the Mecca pilgrimage, came out of the Seventh International Sanitary Conference in 1892. Subsequent conventions evolved to cover cholera (1893), plague (1897), yellow fever (1912) and, into the twentieth century, smallpox (1926) and louse-borne typhus fever (1926); see Table 2.3 and **Figure 2.22**.

The Office International d'Hygiène Publique (1907–46)

The Office International d'Hygiène Publique (OIHP) was born out of the Eleventh International Sanitary Conference, held in Paris in 1903 (Table 2.3 and Figure 2.21). It was founded under the Rome Agreement on 9 December 1907 and based in Paris. Operating on behalf of participating states, the main purpose of the OIHP was to oversee the international codification of procedures for quarantine and associated surveillance activities. Within

this remit, the OIHP served three basic functions (Goodman, 1952):

- as the body with responsibility for the revision and administration of the International Sanitary Conventions and associated Conferences;

- as a technical commission for the study of epidemic diseases;

- as an agency for the rapid exchange of epidemiological information relating to the diseases covered by the International Sanitary Conventions.

The OIHP's Paris headquarters were established at 195 Boulevard Saint-Germain, from which a regular (monthly) report was circulated to participating states under the title *Bulletin Mensuel* (**Figure 2.23**).

Developments in the aftermath of the First World War ushered in a formal collaboration between the OIHP and the newly-created League of Nations. As described more fully later in this section, the Covenant of the League of Nations included an article relating to international concern for the prevention and control of diseases and, to avoid duplication of activities, consideration was given to the continuation of the

Table 2.3 The International Sanitary Conferences and Conventions, 1851–1938

Year	Conference	Place	Outcome/convention
1851	First	Paris	Abortive convention
1859	Second	Paris	Draft convention only
1866	Third	Constantinople	Regulations on Mecca pilgrimages
1874	Fourth	Vienna	Proposal for an International Commission on Epidemics
1881	Fifth	Washington, D.C.	Recommendation for notification of epidemics through international bureaux
1885	Sixth	Rome	Miscellaneous recommendations, primarily concerned with cholera
1892	Seventh	Venice	First effective convention, limited to Mecca pilgrimage
1893	Eighth	Dresden	General convention on cholera
1894	Ninth	Paris	Further convention on cholera and the Mecca pilgrimage (not effective)
1897	Tenth	Venice	New convention, including plague
1903	Eleventh	Paris	Consolidating convention on cholera and plague
1912	Twelfth	Paris	Amended convention, including yellow fever
1926	Thirteenth	Paris	Amended convention, including typhus and smallpox
1938	Fourteenth	Paris	Amendments to the 1926 convention

Source: based on Goodman (1952, Appendix 1, p. 77).

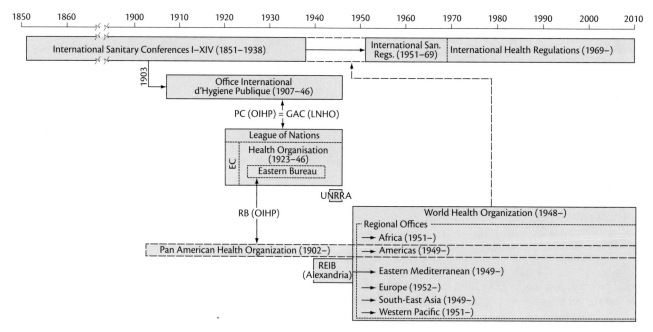

Figure 2.21 Major international health organisations, 1850–2000. EC = League of Nations Epidemic Commission (1920–23). GAC (LNHO) = General Advisory Committee of the League of Nations Health Organisation. International San. Regs. = International Sanitary Regulations. PC (OIHP) = Permanent Committee of the Office International d'Hygiène Publique. RB (OIHP) = Regional Bureau of the Office International d'Hygiène Publique. REIB (Alexandria) = Regional Epidemiological Intelligence Bureau, Alexandria. UNRRA = United Nations Relief and Rehabilitation Administration.

OIHP under the authority of the League. The United States objected to this arrangement and, although a relationship was forged in which the Permanent Committee of the OIHP acted as the General Advisory Council of the League of Nations Health Organisation (**Figure 2.24**), the OIHP and the League's Health Organisation continued as autonomous international health organisations in Paris and Geneva until the post-war period (World Health Organization, 1958).

One of the principal tasks of the OIHP in the early inter-war years was to oversee the revision of the 1912 Sanitary Convention. The resulting International Sanitary Convention of 1926 increased the number of quarantine diseases to five (by the addition of

smallpox and typhus; see Table 2.3 and Figure 2.22), while requiring countries to notify immediately the first cases of plague, cholera and yellow fever and the occurrence of typhus and smallpox in epidemic form. The International Sanitary Conference of 1926 also recommended that certain regional organisations should operate as Regional Bureaux of the OIHP for the provision of epidemiological intelligence. By 1927, arrangements had been made for three such organisations (League of Nations Eastern Bureau at Singapore, Pan American Sanitary Bureau at Washington, D.C. and Sanitary, Maritime and Quarantine Council of Egypt at Alexandria) to operate in this capacity. In turn, the OIHP was required to relay the

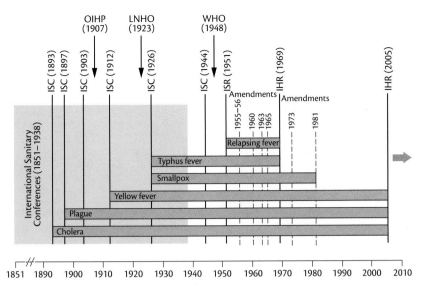

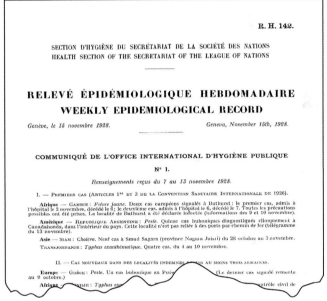

Figure 2.22 **The quarantine diseases.** Time interval for which different diseases were covered by the International Sanitary Conventions (ISC), the International Sanitary Regulations (ISR) and the International Health Regulations (IHR). IHR (2005) ushered in a new regime that requires the notification of all events which may constitute a public health emergency of international concern. The dates of establishment of international organisations with responsibility for overseeing the Conventions and Regulations are indicated: Office International d'Hygiène Publique (OIHP); League of Nations Health Organisation (LNHO); and World Health Organization (WHO).

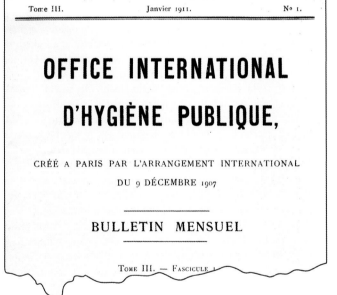

Figure 2.23 **Publications and communiqués of the Office International d'Hygiène Publique.** (*Left*) The *Bulletin Mensuel de l'Office International d'Hygiène Publique*. Article 9 (Annex) of the Rome Agreement of 1903 committed the OIHP to the publication, at least once a month, of a *Bulletin*. The *Bulletin* was to include: "(1) Laws and general or local regulations promulgated in the various countries respecting transmissible diseases; (2) Information respecting the spread of infectious diseases; (3) Information respecting the works executed or the measures taken for improving the healthiness of localities; (4) Statistics dealing with public health; (5) Bibliographical notes" [Rome Agreement, 1930, Article 10 (Annex), reproduced in Goodman, 1952, p. 98]. The *Bulletin* first appeared in 1909 and continued until 1946. (*Right*) Beginning in November 1928, information collected by the OIHP was summarised in a regular communiqué, published in the *Weekly Epidemiological Record* of the League of Nations Health Section.

information received to all countries by weekly telegram or, in urgent instances, immediately. The same information formed the basis of a regular OIHP communiqué that was included in the *Weekly Epidemiological Record* of the League of Nations Health Section from November 1928 (Figure 2.23), while additional information collected from governments was published in the *Annuaire Sanitaire Maritime International* (Goodman, 1952; World Health Organization, 1958).

Over the years, the work of the OIHP extended beyond maritime quarantine to include such issues as quarantine regulations for air traffic (an International Sanitary Convention for Aerial Navigation was drawn up in 1932 and came into force in 1935; see Figure 3.39), venereal diseases in seamen, the international standardisation of anti-diphtheritic serum and the control of narcotic drugs. In 1945, the United Nations Relief and Rehabilitation Administration (UNRRA) assumed responsibility for the OIHP's duties with

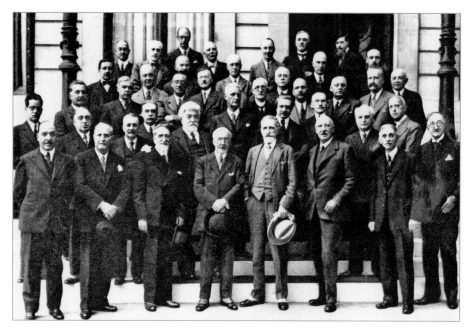

Figure 2.24 The Permanent Committee of the Office International d'Hygiène Publique. The Committee at its session in Paris, May 1933. The bearded gentleman in the centre of the front row, holding a light-coloured hat, is Camille Barrère. As President of the Eleventh International Sanitary Conference, Barrère had put forward the original resolution to create the OIHP in 1903. *Source:* © World Health Organization.

respect to the International Sanitary Conventions; the OIHP was dissolved by protocols signed on 22 July 1946, with the epidemiological service being incorporated into the Interim Commission of the World Health Organization on 1 January 1947 (World Health Organization, 1958).

The International (Pan American) Sanitary Bureau

The International Sanitary Bureau has the distinction of being the first international health bureau with its own secretariat. Established in 1902 as the regional health bureau for the Americas, the organisation's subsequent aliases have included the Pan American Sanitary Bureau, the Pan American Sanitary Organization and, today, the familiar Pan American Health Organization (Figure 2.21). By the 1890s, a movement towards inter-American cooperation had begun to take shape and, at the Second International Conference of American Republics (Mexico City, October 1901–January 1902), a recommendation was made that health representatives of the American republics should come together to formulate sanitary regulations and that a permanent executive board should be formed (International Sanitary Bureau) with headquarters at Washington, D.C. A primary function of the Bureau was to oversee inter-American quarantine regulations and to act as a centre for the international exchange of information on epidemic diseases of international importance. Yellow fever was the dominant concern from the outset, although other health matters (smallpox vaccination, malaria and tuberculosis campaigns, national health legislation and other matters) appeared on the agenda in later years (Goodman, 1952; Howard-Jones, 1981).

A reorganisation of the Bureau was undertaken in the years that followed the First World War. With a change of name to the Pan American Sanitary Bureau, the chief activities of the Bureau evolved to include: (i) the collection and transmission of information on outbreaks of epidemic diseases; (ii) preparation of the agenda for the Pan American Sanitary Conferences; (iii) services as a central consultative agency for improving the efficiency of national public health authorities; and (iv) special studies and investigations for

combating outbreaks and improving sanitary conditions in member states. As noted earlier, the Bureau was appointed as one of the Regional Bureaux of the OIHP under the International Sanitary Convention of 1926 (Goodman, 1952; Howard-Jones, 1981).

With the establishment of the World Health Organization in the early post-war period, the US advocated that the Bureau should continue to promote regional health programmes in the Americas, whilst also serving as the WHO Regional Office for the Americas (Figure 2.21). Accordingly, it was agreed at the XII Pan American Sanitary Conference at Caracas (1947) that the separate identity of the Bureau should to be maintained, with operations reconstituted under the title of the Pan American Sanitary Organization and, from 1958, the Pan American Health Organization (PAHO). Since that time, the PAHO has continued as a functionally (if not legally) integral part of the WHO's system of Regional Offices (Figure 2.21), whilst also maintaining its independent identity as a specialist public health organisation for the Western Hemisphere (Howard-Jones, 1981).

2.6 Wireless Technologies: The League of Nations Health Organisation (1923–46)

The establishment of the League of Nations Health Organisation in the aftermath of the First World War (Figure 2.21) ushered in a new era in international health cooperation (League of Nations Health Organisation, 1931; Goodman, 1952, pp. 101–37). Prompted by a series of devastating epidemics of cholera and typhus fever that spread across Eastern Europe with the population upheavals of the time, a provisional Health Committee of the League was formed in Geneva in 1921. The constitution of the Health Organisation was adopted in September 1923 and, over the next two decades, the remit of the Organisation developed to include the establishment of a Malaria Commission (1923) and a Cancer Commission (1923), along with technical commissions on biological standardisation, housing, physical fitness, typhus, leprosy and rural hygiene, among other health-related issues (World Health Organization, 1958).

The Epidemiological Intelligence Service

The first meeting of the Health Committee of the League of Nations took place in August 1921 to consider "the question of organising means of more rapid interchange of epidemiological information" (League of Nations Health Section, 1922d, p. 3). At this and subsequent meetings, it was emphasised that epidemiological intelligence work should receive immediate attention and that the most important and pressing work in this field was with regard to the submission of epidemiological information in relation to infectious diseases in Eastern Europe in general and Russia in particular. The need for epidemiological information had been forcibly demonstrated in the course of the work of the League of Nations Epidemic Commission (initially the Typhus Commission) that had been established in April 1920 to tackle the ongoing outbreaks of typhus fever in Poland, Soviet Russia and the Ukraine, Latvia and Greece (Figure 2.21). In response, the Epidemiological Intelligence Service was instituted in the Geneva Health Section and started to prepare reports on the health situation of Eastern Europe in 1921. These reports were first published in 1922 and progressively expanded to include not only Eastern Europe, but also Central Europe and all European countries. Details of the reports included in the *Epidemiological Intelligence* (E.I.) series and, running in parallel, other Health Section statistical series [*Weekly (Epidemiological) Record*, R.H.; and *Monthly Epidemiological Report*, R.E.] are provided by Cliff, *et al.* (1998, pp. 389–93). We note here that, during the inter-war period, the breadth and geographical reach of the publications evolved to include regular counts of disease-specific morbidity and mortality for a global sample of countries.

The League of Nations' concern with disease surveillance owes much to Ludwik Rajchman (see Figure 2.25), the first director of the Health Organisation. Rajchman's vision for the Organisation as a global centre for epidemiological information collection and exchange is highlighted in an unpublished memorandum, dated 19 January 1922:

> [N]o institution is undertaking at present the publication of a comprehensive survey of the epidemiological situation of the world. ... On the other hand all national health administrations publish periodical, mostly annual reports concerning health conditions in their respective countries. No institution has yet undertaken a comparative study of the information contained in those valuable reports. No institution is taking the initiative of the study of current epidemics affecting the whole world. ... It is the duty of the Health Section to fill such gaps. ... The Section itself is undertaking the periodical publication of an epidemiological bulletin ... and it is hoped that it will be possible for the Section to evolve a scheme which will allow it to become an international clearing house for such information. ... It may be stated that the Public Health Services of the world are at present far from being united in a common 'esprit de corps' and in an equal realization of the ideas of common service (Ludwik Rajchman, unpublished memorandum, 19 January 1922, cited in Brown, 2006, p. 12).

The surveillance function developed in line with this vision. Between 1927, when collaboration between the Office International d'Hygiène Publique and the League of Nations Health Organisation was defined, and 1939 the reach of the Organisation's Epidemic Intelligence Service expanded to cover 90 percent of the world's population. As Goodman (1952, p. 109) observes:

> By the analysis of reports coming to Geneva directly or from the Paris *Office* and its regional bureaux in Washington, Alexandria, Singapore and Sydney, the Health Organisation could keep a kind

of sphygmographic record of the pulse of the world's epidemics and so keep governments informed of them by cable and wireless and by weekly, monthly, bi-monthly and annual publications.

When surveillance operations began in the early 1920s, the postal service represented the principal mechanism for the submission of epidemiological information from administrations to Geneva. But communications technology was developing rapidly. In October 1923, N.V. Lothian, a Field Epidemiologist in the Health Section of the League of Nations, could assure a meeting of the Section on Vital Statistics of the American Public Health Association that the "question of telegraphing reports to ensure greater promptitude is under discussion" and "that a scheme has been worked out whereby the American weekly summary can be cabled to Geneva by an ingenious code costing us only some 500 francs per year" (Lothian, 1924, p. 289). Just a few years later, the Eastern Bureau of the League of Nations Health Organisation would lead the development of wireless technology as a tool in global disease surveillance. It is to the work of the Eastern Bureau that we now turn.

Expanding Horizons and New Technologies: The Eastern Bureau

While the early work of the League of Nations Health Organisation was directed towards the emergency situation in Eastern Europe – a situation that had begun to wane by 1922 – the Epidemiological Intelligence Service continued to collect and publish data that provided a world view of epidemic diseases of international importance. The relative prevalence of such diseases in Asia prompted the establishment of the Organisation's Eastern Bureau in Singapore in March 1925 (Figure 2.21). Under the initial directorship of Gilbert E. Brooke (**Figure 2.25**), the Eastern Bureau provides an example of the early use of wireless communications in international health cooperation and disease surveillance (Manderson, 1995; Yach, 1998).

Scope of Operations

The Council of the League of Nations agreed to the establishment of the Eastern Bureau at their meeting of June 1924. The scope of the Bureau's operations was defined at the First Meeting of the Advisory Council of the Eastern Bureau, convened in Singapore in early 1925 (Figure 2.25). The "essential task" of the Bureau was to:

> collect information on the prevalence of epidemic disease at ports in an area extending from Cape Town to Vladivostock and Alexandria, including Australia; also, to obtain intelligence on 'infected' ships to classify the information and to re-telegraph ... [the] same in the form of a weekly bulletin, confirmed subsequently by mail by means of a Weekly Fasciculus, which contains also additional information on public health in various districts of the territory (Eastern Bureau of the League of Nations Health Organisation, 1926a, unpaginated).

The area under epidemiological surveillance by the Bureau, occasionally referred to in official publications as the 'Eastern Arena', is mapped in **Figure 2.26**. The vast area extended from approximately 20°E to 150°E of longitude and 40°S to 40°N of latitude and included ports on the East African seaboard, and the Southern and Eastern coast of Asia and Australasia. For administrative purposes, the area was divided into four geographic groups: a Western group (East Coast of Africa and the Asiatic Coast from Egypt to Burma); a Central group (Malaya, Netherlands East Indies and the administrations of Borneo and the Philippine Islands); an Eastern group (Asiatic Coast from Siam to Siberia, including Japan); and a Southern group (Australia, New Zealand, French New Caledonia,

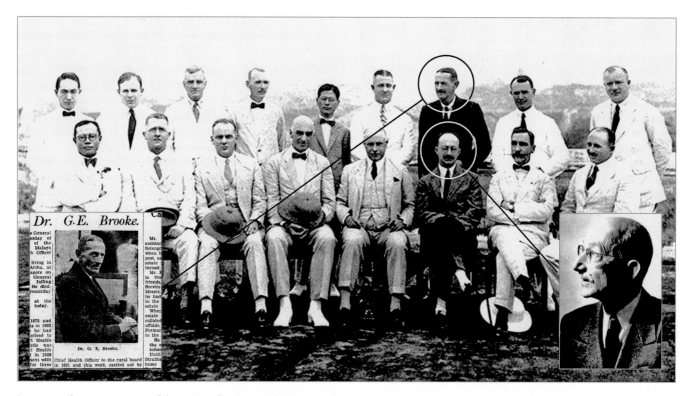

Figure 2.25 The Eastern Bureau of the League of Nations Health Organisation. (*Group photograph*) The First Meeting of the Advisory Council of the Eastern Bureau of the League of Nations Health Organisation, Singapore, 1925. The delegates include: Ludwik Rajchman (seated, third from the right and *inset*), first director of the League of Nations Health Organisation and the chief architect of the Organisation's global disease surveillance function; and Gilbert E. Brooke (standing, third from the right and *inset*), Chief Health Officer of Singapore and the first Director of the Eastern Bureau. As Chief Health Officer, Brooke's name will always be associated with the development of St John's Quarantine Station (see Figure 3.13). Brooke assumed the Directorship of the Eastern Bureau in June 1925 and continued in the position on a part-time basis until October 1926. Brooke was instrumental in the establishment of the Bureau, its scope of operations and the development of the AA code by which the Bureau's Weekly Health Bulletin was routinely transmitted by cable and wireless to corresponding administrations. *Sources:* (*Group photograph*) World Health Organization archives; (*Rajchman, inset*) UNICEF (http://www.unicef.org/about/history/index_leadership_exec_board.html); (*Gilbert, inset*) *The Straits Times*, 16 January 1936 (p. 13).

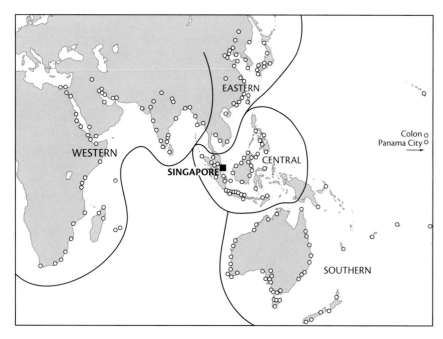

Figure 2.26 The 'Eastern Arena': the area under epidemiological surveillance by the Eastern Bureau of the League of Nations Health Organisation. The dots show the geographical distribution of ports in telegraphic communication with the Bureau's office in Singapore in the sample year of 1938. The Bureau's administrative division of the ports into Central, Eastern, Southern and Western groups is indicated. *Source:* based on League of Nations Health Section (1938, unnumbered figure, p. 583).

Fiji and Honolulu). The logic behind this fourfold division was that maritime communications within each group were mainly self-contained, with connections between the groups being chiefly the concern of larger ports. Beginning with a tentative list of 35 'important ports' that were frequented by foreign trade ships, the number of ports in regular telegraphic communication with the Bureau grew rapidly, to 66 (1926), 135 (1931) and, as illustrated by the dot distribution in Figure 2.26, 147 (1938).

Surveillance operations

Figure 2.27 summarises the routine surveillance operations of the Bureau within the Eastern Arena. As the upper boxes in the diagram show, epidemiological information reached the Bureau through three main channels (cf. Figure 3.6):

(A) *immediate notification by telegram.* All countries were required to submit an immediate telegraphic report to the Bureau on the first appearance of cholera, plague, smallpox, yellow fever or an unusual prevalence of mortality from any other disease in a port frequented by foreign trade ships (designated 'important ports'). On the basis of the epidemiological information received, the Bureau determined which countries were in direct communication with the infected ports and sent a summary of the situation by telegram to their administrations;

(B) *weekly notification by telegram.* All countries were required to submit a weekly telegram, to reach the Bureau by no later than Wednesday (midday), summarising the epidemiological situation in the important ports and other territories in the seven-day period up to the preceding Saturday (midnight);

(C) *letter by first available post.* The weekly telegram in (B) was to be confirmed by a letter, to be sent to the Bureau by the first available post, that contained supplementary information on the epidemiological status of the ports and other territories.

The information collected by the Bureau was to be circulated, as emergency circumstances dictated, in the form of a telegram to concerned countries and, routinely, in the form of a Weekly Bulletin or resumé to all countries in the Eastern Arena and the League of Nations Health Organisation in Geneva. The information so received was to be used by the administrations to inform decisions on how to prevent entry of a given disease by sea and, in later years, by air. As noted in Section 2.5, in addition to these initially prescribed operations, the International Sanitary Convention of 1926 imposed on the Eastern Bureau the additional role of regional bureau to the Office International d'Hygiène Publique. The Convention came into force in 1928 and, from thereon, the Bureau

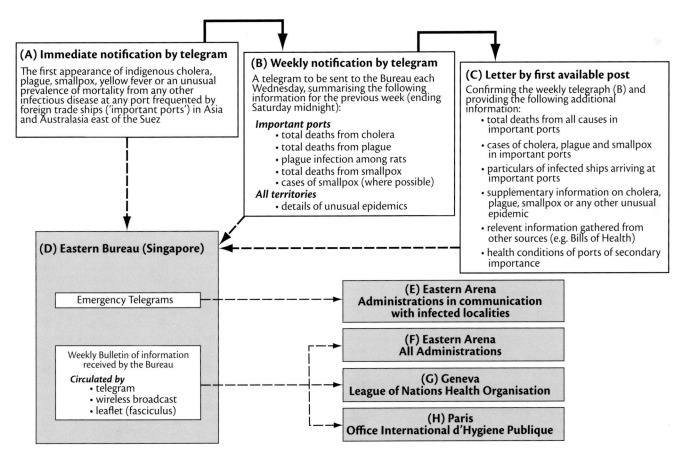

Figure 2.27 Core surveillance operations of the Eastern Bureau of the League of Nations Health Organisation. Disease-related information (summarised in boxes A–C) transmitted by participating countries to the Eastern Bureau at Singapore (D). The information was then circulated by the Eastern Bureau as (i) emergency telegrams to administrations in the Eastern Arena that were in communication with infected localities (E) and (ii) summary Weekly Bulletins to all administrations in the Eastern Arena (F), to the League of Nations Health Organisation, Geneva (G) and, under the International Sanitary Convention of 1926, to the Office International d'Hygiène Publique, Paris (H). *Source*: based on information in Eastern Bureau of the League of Nations Health Organisation (1926b, pp. 2–4).

also operated as the Paris Office's reporting agency in the Far East (Manderson, 1995).

Telecommunications: cable and wireless

When the Eastern Bureau was first established, it was envisaged that the Bureau's Weekly Bulletin would be communicated to governments and Geneva by way of a telegram, supplemented by additional information in a printed leaflet or *Weekly Fasciculus* (**Figure 2.28**). Routine telegraphic communications, however, were a significant financial liability. As the Bureau's *Annual Report* for 1925 explained, "The despatch of telegrams is the basic activity of the Bureau and is an item which will not readily admit of retrenchment without unduly stultifying such activity" and, as such, "The cables will always be the chief item of the Bureau's expenditure" (Eastern Bureau of the League of Nations Health Organisation, 1926b, p. 9). The same report recognised that wireless broadcasts would be much more economical, with the Governments of French Indo-China and the Dutch East Indies having offered to broadcast the Bureau's Weekly Bulletin via the powerful radio transmitters at Saigon (French Indo-China) and Malabar (Dutch East Indies) at no cost. Through these facilities, wireless broadcasting of the Weekly Bulletin began in early April 1925:

> The first general return was despatched by the Bureau to Saigon on Thursday April 2nd, in clear [uncoded], and was broadcasted by

their powerful wireless installation and has continued to transmit the weekly message in code, ever since, each Friday at 01:30 G.M.T. on a wave-length of 20,800 metres, and the message is picked-up by Paris and telegraphed to Geneva (Eastern Bureau of the League of Nations Health Organisation, 1926b, p. 10).

But wireless transmission of the Weekly Bulletin was not without its difficulties:

> Most unfortunately the atmospherics of the East would appear to be indifferently good, and the messages can only be picked up by Japan, British North Borneo, and Bandong. The matter is being considered by the Bureau with a view to possible extension of the wireless messages. Were a large number of administrations of the Arena able to get the broadcast, much expense would be saved by the Bureau (Eastern Bureau of the League of Nations Health Organisation, 1926b, p. 10).

Throughout 1926, improvements in the wireless reception of the Weekly Bulletin were pursued, with increasing numbers of stations being able to pick up the Saigon and Malabar broadcasts. In January 1926, Noumea (New Caledonia) confirmed the establishment of a weekly connection with Saigon; Hong Kong followed suit in February, along with India (March), Ceylon (March), Shanghai (June), Australia (June), Fiji (August), Manila (September), Djibouti (September) and Rabaul on the New Britain Archipelago (October) (Eastern Bureau of the League of Nations

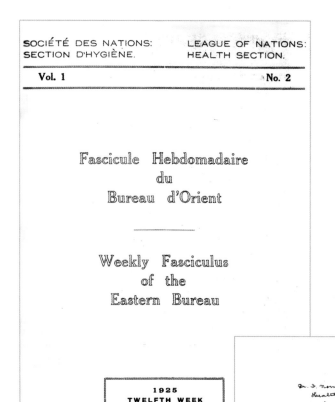

SOCIÉTÉ DES NATIONS: SECTION D'HYGIÈNE.   LEAGUE OF NATIONS: HEALTH SECTION.

Vol. 1   No. 2

Fascicule Hebdomadaire
du
Bureau d'Orient

Weekly Fasciculus
of the
Eastern Bureau

1925
TWELFTH WEEK
ENDING
SATURDAY, MARCH 21st
AT MIDNIGHT

Published for the Eastern Bureau
by
C. A. Ribeiro & Co., Ltd.
Singapore.

Figure 2.28 *Weekly Fasciculus of the Eastern Bureau.* The *Weekly Fasciculus* provided a printed summary of epidemiological intelligence gathered by the Eastern Bureau from 'important ports' and their associated administrations in a given week to Saturday (midnight). The handwritten address that appears on the rear of the original document (reproduced *lower right*) shows the copy illustrated (Volume 1, No. 2, 1925) to have been sent to Norman F. White, former Commissioner of the League of Nations Epidemic Commission and the Health Section official on whose recommendation the Eastern Bureau was established. *Source*: World Health Organization archives.

Health Organisation, 1927). By 1927, the Director of the Eastern Bureau could note that:

> The development of our wireless service has been satisfactory. Its network has become denser and has greatly extended through the rebroadcast by new stations of our weekly wireless bulletin. We consider it a sound policy to use powerful stations with wide range of action for the broadcast of our bulletin in code, and to leave to stations of less range the broadcast of the bulletin in clear intended for shipping at sea (Eastern Bureau of the League of Nations Health Organisation, 1928, p. 3).

A total of 30 health administrations in the Eastern Arena were able to pick up the weekly wireless transmission in 1929 and, through the 1930s, a fully functional broadcast system for the Weekly Bulletin became established (**Figure 2.29**). As hostilities in Europe and Asia intensified, however, there was a decline in the regularity and quality of information being remitted to the Bureau, while wireless broadcasts became impossible. French Indo-China halted

communications with Singapore in early 1940, while similar developments in relation to India and other British colonies resulted in the suspension of the Bureau's operations at the end of 1941.

2.7 Wireless to Internet: The World Health Organization (1946–)

Histories of the origin and development of the World Health Organization (WHO) are provided by Goodman (1952, pp. 152–233) and World Health Organization (1958, 1968, 2008a). The establishment of a specialised health agency within the United Nations was first proposed by the Brazilian and Chinese delegates at the United Nations Conference on International Organization held in San Francisco (April–June 1945). The Constitution of the WHO was drafted and agreed at an International Health Conference held in New York (June–July 1946) and came into force on 7 April 1948. In preparation for the establishment of the permanent WHO,

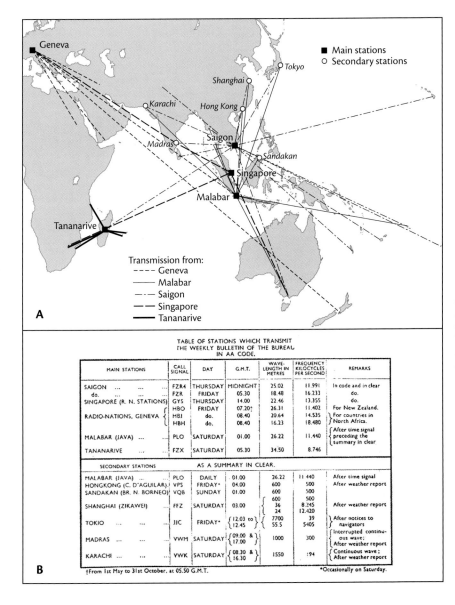

Figure 2.29 Broadcast network for the Eastern Bureau of the League of Nations Health Organisation.
(A) Network of wireless stations through which the Eastern Bureau's Weekly Bulletin was broadcast to corresponding administrations in the sample year of 1939. Information for a given week was transmitted by cable from the Bureau's office (Singapore) to Saigon (French Indo-China) every Thursday morning. The message was then broadcast in code from the powerful Saigon wireless station, courtesy of the Government of French Indo-China, each Friday morning. The east coast of Africa received the message indirectly through the intermediary station at Tananarive (Madagascar) which picked it up and re-transmitted it each Saturday morning. The Saigon message was also picked up by the Malabar (Dutch East Indies) station, which transmitted it each Saturday morning. Radio Nations, Geneva, transmitted the message to North African countries and New Zealand. In addition, certain administrations summarised the decoded message and re-transmitted it in abbreviated form on a daily (Malabar) or weekly (Hong Kong, Karachi, Madras, Sandakan, Shanghai, Tokyo) basis. (B) Broadcast schedule for the Weekly Health Bulletin in code (AA code) and in clear by transmitting station. *Source*: redrawn from Eastern Bureau of the League of Nations Health Organisation (1939, unnumbered figure, between pp. 2–3).

an Interim Commission was appointed to continue and unify the epidemiological functions of the League of Nations Health Organisation (October 1946), the Health Division of the United Nations Relief and Rehabilitation Administration (December 1946) and the Office International d'Hygiène Publique (January 1947). The First World Health Assembly (June 1948) resolved that the Interim Commission should cease to exist at midnight on 31 August 1948, with the functions of the Commission passing to the WHO in Geneva on 1 September 1948 (**Figure 2.30**).

Articles 63–65 of the Constitution of the WHO (World Health Organization, 2006) laid down that:

Article 63: *Each Member [State] shall communicate promptly to the Organization important laws, regulations, official reports and statistics pertaining to health which have been published by the State concerned;*

Article 64: *Each Member shall provide statistical and epidemiological reports in a manner to be determined by the Health Assembly; and*

Article 65: *Each Member shall transmit upon the request of the Board such additional information pertaining to health as may be practicable.*

Chapter XI of the Constitution determined that activities should be decentralised along regional lines, with the First World Health Assembly agreeing to the delineation of six world regions: Africa, Americas, Eastern Mediterranean, Europe, South-East Asia and Western Pacific (Figure 2.21). The six Regional Offices had come into being by 1952, with the long-established Pan American Sanitary Bureau (Section 2.5) assuming the role of the Office for the Americas. This regional structure has continued through to the present day (**Figure 2.31**).

Epidemiological Intelligence and Surveillance, 1940s–1970s

The inheritance of the newly-created WHO included responsibility for international epidemic control in terms of: (i) quarantine and the International Sanitary Conventions; and (ii) epidemic intelligence and epidemiological services. One of the first major tasks of the WHO was to revise and reform the existing International Sanitary Conventions (Table 2.3) and these came into force under the new title of the International Sanitary Regulations in 1952. Further details are provided in Section 3.2, but we note here that the 1952 Regulations represented a synthesis of existing Conventions dealing with maritime, land and air traffic in relation to a total of six quarantine diseases (Figure 2.22). The Regulations continued to require national health administrations to notify the WHO by telegram (or, in some instances, airmail) of the appearance of quarantinable diseases in their territories. Information received under the Regulations was collated by the four WHO quarantine and

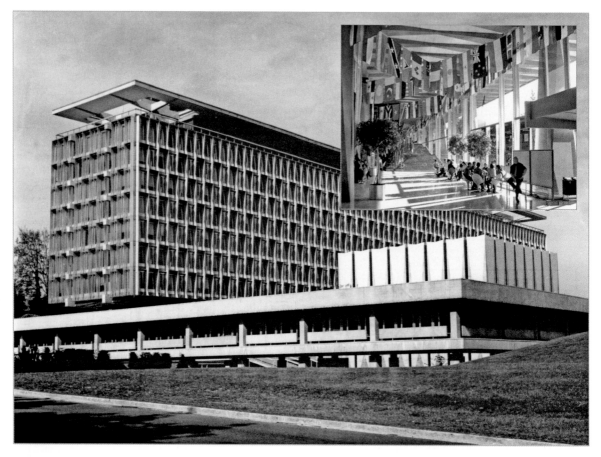

Figure 2.30 Headquarters of the World Health Organization, Geneva. The WHO moved into its own dedicated headquarters in 1966, having originally been based at the Palais des Nations, Geneva. (*Inset*) Interior (ground floor), bedecked in the national flags of WHO Member States to celebrate the Fortieth Anniversary of the opening of the building. *Sources:* © World Health Organization/Tibor Farkas and (*inset*) the authors.

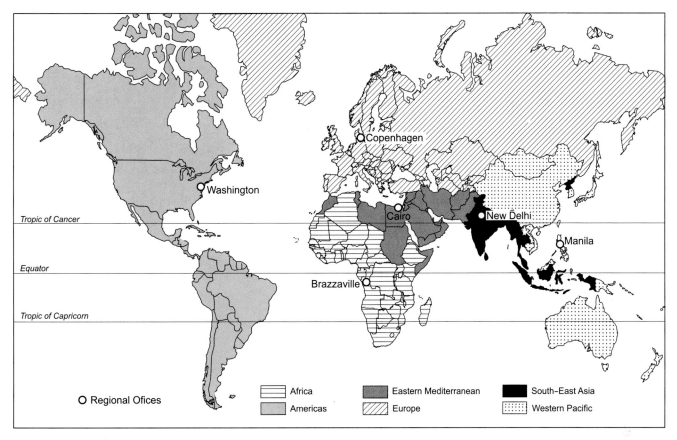

Figure 2.31 Standard regions of the World Health Organization (WHO).

information services (Geneva, Singapore, Washington, D.C. and Alexandria), with urgent information distributed worldwide by a system of radio bulletins (**Figure 2.32**). The radio bulletins, in turn, were confirmed via weekly publications. The *Weekly Epidemiological Record* formed the main WHO publication for this purpose, containing notifications of quarantinable diseases, information on international sanitary legislation and notes on the incidence of non-quarantinable diseases whenever their prevalence became of international importance. In 1961, the functions of the WHO Epidemiological Intelligence Stations at Alexandria, Singapore and Washington were transferred to WHO HQ at Geneva and, from that time, administration of the International Sanitary Regulations was totally centralised with direct communications between the various national health administrations and Geneva (World Health Organization, 1958, 1968).

Increasingly, the WHO's work extended beyond surveillance functions for the quarantine diseases to include other communicable diseases through various programmes and an expanding network of collaborators in the field and laboratories. Important developments included the establishment in 1958 of a WHO study group to advise on the collection of immunological information through immunological and haematological surveys. WHO serum reference banks were established and antibody studies of a range of diseases (including poliomyelitis, measles, rubella, influenza, arbovirus infections, rickettsial infections, pertussis, typhoid and diphtheria, among other diseases) were undertaken in the 1960s in Africa, the Americas, Asia and Europe. Alongside diseases for

which surveillance activities were already in place (including cholera, influenza, malaria, smallpox and tuberculosis), surveillance of a range of other diseases was initiated, including: dengue haemorrhagic fever (started in 1964), salmonellosis (started in 1965) and, in cooperation with the Food and Agriculture Organization (FAO) and the World Organisation for Animal Health (OIE), rabies.

In the late 1960s, the WHO replaced 'epidemiological intelligence' with 'epidemiological surveillance' as an approach to disease control. The new approach had grown out of improved epidemiological methods (including data processing and analysis, laboratory and field studies) and was defined as

> The exercise of continuous scrutiny of and watchfulness over the distribution and spread of infections and factors related thereto, of sufficient accuracy and completeness to be pertinent to effective control (World Health Organization, 2008a, p. 175).

With this development, the Unit of Quarantine was merged with the Unit of Epidemiological Surveillance in 1968 and, by 1970, the programme was referred to as Epidemiological Surveillance. This strategy was adopted as a means of moving away from the concept that disease prevention and control could only be achieved through the application of quarantine measures. As a consequence of this development, the existing International Sanitary Regulations (1952) were revised and adopted as the International Health Regulations in 1969 (Figure 2.22). Accordingly, the Committee on International Quarantine changed its name to the Committee on International Surveillance of Communicable Diseases. Information collected by

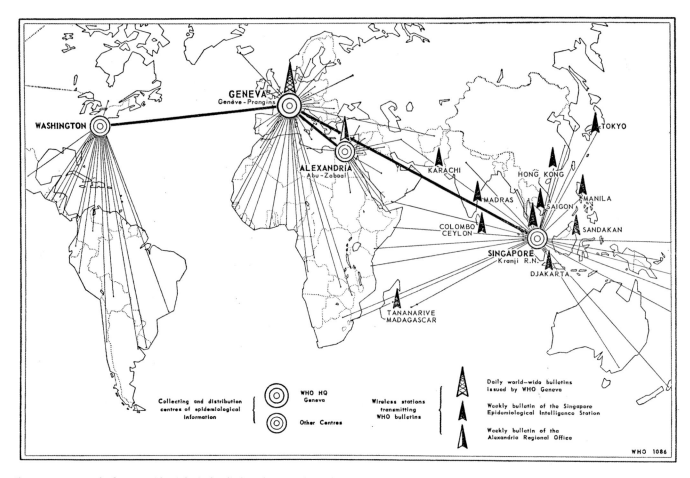

Figure 2.32 Network of WHO epidemiological radio broadcasts in the mid-twentieth century. The radio broadcast web, pioneered by the Eastern Bureau at Singapore and depicted for the 1930s in Figure 2.29, expanded to include: (i) daily epidemiological broadcasts worldwide from Geneva, relayed to the Americas via the Pan American Sanitary Bureau at Washington; (ii) weekly epidemiological broadcasts to the Eastern Mediterranean by the Alexandria Regional Office. *Source*: Goodman (1952, Figure 36, p. 172).

the Epidemiological Surveillance programme was disseminated daily through the WHO epidemiological radiotelegraphic (later telex) bulletin and the *Weekly Epidemiological Report*. Additionally, the Epidemiological Surveillance programme placed emphasis on the strengthening of national surveillance; training of epidemiologists in Member States in surveillance methods was provided, along with the availability of technicians and allied health personnel to observe and report on outbreaks. Inter-country centres for epidemiological surveillance were established in the WHO Africa (Abidjan, Nairobi and Brazzaville in 1974) and Americas (Caribbean Epidemiology Centre, Port-of-Spain, in 1975) Regions. Technical manuals were prepared for the surveillance of four diseases under the international health regulations (cholera, plague, smallpox and yellow fever) and five other diseases (influenza, louse-borne typhus fever, louse-borne relapsing fever, malaria and paralytic poliomyelitis), while a general guide on disease surveillance was prepared in 1975. This same period witnessed great strides in disease prevention and control through the eradication of smallpox (see Section 5.2) and, from 1973, the implementation of the Expanded Programme on Immunization (see Section 4.4) (World Health Organization, 2008a).

With the advent of computer technology, a computer was installed at the WHO HQ in the mid-1960s and computerisation of

statistical work was undertaken. Data received by the WHO from Member States since 1950 was stored in digital format. Computers, in turn, permitted information processing and the development of epidemiological models in relation to such diseases as typhoid, cholera, tetanus and diphtheria (Uemura, 1988).

International Patterns of Communicable Disease Surveillance, 1923–83

What was the practical reality on the ground of all this international disease surveillance activity in the six decades from the formation of the League of Nations Health Organisation? Which communicable diseases were recorded by which countries? To address these questions, Cliff, Smallman-Raynor, Haggett, *et al.* (2009, pp. 112–32) have used three main League of Nations/WHO sources of international morbidity and mortality data (*Annual Epidemiological Report*, 1923–38; *Annual Epidemiological and Vital Statistics*, 1939–61; and *World Health Statistics Annual*, 1962–83) to construct a worldwide (year × disease × country) matrix of diseases subject/not subject to globally documented surveillance, 1923–83. While details of the data matrix are given by Cliff and colleagues, we note here that it is based on two categories of data:

(1) *notifiable diseases (1923–58).* For the period 1923–58, *Annual Epidemiological Report* and its successor publication, *Annual*

Epidemiological and Vital Statistics, included a chart or table which recorded in matrix format (diseases × countries) which diseases were *notifiable* in each region of the world. **Figure 2.33** shows a detail of one such chart for 1930;

(2) *reported diseases (1959–83)*. Between 1959 and 1983, the matrices of notifiable diseases were not published, but equivalent matrices of *reported* diseases by country can be constructed from the raw returns of recorded (non-zero) mortality and morbidity published in later issues of *Annual Epidemiological and Vital Statistics* and its successor publication, *World Health Statistics Annual*.

For 29 sample years (1923–37, 1946, 1949–55, 1958, 1963, 1965, 1970, 1975, 1980 and 1983; see Cliff, *et al.*, 2009, pp. 112–32), data types (1) and (2) yielded a 29 (years) × 123 (communicable diseases) × 193 (Member States) 1/0 matrix of communicable diseases subject/not subject to globally documented surveillance. The geographical sample included 100 percent of WHO Member States (2008 status), distributed according to the six standard WHO regions in Figure 2.31. The 123 sample communicable diseases, categorised according to Chapter I (Certain Infectious and Parasitic Diseases, A00–B99) of *ICD*-10, are given in Appendix 2.1.

Global Trends

Figure 2.34A plots, by annual period, the number of sample communicable disease categories (lower line trace) and the associated number of WHO Member States (upper line trace) for which surveillance activities were documented in the League of Nations/WHO data set. As the graph shows, the number of disease categories under surveillance by WHO Member States varied between 40–60 per annum for much of the observation period, but with a rapid increase to > 80 in the early 1980s. The same interval was associated with a steady and progressive increase in the number of WHO Member States for which surveillance activities for the sample disease categories were documented, from 85 (44 percent of WHO Member States) at the start of the observation period to a peak of 160 (83 percent of WHO Member States) in the early 1970s.

The time series of diseases in Figure 2.34A is based on the count of disease categories for which surveillance activities were documented across the set of Member States. It is important to recognise that not all countries undertook surveillance for all the diseases, and Member States varied in terms of the number of disease categories under surveillance in any given year. To capture this variability, the heavy line trace in Figure 2.34B plots, by annual period, the median

MALADIES A DÉCLARATION OBLIGATOIRE DANS DIFFÉRENTS PAYS EN 1930.
NOTIFIABLE DISEASES IN VARIOUS COUNTRIES IN 1930.

Le signe ◆ indique que la déclaration de la maladie est obligatoire. — The sign ◆ indicates that the disease is notifiable.

Maladies	Actinomycose / Actinomycosis	Angine fuso-spirillaire de Vincent / Vincent's angina	Angine à streptocoques / Septic sore-throat	Angine tonsillaire / Angina tonsillaris	Ankylostomiase / Ankylostomiasis	Béribéri / Beri-beri	Bilharziose / Bilharziasis	Blennorragie / Gonorrhœa	Botulisme / Botulism	Bronchite aiguë / Acute bronchitis	Broncho-pneumonie / Broncho-pneumonia	Cancer / Cancer	Chancre mou / Soft chancre	Charbon / Anthrax	Choléra asiatique / Cholera	Coqueluche / Whooping-cough	Delirium tremens / Delirium tremens	Dengue / Dengue fever	Diarrhée et entérite, 0-2 ans / Diarrhœa and enteritis, 0-2 years	Diarrhée et entérite, 2 ans et plus / Diarrhœa and enteritis, 2 years and over	Diphtérie et croup / Diphtheria and croup	**Dysenterie, non spécifiée / Dysentery, unspecified	Dysenterie amibienne / Dysentery, amœbic	Dysenterie bacillaire / Dysentery, bacillary	Echinococcose / Hydatid disease	Empoisonnement chronique par le phosphore / Chronic phosphorus poisoning	Empoisonnement chronique par le plomb / Chronic lead poisoning	Encéphalite léthargique / Encephalitis lethargica	Erysipèle / Erysipelas	Favus / Favus	Fièvre bilieuse hémoglobinurique / Blackwater fever	Fièvre continue / Continued fever	Fièvre des tranchées / Trench fever	Fièvre jaune / Yellow fever	Fièvre ondulante / Undulant fever	Fièvres paratyphoïdes / Paratyphoid fevers	Fièvre puerpérale / Puerperal fever	Fièvres récurrentes / Relapsing fevers	Fièvre tachetée des Montagnes Rocheuses / Rocky Mountain spotted fever	Fièvre typhoïde / Typhoid fever	Filariose / Filariasis	Gale / Scabies	Gingivite nécrosante / Necrotic gingivitis (Trench mouth)	Goitre / Goitre	Grippe / Influenza	Diseases
Numéros de la nomenclature internat. détaillée revisée en 1929	43 B	115 B	115 B	115 B	40	61	42	35	177	106 a	107	53	35	20	12	9	75	44	119	120	10	13	13 a	13 b	41 a	77	77	17	15	43	44	200	44	37	5	2	145 a	4	44	1	42	153 b	115 A	66 a	11	Detailed International List Nos., as revised in 1929
Pays																																														Countries
Afrique :																																														**Africa :**
Afrique-Occidentale française	—	—	—	—	—	—	—	—	—	—	—	—	—	—	◆	—	—	—	—	—	◆	◆	—	—	—	—	—	—	—	—	—	—	—	◆	—	—	—	◆	—	◆	—	—	—	—	—	French West Africa
Algérie	—	—	—	—	—	—	—	—	—	—	◆	—	—	—	◆	◆	—	—	—	—	◆	◆	—	—	—	—	—	◆	◆	—	—	—	—	◆	◆	◆	—	◆	—	◆	—	—	—	—	◆	Algeria
Angola	◆	—	—	—	◆	◆	◆	◆	—	—	—	—	—	◆	◆	◆	—	◆	—	—	◆	◆	—	—	—	—	—	◆	◆	—	◆	—	—	◆	◆	◆	◆	◆	—	◆	—	◆	—	—	◆	Angola
Bassoutoland	—	—	—	—	—	—	—	—	—	—	—	—	—	—	◆	—	—	—	—	—	—	—	—	—	—	—	—	—	—	—	—	—	—	◆	—	—	—	—	—	—	—	—	—	—	—	Basutoland
Cameroun *(mandat français)*	—	—	—	—	—	—	—	—	—	—	—	—	—	—	◆	—	—	—	—	—	◆	◆	—	—	—	—	—	—	—	—	—	—	—	◆	—	—	—	◆	—	◆	—	—	—	—	—	Cameroons *(French Mand.)*
Congo belge	—	—	—	—	—	—	—	◆	—	—	—	—	◆	◆	◆	—	—	◆	—	—	◆	—	◆	◆	—	—	—	◆	◆	—	—	—	—	◆	◆	◆	◆	◆	—	◆	—	—	—	—	◆	Belgian Congo
Côte de l'Or	—	—	—	—	—	—	—	—	—	—	—	—	—	◆	◆	—	—	—	—	—	—	—	—	—	—	—	—	◆	—	—	—	—	—	◆	—	—	—	—	—	—	—	—	—	—	◆	Gold Coast
Cyrénaïque	—	—	—	—	—	—	—	—	—	—	—	—	—	◆	◆	—	—	—	—	—	◆	—	◆	◆	—	—	—	◆	—	—	—	—	—	◆	—	◆	—	—	—	◆	—	—	—	—	—	Cyrenaica
Egypte	—	—	—	—	—	—	—	—	—	—	—	—	—	◆	◆	◆	—	◆	—	—	◆	◆	—	—	—	—	—	◆	◆	—	—	—	—	—	◆	—	◆	◆	—	◆	—	—	—	—	◆	Egypt
Erythrée	—	—	—	—	—	—	—	—	—	—	—	—	—	—	◆	—	—	—	—	—	—	—	—	—	—	—	—	—	—	—	—	—	—	◆	—	—	—	—	—	—	—	—	—	—	—	Eritrea
Kénia	—	—	—	—	—	◆	—	—	—	—	—	—	—	◆	◆	◆	—	—	—	—	◆	—	—	—	—	—	—	◆	◆	—	—	—	—	◆	◆	◆	◆	—	—	◆	—	—	—	—	—	Kenya
Madagascar	—	—	—	—	—	—	—	—	—	—	—	—	—	—	◆	—	—	—	—	—	◆	◆	—	—	—	—	—	—	—	—	—	—	—	◆	—	—	—	◆	—	◆	—	—	—	—	—	Madagascar
Maroc, Protectorat français	—	—	—	—	—	—	—	—	—	—	—	—	—	—	◆	—	—	—	—	—	◆	—	◆	◆	—	—	—	◆	—	—	—	—	—	◆	◆	◆	◆	◆	—	◆	—	—	—	—	—	French Protectorate of Morocco
Maurice, Ile	—	—	—	—	—	—	—	—	—	—	—	—	—	◆	◆	—	—	—	—	—	◆	—	—	—	—	—	—	◆	◆	—	—	—	—	◆	◆	◆	◆	—	—	◆	—	—	—	—	—	Mauritius
Mozambique	—	—	—	—	—	—	—	—	—	—	—	—	—	—	◆	◆	—	—	—	—	—	—	◆	◆	—	—	—	—	◆	—	◆	—	—	◆	—	◆	—	—	—	◆	—	—	—	—	◆	Mozambique
Nigéria	—	—	—	—	—	—	—	—	—	—	—	—	—	—	◆	—	—	—	—	—	◆	—	—	—	—	—	—	—	—	—	—	—	—	◆	—	◆	—	—	—	◆	—	—	—	—	—	Nigeria
Nyassaland, Prot.	—	—	—	—	—	—	—	—	—	—	—	—	—	—	◆	◆	—	—	—	—	◆	—	—	—	—	—	—	—	—	—	—	—	—	◆	—	◆	—	—	—	◆	—	—	—	—	—	Nyasaland Protect.
Ouganda	—	—	—	—	—	—	—	—	—	—	—	—	—	—	◆	◆	—	—	—	—	◆	—	—	—	—	—	—	—	◆	—	—	—	—	◆	—	◆	◆	◆	—	◆	—	—	—	—	—	Uganda
Réunion	—	—	—	—	—	—	—	—	—	—	—	—	—	—	◆	—	—	—	—	—	◆	◆	—	—	—	—	—	—	—	—	—	—	—	◆	—	—	—	◆	—	◆	—	—	—	—	—	Reunion
Rhodésie du Nord	—	—	—	—	—	—	—	—	—	—	—	—	—	◆	◆	◆	—	—	—	—	◆	◆	—	—	—	—	—	—	◆	—	◆	—	—	◆	◆	◆	◆	◆	—	◆	—	—	—	—	—	Northern Rhodesia
Rhodésie du Sud	—	—	—	—	—	—	—	—	—	—	—	—	—	◆	◆	—	—	—	—	—	◆	—	—	—	—	—	—	—	◆	—	—	—	—	—	◆	◆	◆	—	—	◆	—	—	—	—	—	Southern Rhodesia
Sierra-Leone	—	—	—	—	—	◆	—	—	—	—	—	—	—	—	◆	—	—	—	—	—	◆	◆	—	—	—	—	—	—	◆	—	—	—	—	◆	—	◆	◆	◆	—	◆	—	—	—	—	◆	Sierra Leone
Somalie britann.	—	—	—	—	—	—	—	—	—	—	—	—	—	—	◆	—	—	—	—	—	◆	—	—	—	—	—	—	—	—	—	—	—	—	◆	—	◆	—	—	—	◆	—	—	—	—	—	British Somaliland
Somalie française	—	—	—	—	—	—	—	—	—	—	—	—	—	—	◆	—	—	—	—	—	◆	◆	—	—	—	—	—	—	—	—	—	—	—	◆	—	—	—	◆	—	◆	—	—	—	—	—	French Somaliland
Soudan anglo-égyptien	—	—	—	—	—	—	—	—	—	—	—	—	—	—	◆	—	—	—	—	—	◆	—	—	—	—	—	—	—	—	—	—	—	—	—	—	◆	—	◆	—	◆	—	—	—	—	—	Anglo-Egyptian Sudan
Tanganyika, Territoire du *(mandat britannique)*	—	—	—	—	—	◆	—	—	—	—	—	—	—	◆	◆	—	—	—	—	—	◆	—	—	—	—	—	—	◆	—	—	—	◆	—	◆	—	◆	—	◆	—	◆	—	—	—	—	◆	Tanganyika Territory *(British Mandate)*
Togo *(mandat français)*	—	—	—	—	—	—	—	—	—	—	—	—	—	—	◆	—	—	—	—	—	◆	◆	—	—	—	—	—	—	—	—	—	—	—	◆	—	—	—	◆	—	◆	—	—	—	—	—	Togo *(French Mandate)*
Tripolitaine	—	—	—	—	—	—	—	—	—	—	—	—	—	◆	◆	—	—	—	—	—	◆	—	◆	◆	—	—	—	◆	—	—	—	—	—	◆	—	◆	—	—	—	◆	—	—	—	—	—	Tripolitania
Tunisie	—	—	—	—	—	—	—	—	—	—	—	—	—	—	◆	—	—	—	—	—	◆	—	◆	◆	—	—	—	—	—	—	—	—	—	◆	◆	◆	—	◆	—	◆	—	—	—	—	—	Tunis
Union de l'Afrique du Sud	—	—	—	—	—	—	—	—	—	—	—	—	—	◆	◆	—	—	—	—	—	◆	—	—	—	—	—	—	◆	◆	—	—	—	—	◆	◆	◆	◆	—	—	◆	—	—	—	—	—	Union of South Africa
Zanzibar	—	—	—	—	—	◆	—	—	—	—	—	—	—	◆	◆	◆	—	—	—	—	◆	◆	—	—	—	—	◆	◆	◆	—	—	—	—	◆	◆	◆	◆	◆	—	◆	—	—	—	—	—	Zanzibar

Figure 2.33 League of Nations Health Organisation. Country-by-disease matrix showing those countries of Africa (rows) in which specified diseases (columns) were subject to mandatory notification in the sample year of 1930. Diseases subject to mandatory notification are identified by the diamond-shaped pips. *Source*: League of Nations Health Organisation (1932, pp. 54–65, detail).

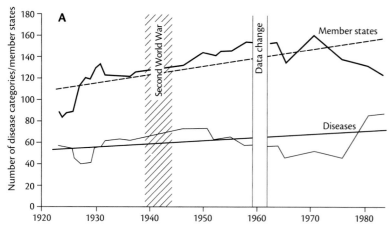

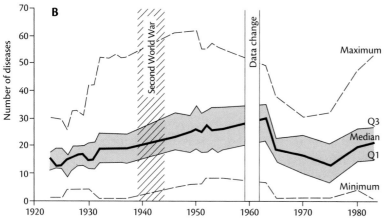

Figure 2.34 Trends in global surveillance for 123 sample communicable disease categories, 1923–83. (A) Plot of the number of disease categories (lower line trace) and the associated number of WHO Member States (upper line trace) for which surveillance activities were documented in the League of Nations/WHO data set. Trends are shown by linear regression lines fitted to the data by ordinary least squares. (B) Number of disease categories per WHO Member State for which surveillance activities were documented in the League of Nations/WHO data set. The graph plots the median (heavy line trace), inter-quartile range (Q1, Q3; shaded envelope) and maximum and minimum counts (broken line traces) of disease categories for sample years. Graphs (A) and (B) have been formed on the basis of the notifiable status of diseases (1923–58) and published disease reports (1959–83); the hinge period marking the change in data type is indicated. *Source*: redrawn from Cliff, Smallman-Raynor, Haggett, *et al.* (2009, Figures 3.2 and 3.3A, pp. 118, 120).

number of sample communicable disease categories for which surveillance activities were documented by Member States, along with the inter-quartile range (Q1 and Q3; shaded envelope) and maximum and minimum (broken line traces) counts. As the graph shows, the first four decades of the observation period were associated with a steady increase in the median number of disease categories, rising from 15 (1923) to 30 (1963), but with a sharp reduction thereafter. As judged by the inter-quartile range, many WHO Member States approximated this general surveillance pattern.

Emerging Diseases in the Global Surveillance Record

Of the 123 sample disease categories under consideration, 53 were included in the League of Nations/WHO records for the 1920s. For the remaining 70, **Figure 2.35** shows the number first included in the surveillance records by decadal period, 1930s, … , 1980s; the associated diseases are given in **Table 2.4**. While 'new' disease categories were added to the surveillance records at various stages during the six-decade interval, some 25 percent of the 123 categories included in the analysis were recorded for the first time in the 1980s. As a rule, this latter development reflected the extension of *ICD* recording classes, graphed in Figure 2.4, to include 'other', 'unspecified' and 'not elsewhere classified' disease categories associated with a broad range of bacterial, fungal, helminthic, protozoal and viral diseases.

World Regional Disease Patterns

One important geographical question that can be asked of the data set relates to the regional specificity of disease surveillance activities. More particularly, is it possible to identify distinctive regional concentrations of disease categories for which surveillance was undertaken and, if so, did these regional concentrations change over time? **Table 2.5** is based on Cliff, Smallman-Raynor, Haggett, *et al.* (2009, pp. 126–32) and identifies those communicable disease categories for which each of the six WHO Regions displayed a particular concentration of surveillance activities, relative to the global pattern, in a given decadal period (1920s, … , 1980s). Up to five diseases with the highest regional concentrations of surveillance activities (rank 1 = highest concentration) are shown.

The table identifies a series of distinctive marker diseases for several of the world regions. In Africa, for example, African trypanosomiasis (1920s–80s), schistosomiasis (1920s–60s) and relapsing fever (1940s–70s) feature in the list in three or more decadal periods. Likewise, spotted fever (1920s–70s), coccidioidomycosis (1930s–50s) and yellow fever (1960s–80s) are prominent in the Americas, as are trench fever (1920s–50s), tularemia (1950s–70s) and Brill's disease (1960s–80s) in Europe and echinococcosis (1920s–40s) and diarrhoea and gastroenteritis (1940s–60s) in the Western Pacific. Only in relatively rare instances, however, does a single disease category remain important throughout the entire observation period.

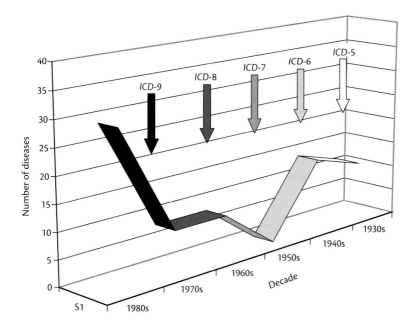

Figure 2.35 Emergence of sample communicable diseases in the global surveillance record: newly recorded disease categories by decade, 1930s–1980s. The graph plots the number of disease categories first included in the League of Nations/WHO data set in a given decade, 1930s, … , 1980s. The timings of successive revisions of the *International Classification of Diseases (ICD)*, described in Section 2.2, are indicated for reference. *Source*: redrawn from Cliff, Smallman-Raynor, Haggett, *et al.* (2009, Figure 3.5, p. 123).

Table 2.4 League of Nations/WHO: communicable disease categories included for the first time in global surveillance records, 1930s–80s

Decade of first inclusion	Disease category (*ICD*-10 code)
1930s	Shigellosis (A03); amoebiasis (A06); tularemia (A21); rat-bite fevers (A25); rhinoscleroma (A48); other spirochaetal infections (A69); psittacosis (A70); foot-and-mouth disease (B08); coccidioidomycosis (B38); other fluke infections (B66); other helminthiases (B83).
1940s	Bartonellosis (A44); gas gangrene (A48); colibacillosis (A49); chlamydial lymphogranuloma (venereum) (A55); typhus, endemic (murine typhus) (A75); Q fever (A78); trench fever (A79); unspecified viral encephalitis (A86); other arthropod-borne viral fevers, not elsewhere classified (A93); zoster (B02); viral hepatitis (B15–B19); infectious mononucleosis (B27); Chagas' disease (B57); ascariasis (B77).
1950s	None.
1960s	Other tetanus (A35); congenital syphilis (A50); early syphilis (A51); late syphilis (A52); other and unspecified syphilis (A53); relapsing fever, tick-borne (A68); Brill's disease (A75); unspecified malaria (B54).
1970s	Other zoonotic bacterial diseases, not elsewhere classified (A28); infection due to other mycobacteria (A31); Boutonneuse fever (A77); tick-borne viral encephalitis (A84); acute hepatitis B (B16); other acute viral hepatitis (B17); chronic viral hepatitis (B18); other and unspecified infectious diseases (B99).
1980s	Other salmonella infections (A02); other bacterial intestinal infections (A04); other bacterial foodborne intoxications (A05); other protozoal intestinal diseases (A07); viral and other specified intestinal infections (A08); trichomoniasis (A59); unspecified sexually transmitted disease (A64); atypical virus infections of central nervous system (A81); mosquito-borne viral encephalitis (A83); viral meningitis (A87); other viral infections of central nervous system, not elsewhere classified (A88); unspecified viral infection of central nervous system (A89); sandfly fever (A93); unspecified arthropod-borne viral fever (A94); arenaviral haemorrhagic fever (A96); other viral haemorrhagic fevers, not elsewhere classified (A98); unspecified viral haemorrhagic fever (A99); viral conjunctivitis (B30); candidiasis (B37); histoplasmosis (B39); blastomycosis (B40); other mycoses, not elsewhere classified (B48); toxoplasmosis (B58); other predominantly sexually transmitted diseases, not elsewhere classified (B63); unspecified protozoal disease (B64); other cestode infections (B71); other intestinal helminthiases, not elsewhere classified (B81); unspecified intestinal parasitism (B82); unspecified parasitic disease (B89).

Source: Cliff, Smallman-Raynor, Haggett, *et al.* (2009, Table 3.3, p. 124).

Rather, the general tendency is for a disease category newly to enter the list for a given region, remain for one, two or three decades, to be succeeded by other disease categories in subsequent periods.

A further feature of Table 2.5 is the way in which documented surveillance activities have evolved as both surveillance capacity and the number of recognised disease categories has expanded over time. During the 1930s and 1940s, Cliff, Smallman-Raynor, Haggett, *et al.* (2009) observe that the regional lead in the monitoring of 'new' disease categories was taken by the Americas (coccidioidomycosis, colibacillosis, gas gangrene, Q fever and rat-bite fevers), Europe (infectious mononucleosis) and the Western Pacific (other helminthiases, chlamydial lymphogranuloma and viral hepatitis). From the 1960s, the geographical focus of monitoring activities for newly-defined disease categories evolved to include Africa, Eastern Mediterranean and South-East Asia. Especially prominent in this latter development were a range of unspecified and atypical arthropod-borne viral fevers and infections of the CNS, viral haemorrhagic fevers, bacterial, fungal, helminthic and protozoal infections that were first included in the League of Nations/WHO surveillance records in the 1980s.

Table 2.5 Regional specificity of communicable disease categories most commonly subject to monitoring in WHO member states, 1920s–1980s

World region	Decade	Disease[1]				
		Rank 1	Rank 2	Rank 3	Rank 4	Rank 5
Africa	1920s	African trypanosomiasis (B56)	Schistosomiasis (B65)	Brucellosis (A23)	---	---
	1930s	African trypanosomiasis (B56)	Yaws (A66)	---	---	---
	1940s	African trypanosomiasis (B56)	Yaws (A66)	Relapsing fever, unspecified (A68)	Schistosomiasis (B65)	---
	1950s	African trypanosomiasis (B56)	Leishmaniasis (B55)	---	---	---
	1960s	African trypanosomiasis (B56)	Relapsing fever, tick-borne (A68)	Smallpox (B03)	Schistosomiasis (B65)	Leishmaniasis (B55)
	1970s	Tick-borne viral encephalitis (A84)	Rubella (B06)	Chronic viral hepatitis (B18)	Relapsing fever, tick-borne (A68)	Pediculosis (B85)
	1980s	Unspecified viral infection of the CNS (A89)	Unspecified arthropod-borne viral fever (A94)	Coccidioidomycosis (B38)	Histoplasmosis (B39)	African trypanosomiasis (B56)
Americas	1920s	Filariasis (B74)	Spotted fever (A77)	Dengue fever (A90)	Syphilis (A50–A53)	Leptospirosis (A27)
	1930s	Rat-bite fevers (A25)	Coccidioidomycosis (B38)	Spotted fever (A77)	Pediculosis (B85)	Tularemeia (A21)
	1940s	Rat-bite fevers (A25)	Gas gangrene (A48)	Colibacillosis (A49)	Q fever (A78)	Coccidioidomycosis (B38)
	1950s	Spotted fever (A77)	Q fever (A78)	Coccidioidomycosis (B38)	Other fluke infections (B66)	Ascariasis (B77)
	1960s	Spotted fever (A77)	Granuloma inguinale (A58)	Other spirochaetal infections (A69)	Unspecified mycosis (B49)	Yellow fever (A95)
	1970s	Diarrhoea and gastroenteritis (A09)	Infection due to other mycobacteria (A31)	Spotted fever (A77)	Other and unspecified infectious diseases (B99)	Yellow fever (A95)
	1980s	Yellow fever (A95)	Erysipelas (A46)	Dengue fever (A90)	Plague (A20)	Viral hepatitis (B15–B19)
Eastern Mediterranean	1920s	Dermatophytosis (B35)	---	---	---	---
	1930s	---	---	---	---	---
	1940s	Schistosomiasis (B65)	Echinococcosis (B67)	---	---	---
	1950s	Pediculosis (B85)	Echinococcosis (B67)	---	---	---
	1960s	Congenital syphilis (A50)	Cholera (A00)	---	---	---
	1970s	Typhus, endemic (murine typhus) (A75)	Acute hepatitis B (B16)	Other acute viral hepatitis (B17)	Pediculosis (B85)	Malaria (B50–B54)
	1980s	Unspecified protozoal disease (B64)	Blastomycosis (B40)	Leishmaniasis (B55)	Other intestinal helminthiases, NEC (B81)	Other fluke infections (B66)
Europe	1920s	Trench fever (A79)	Unspecified mycosis (B49)	Pediculosis (B85)	Scabies (B86)	Other viral diseases, NEC (B33)
	1930s	Other specified bacterial diseases (A48)	Trench fever (A79)	Other viral diseases, NEC (B33)	Leptospirosis (A27)	Glanders (A24)
	1940s	Other specified bacterial diseases (A48)	Other rickettsioses (A79)	Trench fever (A79)	Sandfly fever (A93)	Infectious mononucleosis (B27)
	1950s	Trench fever (A79)	Other arthropod-borne diseases, NEC (A93)	Botulism (A05)	Tularemia (A21)	Infectious mononucleosis (B27)
	1960s	Late syphilis (A52)	Brill's disease (A75)	Q fever (A78)	Tularemia (A21)	Echinococcosis (B67)

Table 2.5 *(Continued)*

World region	Decade	Disease[1]				
		Rank 1	**Rank 2**	**Rank 3**	**Rank 4**	**Rank 5**
	1970s	Other zoonotic bacterial diseases, NEC (A28)	Brill's disease (A75)	Boutonneuse fever (A77)	Tularemia (A21)	Psittacosis (A70)
	1980s	Brill's disease (A75)	Infection due to other mycobacteria (A31)	Unspecified sexually transmitted disease (A64)	Q fever (A78)	Zoster (B02)
South-East Asia	1920s	Leishmaniasis (B55)	Diarrhoea and gastroenteritis (A09)	---	---	---
	1930s	Diarrhoea and gastroenteritis (A09)	Filariasis (B74)	---	---	---
	1940s	---	---	---	---	---
	1950s	---	---	---	---	---
	1960s	Cholera (A00)	Plague (A20)	---	---	---
	1970s	Smallpox (B03)	---	---	---	---
	1980s	Relapsing fever, tick-borne (A68)	Atypical virus infections of the CNS (A81)	Arenaviral haemorrhagic fever (A96)	Other mycoses, NEC (B48)	Unspecified viral haemorrhagic fever (A99)
Western Pacific	1920s	Echinococcosis (B67)	Dermatophytosis (B35)	Botulism (A05)	Actinomycosis (A42)	Granuloma inguinale (A58)
	1930s	Other heminthiases (B83)	Echinococcosis (B67)	Other fluke infections (B66)	Schistosomiasis (B65)	Other septicaemia (A41)
	1940s	Chlamydial lymphogranuloma (venereum) (A55)	Echinococcosis (B67)	Diarrhoea and gastroenteritis (A09)	Viral hepatitis (B15–B19)	Filariasis (B74)
	1950s	Diarrhoea and gastroenteritis (A09)	Filariasis (B74)	Rubella (B06)	Dengue fever (A90)	Viral hepatitis (B15–B19)
	1960s	Diarrhoea and gastroenteritis (A09)	Cholera (A00)	Yaws (A66)	Dengue fever (A90)	Filariasis (B74)
	1970s	Other acute viral hepatitis (B17)	Leptospirosis (A27)	Syphilis (A50–A53)	Unspecified viral encephalitis (A86)	Gonococcal infection (A54)
	1980s	Unspecified parasitic disease (B89)	Mosquito-borne viral encephalitis (A83)	Arenaviral haemorrhagic fever (A96)	Candidiasis (B37)	Other acute viral hepatitis (B17)

Notes: [1]Up to five disease categories with a marked regional concentration of surveillance activities are shown (rank 1 = highest concentration); the associated three-character *ICD*-10 codes are given in parentheses. CNS = central nervous system. NEC = not elsewhere classified.
Source: Cliff, Smallman-Raynor, Haggett, *et al.* (2009, Table 3.4, pp. 128–31).

Developments in Programme-Oriented Surveillance

From the mid-1980s, the character of international recording of communicable disease morbidity and mortality changed fundamentally from systematic time period × disease × country surveillance of a large basket of infectious conditions to a targeted surveillance related to international health programmes. And so, in 1982, the WHO programmes on Health Statistics and Epidemiological Surveillance were merged to form the Health Situation and Trend Assessment Programme. This new programme placed emphasis on a target-oriented approach to information, with priority given to only the most essential information for the improvement of health systems (Uemura, 1988). This approach, built around vaccine-controllable and potentially globally-eradicable diseases, had been presaged by the Smallpox Eradication Programme in the 1960s and 1970s and was followed by the Expanded Programme on Immunization from 1974 and the Global Polio Eradication Initiative from 1988. Here,

we examine aspects of programme-oriented surveillance in relation to the global smallpox and poliomyelitis eradication campaigns. Overviews of the eradication campaigns are provided in Sections 5.2 (smallpox) and 5.3 (poliomyelitis).

Active Search Operations: The Intensified Smallpox Eradication Programme (1967–77)

As described in Section 5.2, the Nineteenth World Health Assembly committed the WHO to an intensified 10-year global Smallpox Eradication Programme which was launched in 1967. The eradication campaign started with mass vaccination, but rapidly recognised the importance of selective control. As Fenner, *et al.* (1988, pp. 473–4) explain, the issue of smallpox surveillance at the national or international levels had received little attention prior to the onset of the eradication campaign and, although the disease was subject to reporting under international quarantine agreements (Figure 2.22), endemic countries lacked formal programmes to investigate and contain outbreaks. From the outset of the campaign, however, the number of reported cases of smallpox and the number of endemic countries became the key indicators of the campaign's progress:

> The primary objective of the smallpox programme is the eradication of this disease. Surveillance is thus an essential component of the programme since the term 'eradication' implies that the number of indigenous cases of smallpox reach '0' … (WHO Handbook, cited in Fenner, *et al.*, 1988, p. 474).

Fully satisfactory networks of notification took 1–2 years to develop. Initially, reliance was placed on surveillance of those attending health units. From September 1973, however, the nature of both surveillance and containment began to change. At this stage, surveillance-containment operations and mass vaccination had halted transmission of smallpox in all but five countries (Bangladesh, Ethiopia, India, Nepal and Pakistan). In the summer of 1973, WHO devised an intensified system of case detection and (later) containment, applied first in India and, subsequently in Pakistan (late 1973), Bangladesh (early 1975), Ethiopia (late 1975) and Somalia (mid 1977). This intensified system rested with the more complete and prompt detection of outbreaks and involved supplementing the existing notification system by engaging health staff from other programmes in national village-by-village and house-to-house searches. Echoing aspects of the local detective work undertaken by searchers employed in the compilation of the London *Bills*

centuries earlier (Section 2.3), the smallpox searches involved many tens of thousands of workers and were conducted at different intervals in different areas (typically, every 4–8 weeks in endemic areas and every 2–3 months in non-endemic areas). When a suspected smallpox case was found, the search worker notified the supervisor or nearest health unit so that containment staff could move in. Searches were accompanied by an intensive publicity campaign, and rewards were offered to the populace for information on cases. Special search programmes were implemented for areas that were difficult to access (Fenner, *et al.*, 1988).

Active search operations in India

Active search operations for smallpox in India are described by Basu, *et al.* (1979, pp. 135–86). The first village-to-village search for smallpox cases was undertaken in West Bengal in September 1973 and, in subsequent months, in the highly endemic states of Bihar, Madhya Pradesh and Uttar Pradesh. The search operations were later extended beyond the four endemic states to include 11 low incidence states in November–December 1973 and 16 smallpox-free states from December 1973. Search operations continued until the last all-India search in October–November 1976 (**Figure 2.36**). Searches involved the questioning of households and people in prominent places (e.g. markets, tea shops and schools) and positions (e.g. village leaders, teachers and postmen) for information on cases of rash with fever; smallpox recognition cards were also shown to illustrate the disease. All told, these operations involved

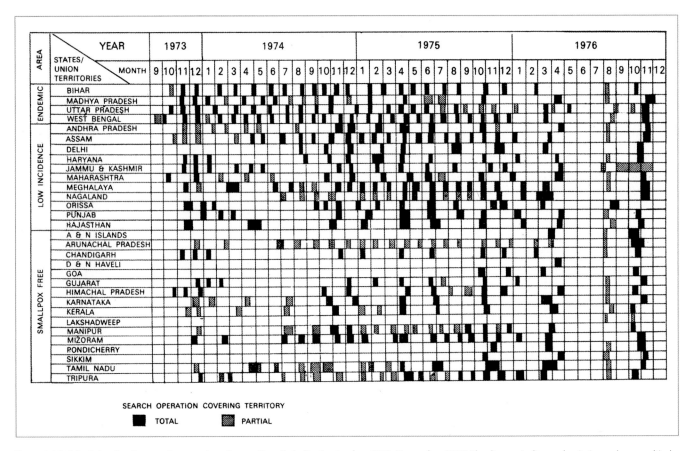

Figure 2.36 Schedule of active search operations for smallpox in India, September 1973–December 1976. The diagram indicates the timing and geographical coverage of search operations in the four endemic states (Bihar, Madhya Pradesh, Uttar Pradesh and West Bengal) and 27 low incidence and smallpox-free states. *Source*: Basu, *et al.* (1979, Figure 7.12, p. 156).

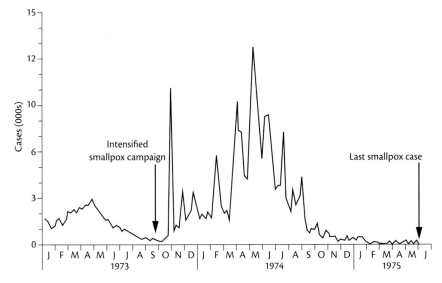

Figure 2.37 Weekly series of reported smallpox cases, India, January 1973–June 1975. Active search operations, implemented under the intensified smallpox campaign from September 1973, had a considerable impact on the number of reported smallpox cases in the country. *Source*: redrawn from Basu, *et al.* (1979, Figure 7.10, p. 154).

a total of 463 searches and 11.27 million village visits between September 1973 and November 1976. The active search operations yielded evidence of 20,835 outbreaks and 77,704 smallpox cases in the entire search period to November 1976; the last detected smallpox case was discharged from hospital in July 1975 and India was declared free of smallpox by an International Commission in April 1977 (Basu, *et al.*, 1979); see **Figure 2.37**.

Syndromic Surveillance: The Global Polio Eradication Initiative (1988–)

Methods of *syndromic surveillance* are frequently adopted where early detection of a disease event is considered a high priority. Syndromic surveillance focuses on the monitoring of health indicators that are available prior to the confirmation of diagnosis or laboratory confirmation of infection. The information is in near-real time and is often available sooner than a laboratory test can be completed.

Sensitive syndromic surveillance for acute flaccid paralysis (AFP) has formed a major strand of the Global Polio Eradication Initiative (Hull, *et al.*, 1997), to which the WHO was committed by the Forty-first World Health Assembly in May 1988 (Section 5.3). Acute flaccid paralysis is the principal clinical syndrome of paralytic poliomyelitis and is characterised by paralysis, muscle flaccidity and sudden onset. Although AFP is a feature of all cases of paralytic poliomyelitis, the syndrome has a number of aetiologies. These range from other neurotropic viruses to trauma and chemical exposure. Surveillance for AFP is considered the gold standard for detecting cases of poliomyelitis and involves four steps: (i) finding and reporting children with AFP; (ii) transporting stool samples for analysis; (iii) isolating and identifying poliovirus in the laboratory; and (iv) mapping the virus to determine the origin of the virus strain.

The syndromic surveillance strategy adopted by the Global Polio Eradication Initiative requires the immediate reporting and rapid laboratory-based investigation of all cases of AFP in children aged < 15 years. This serves in the detection of typical and atypical cases of poliomyelitis due to both wild and vaccine-derived strains of poliovirus. Laboratory-based investigation of samples is coordinated through the Global Polio Laboratory Network, a global and interdependent network of laboratories that was formalised in 1992–93 (**Figure 2.38**). AFP surveillance provides a basis for assessment of the quality of disease surveillance for certification purposes (**Table 2.6**). Molecular epidemiologic methods have enhanced the precision and reliability of laboratory-based poliomyelitis surveillance, allowing wild viruses to be classified into genetic families from which inferences on the geographical source of isolates can be drawn (Cochi, *et al.*, 1997; World Health Organization, 1998b).

Twenty-First-Century Approaches: Electronic Network Systems for Global Disease Detection

Surveillance changed radically from the mid-1980s as a result of technological developments – the rapid and widespread growth in cheap desktop computing power and software replacing a few massive mainframes, and the growth of the communications and information-rich Internet. Recent developments in this area have been shaped by the International Health Regulations which were revised in 2005 to update capacity and standards of the reporting of disease events. The 2005 Regulations expanded the traditional concerns of the International Health Regulations and provided a new framework for the management of events that may constitute a public health emergency of international concern (Figure 2.22). Under the revised Regulations, Member States are required to notify the WHO of *all events which may constitute a public health emergency of international concern* (Article 6.1), whether naturally occurring, intentionally created or unintentionally caused. Four diseases are subject to notification under *all* circumstances: human influenza caused by a new subtype; poliomyelitis due to wild-type poliovirus; severe acute respiratory syndrome (SARS); and smallpox. The revised International Health Regulations set minimum requirements for developing and maintaining core capacity for the detection of, and response to, public health emergencies of international concern ('core capacity requirements for surveillance response'). Internet-based systems of real-time disease surveillance lie at the heart of these developments.

The WHO Global Outbreak Alert and Response Network (GOARN)

The rise of newly emerging diseases, the pandemic spread of influenza and the threat of bioterrorism have highlighted the essential

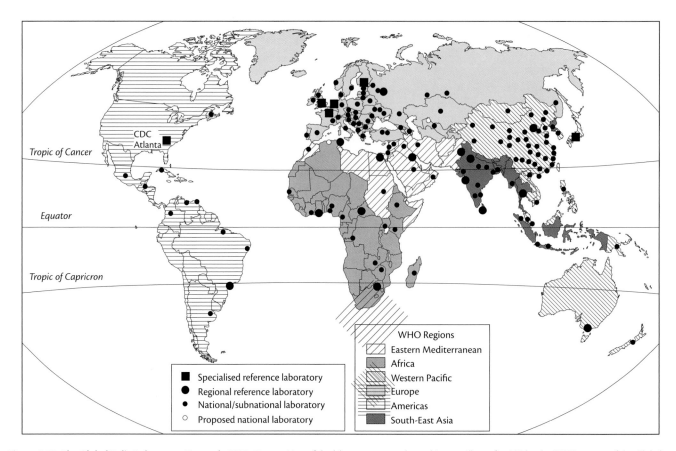

Figure 2.38 **The Global Polio Laboratory Network, 2000.** Composition of the laboratory network, used in surveillance for AFP by the WHO, as part of the Global Polio Eradication Initiative. *Source*: redrawn from Cliff, Smallman-Raynor, Haggett, *et al.* (2009, Figure 11.23, p. 664), originally from World Health Organization (2000a, Map 1, p. 71).

Table 2.6. Principal performance indicators for acute flaccid paralysis (AFP) surveillance

Criterion	Performance measure
Completeness of reporting	≥ 80 percent of expected routine (weekly or monthly) AFP surveillance reports should be received on time, including zero reports where no AFP cases are seen. The distribution of reporting sites should be representative of the geography and demography of the country.
Sensitivity of surveillance	≥ 1 case of non-poliomyelitis AFP should be detected annually per 100,000 population aged < 15 years.
Completeness of case investigation	All AFP cases should have a full clinical and virological investigation with ≥ 80 percent of AFP cases having adequate stool specimens collected for enterovirus studies. (Adequate stool specimens are defined as: two specimens of sufficient quantity for laboratory analysis, collected at least 24 hours apart, within 14 days after the onset of paralysis, and arriving in the laboratory by reverse cold chain and with proper documentation.)
Completeness of follow-up	≥ 80 percent of AFP cases should have a follow-up examination for residual paralysis at 60 days after the onset of paralysis.
Laboratory performance	All virologic studies of AFP cases must be performed in a laboratory accredited by the Global Poliomyelitis Laboratory Network.

Source: abstracted from World Health Organization (1998b, pp. 113–14).

function of global disease surveillance in the maintenance and promotion of international health in the early twenty-first century (Castillo-Salgado, 2010). To this end, the Global Outbreak Alert and Response Network (GOARN) for the early detection of, and rapid response to, outbreaks of diseases of international importance was formalised by the WHO in April 2000 (Heymann, *et al.*, 2001). Conceived as a "network of networks" (Lemon, *et al.*, 2007, p. 19), and formed as an international collaboration of some 140 public, private, non-governmental and intergovernmental institutions and organisations worldwide, GOARN is overseen by the WHO Global Alert and Response (GAR) programme as the principal WHO surveillance network for international outbreak alert and response (**Figure 2.39**).

GOARN operations

GOARN operates in three key areas: outbreak alert (detection, verification and communication); outbreak response (risk assessment, technical advice and support, field investigation, research and communication); and preparedness (assessment, planning, training,

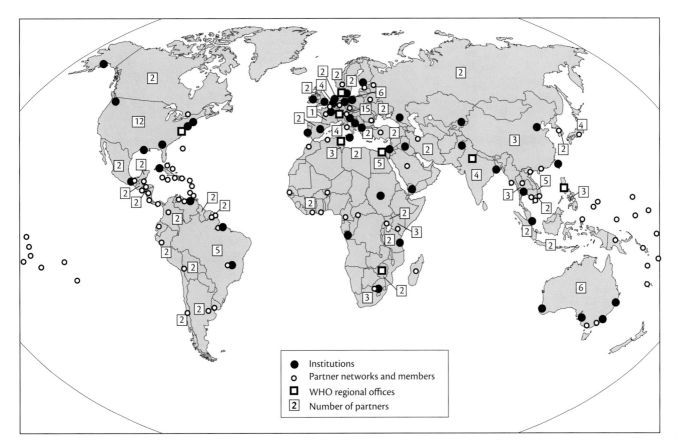

Figure 2.39 The Global Outbreak Alert and Response Network (GOARN). GOARN is formed as an international collaboration of technical associates in the field of epidemic alert and response. The map shows the distribution of GOARN partners. Where locations have more than one partner, the number of partners is identified in the boxes. *Source*: redrawn from World Health Organization (2005e).

stockpiles, research and communication). For these purposes, GOARN connects both formal and informal sources of outbreak information. Formal sources include a range of governmental agencies, universities, laboratories and other institutions that form part of the global network of WHO collaborating centres, along with international agencies and WHO regional and country offices. Informal sources include non-governmental organisations (such as the United Nations Children's Fund (UNICEF), the United Nations High Commissioner for Refugees (UNHCR), the International Committee of the Red Cross, the International Federation of Red Cross and Red Crescent Societies and international humanitarian non-governmental organisations such as Médecins sans Frontières), along with informal Internet-based disease surveillance and scanning systems such as the Global Public Health Intelligence Network (GPHIN) described in Section 2.8.

Real-time information gathered by GOARN is examined on a daily basis by the WHO Outbreak Verification Team. Daily reports on suspected and verified events are then distributed to specified WHO staff at Geneva and in the Regional Offices, while a weekly electronic Outbreak Verification List (including summary details of the disease, location, source of report, number of cases and deaths and investigation status) is distributed throughout the GOARN network. Once an outbreak has been verified, situation reports are posted on the WHO website and in *Weekly Epidemiological Record*. Outbreak responses are implemented by GOARN partners, while WHO HQ has investigative teams for rapid dispatch to outbreak sites (Heymann, *et al.*, 2001).

Global Laboratory Networks and Electronic Surveillance Systems

The WHO maintains programmes for the monitoring and control of a number of well-established diseases and coordinates a number of electronic systems and databases that link networks of laboratories and other facilities worldwide. Examples of such systems include DengueNet (dengue), Global Foodborne Infections Network (foodborne infections) and, for the purposes of illustration here, GISRS and FluNET (influenza).

Global Influenza Surveillance and Response System (GISRS) and FluNET

The Global Influenza Surveillance and Response System (GISRS) (formerly known as the Global Influenza Surveillance Network) was originally established in 1952 as a network of laboratories to provide the WHO and its Member States with information on which to implement influenza control measures. As of 2011, the network was comprised of six WHO Collaborating Centres (Atlanta, USA; Beijing, China; London, UK; Melbourne, Australia; Memphis, USA; and Tokyo, Japan), four Essential Regulatory Laboratories (Woden, Australia; Potters Bar, UK; Rockville, USA; and Tokyo, Japan) and 136 institutions that are recognised by the WHO as National Influenza Centres (**Figure 2.40**). The GISRS monitors the evolution of influenza viruses and provides recommendations on issues that include laboratory diagnostics, vaccines, antiviral susceptibility and risk assessment. The GISRS also serves as a global alert mechanism for the emergence of influenza viruses with pandemic potential.

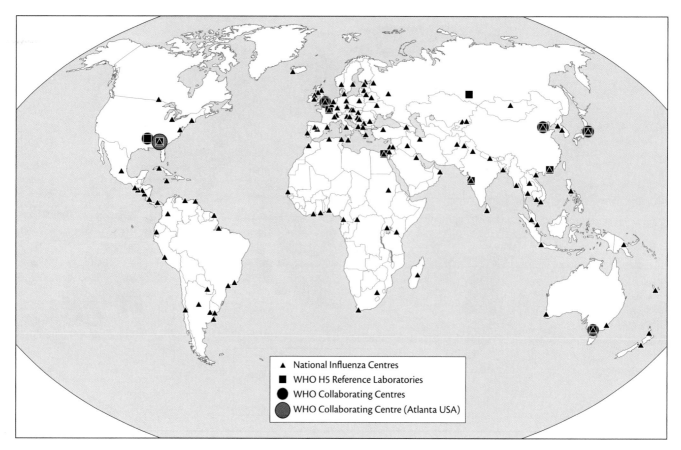

Figure 2.40 Institutional network of the WHO Global Influenza Surveillance and Response System (GISRS). The map shows the location of National Influenza Centres, WHO Collaborating Centres and WHO Reference Laboratories that formed the GISRS network in 2011. *Source*: GISRS, WHO (www.who.int).

Within the framework of GISRS, FluNET provides an electronic system that monitors emerging strains and subtypes of influenza virus and uses this information for the production of seasonal influenza vaccines. The data are provided remotely by National Influenza Centres and other national influenza reference laboratories collaborating actively with GISRS, or are uploaded from WHO regional databases. This system provided early alert of human cases of influenza A/H5N1 in Hong Kong in 1997.

2.8 Evolving Surveillance Practices

Informal Internet-Based Global Reporting Systems

Recent years have seen the development of a spectrum of ad hoc informal Internet-based international and global disease surveillance systems and platforms. These have opened up alternative channels for the rapid detection and reporting of communicable disease outbreaks. Such Internet resources also have the potential to reduce costs and to increase the transparency of reporting. We have already referred to one such 'informal' system, GPHIN, in our discussion of the WHO's GOARN (Section 2.7). Here, we provide a brief review of GPHIN and two other prominent informal systems, ProMED-mail and HealthMap. An overview of the broad range of operative systems and platforms is provided by Castillo-Salgado (2010).

The Global Public Health Intelligence Network (GPHIN)

The Global Public Health Intelligence Network (GPHIN) was established in 1998 by the WHO in partnership with the Public

Health Agency, Canada, as a web-based network for the scanning of Internet media (including news wires, online newspapers and public health email services such as ProMED-mail) with a view to detecting potential disease outbreaks globally. The information is filtered for relevancy by an automated process, and then analysed by GPHIN officials. Notifications about public health events that may have serious public health consequences are verified by the WHO and then forwarded to users (Mykhalovskiy and Weir, 2006).

ProMED-mail

ProMED-mail was established by the Federation of American Scientists' Program for Monitoring Emerging Infectious Diseases (ProMED) in 1994 and has operated as a programme of the International Society for Infectious Diseases since 1999. ProMED-mail is an Internet-based system for the rapid global dissemination of information on outbreaks of communicable diseases and acute exposures to toxins that affect human health. It is a non-hierarchical system that promotes the electronic exchange of information on diseases among a variety of sources, including international organisations, ministries of health, laboratories, practitioners and the public. Submitted reports are screened, reviewed and moderated, before being posted to the network and distributed to subscribers by email. As already noted, ProMED-mail forms one of the sources on which GPHIN draws. Further details of ProMED-mail are available at http://www.promedmail.org.

HealthMap

HealthMap, founded in September 2006 and affiliated to the Children's Hospital Informatics Program at the Harvard-

Massachusetts Institute of Technology (MIT) Division of Health Sciences and Technology, utilises online informal sources for disease outbreak monitoring and mapping within a geographical information system (GIS) framework. As described by Freifeld, *et al.* (2008), HealthMap provides a global view of communicable disease outbreaks as reported by the WHO, ProMED-mail, Google News and Eurosurveillance. The automated system operates to monitor, organise and filter information with a view to providing real-time intelligence on emerging diseases via a website (www.healthmap.org) and a mobile app ('Outbreaks Near Me').

Regional Disease Threat Tracking Tools: The European Commission

An Early Warning and Response System (EWRS) was implemented by the European Commission in 1998 as a means of gathering and analysing data on emerging public health threats to the member states of the European Community. Since 2007, the system has been hosted in Stockholm, Sweden, by the European Centre for Disease Prevention and Control (ECDC). Notifications received from member states through the EWRS and through other epidemic surveillance activities (including the active screening of national epidemiological bulletins and informal sources such as ProMED-mail,

GPHIN and the media) are documented and monitored through a dedicated database (Threat Tracking Tool, or TTT) that was first activated in June 2005. Between June 2005 and December 2009, a total of 806 threats were monitored through the TTT, representing an average of 13 threats per month (range 5–39) and with distinct seasonal peaks in the summer and autumn (**Figure 2.41**). Of these threats, 582 were initially identified through confidential sources (including 233 through EWRS) and 224 through public channels. Of the latter, ProMED-mail (85 threats) and GPHIN (32 threats) were the single most important sources of information (European Centre for Disease Prevention and Control, 2010).

Sentinel Practices

The legal requirements to notify critical infectious diseases are tending to be left behind by the reality of disease proliferation. As a result, blanket reporting is increasingly replaced by sampling systems in which sentinel practices are used to pick up trends in disease prevalence. Some cities have pioneered local monitoring, of which the Seattle Virus Watch Program of the 1960s is an outstanding early example (Hall, *et al.*, 1970). In the developing world, sentinel surveillance is the only cost-effective way of monitoring popula-

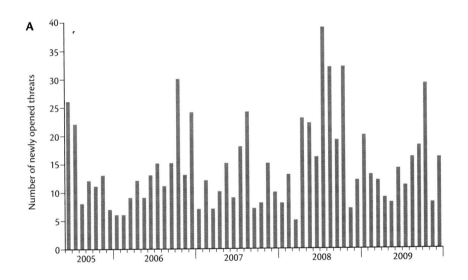

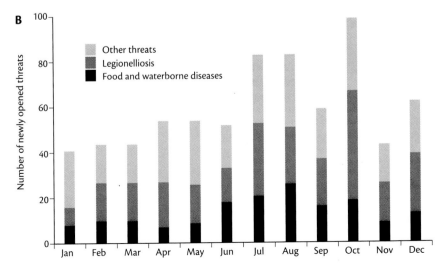

Figure 2.41 Emerging threats to public health in the European Community as monitored through the Threat Tracking Tool (TTT). (A) Time series of newly identified threats by month, June 2005–December 2009. (B) Distribution of newly identified threats by calendar month of report, 2006–9. *Source*: redrawn from European Centre for Disease Prevention and Control (2010, Figures 1, 2, p. 5).

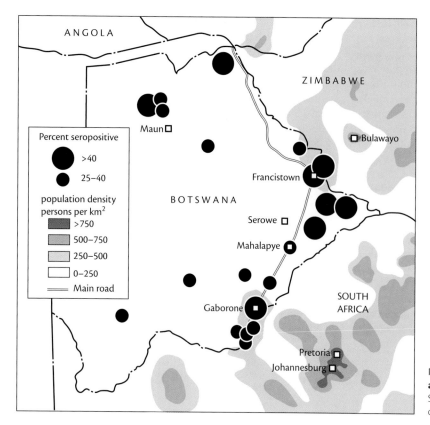

Figure 2.42 Botswana: HIV sentinel surveillance rates among pregnant women, 2002–5. *Source*: redrawn from Cliff, Smallman-Raynor, Haggett, *et al.* (2009, Figure 11.24, p. 666), originally from World Health Organization (2007, p. 12).

tion health. As an example, **Figure 2.42** maps the HIV sentinel surveillance rates for pregnant women in Botswana, 2002–5.

2.9 Conclusion

Timely and accurate surveillance data which are geographically and temporally coded lie behind any control strategy which attempts to interrupt the spatial propagation of communicable disease from one area to another. For, without such information, the development of appropriate control strategies to inhibit epidemic upturns rapidly descends into a Delphic art. Public health surveillance is the ongoing, systematic collection, analysis and interpretation of health data essential to (i) the planning, implementation and evaluation of public health practice and (ii) disease prevention and control. For control purposes, public health surveillance data systems should have the capacity to collect and analyse data, disseminate data to public health programmes (Langmuir, 1963; McNabb, *et al.*, 2002), and regularly evaluate the effectiveness of the use of the disseminated data (Miller, *et al.*, 2004; Regidor, *et al.*, 2007). Public health information systems may include data collected for other purposes, but which are essential to public health and are often used for surveillance. But such data often lack critical elements of surveillance

systems (Choi, *et al.*, 2002). For example, vital statistics data are critical to surveillance, particularly for chronic conditions. But they do not focus on specific outcomes and are often collected for other purposes (for example, legal burial or cremation), and they may not be timely (Stroup, *et al.*, 2003).

In this chapter, we have examined the development of surveillance systems across a variety of geographical scales from the local (bills of mortality), through the national (the US NEDSS framework) to the global (WHO epidemiological surveillance), as well as through time from the seventeenth to the twenty-first centuries. Our analysis of the ways in which surveillance data feed into control strategies begins in the next chapter with quarantine and isolation.

Appendix 2.1: Communicable Disease Categories

Table A2.1 gives the 123 sample communicable disease categories, along with their associated *ICD*-10 codes, analysed in *International Patterns of Communicable Disease Surveillance, 1923–83* (Section 2.7).

Table A2.1 Sample communicable disease categories for analysis: Certain Infectious and Parasitic Diseases (*ICD*-10 A00–B99)

ICD-10 code	Title of category	Diseases[1]
A00–A09	Intestinal infectious diseases	Cholera (A00); typhoid and paratyphoid fevers (A01); other salmonella infections (A02); shigellosis (A03); other bacterial intestinal infections (A04); botulism (A05); other bacterial foodborne intoxications (A05); amoebiasis (A06); other protozoal intestinal diseases (A07); viral and other specified intestinal infections (A08); diarrhoea and gastroenteritis (A09).
A15–A19	Tuberculosis	Respiratory tuberculosis (A15–A16); tuberculosis, non-respiratory (A17–A19).
A20–A28	Certain zoonotic bacterial diseases	Plague (A20); tularemia (A21); anthrax (A22); brucellosis (A23); glanders (A24); rat-bite fevers (A25); leptospirosis (A27); other zoonotic bacterial diseases, not elsewhere classified (A28).
A30–A49	Other bacterial diseases	Leprosy (A30); infection due to other mycobacteria (A31); tetanus (A33–A35); other tetanus (A35); diphtheria (A36); whooping cough (A37); scarlet fever (A38); meningococcal infection (A39); other septicaemia (A41); actinomycosis (A42); bartonellosis (A44); erysipelas (A46); gas gangrene (A48); rhinoscleroma (A48); colibacillosis (A49).
A50–A64	Infections with a predominantly sexual mode of transmission	Congenital syphilis (A50); syphilis (A50–A53); early syphilis (A51); late syphilis (A52); other and unspecified syphilis (A53); gonococcal infection (A54); chlamydial lymphogranuloma (venereum) (A55); chancroid (A57); granuloma inguinale (A58); trichomoniasis (A59); unspecified sexually transmitted disease (A64).
A65–A69	Other spirochaetal diseases	Yaws (A66); relapsing fever, tick-borne (A68); relapsing fever, unspecified (A68); other spirochaetal infections (A69).
A70–A74	Other diseases caused by chlamydiae	Psittacosis (A70); trachoma (A71).
A75–A79	Rickettsioses	Typhus fever (A75); Brill's disease (A75); typhus, endemic (murine typhus) (A75); spotted fever (A77); Boutonneuse fever (A77); Q fever (A78); other rickettsioses (A79); trench fever (A79).
A80–A89	Viral infections of the CNS	Poliomyelitis (A80); atypical virus infections of central nervous system (A81); rabies (A82); mosquito-borne viral encephalitis (A83); tick-borne viral encephalitis (A84); encephalitis lethargica (A85); unspecified viral encephalitis (A86); viral meningitis (A87); other viral infections of central nervous system, not elsewhere classified (A88); unspecified viral infection of central nervous system (A89).
A90–A99	Arthropod-borne viral fevers and viral haemorrhagic fevers	Dengue fever (A90); other arthropod-borne viral fevers, not elsewhere classified (A93); sandfly fever (A93); unspecified arthropod-borne viral fever (A94); yellow fever (A95); arenaviral haemorrhagic fever (A96); other viral haemorrhagic fevers, not elsewhere classified (A98); unspecified viral haemorrhagic fever (A99).
B00–B09	Viral infections characterised by skin and mucous membrane lesions	Chickenpox (B01); zoster (B02); smallpox (B03); measles (B05); rubella (B06); foot-and-mouth disease (B08).
B15–B19	Viral hepatitis	Viral hepatitis (B15–B19); acute hepatitis B (B16); other acute viral hepatitis (B17); chronic viral hepatitis (B18).
B25–B34	Other viral diseases	Mumps (B26); infectious mononucleosis (B27); viral conjunctivitis (B30); other viral diseases, not elsewhere classified (B33).
B35–B49	Mycoses	Dermatophytosis (B35); candidiasis (B37); coccidioidomycosis (B38); histoplasmosis (B39); blastomycosis (B40); other mycoses, not elsewhere classified (B48); unspecified mycosis (B49).
B50–B64	Protozoal diseases	Malaria (B50–B54); unspecified malaria (B54); leishmaniasis (B55); African trypanosomiasis (B56); Chagas' disease (B57); toxoplasmosis (B58); other predominantly sexually transmitted diseases, not elsewhere classified (B63); unspecified protozoal disease (B64).
B65–B83	Helminthiases	Schistosomiasis (B65); other fluke infections (B66); echinococcosis (B67); other cestode infections (B71); filariasis (B74); trichinellosis (B75); ancylostomiasis (B76); ascariasis (B77); other intestinal helminthiases, not elsewhere classified (B81); unspecified intestinal parasitism (B82); other helminthiases (B83).
B85–B89	Pediculosis, acariasis and other infestations	Pediculosis (B85); scabies (B86); unspecified parasitic disease (B89).
B99	Other infectious diseases	Other and unspecified infectious diseases (B99).

Notes: [1] Three-character *ICD*-10 codes in parentheses.
Source: Cliff, Smallman-Raynor, Haggett, *et al.* (2009, Table 3.1, pp. 116–17).

CHAPTER 3

Quarantine: Spatial Strategies

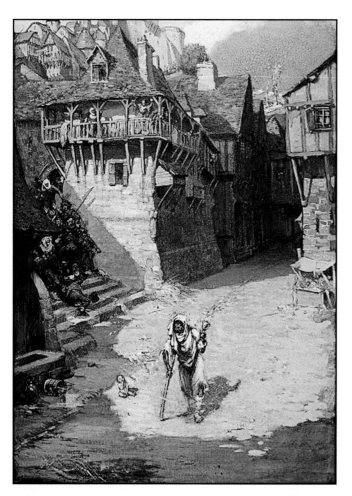

Figure 3.1 Historic attitudes to communicable diseases. Many infections, of which leprosy is the prime example, often caused sufferers to be stigmatised socially and to be physically isolated. In this watercolour by Richard Tennant, a leper warns of his approach by ringing a bell. Supported by his pointing pole, he has cleared a village street of adults leaving only an unknowing infant by the roadside to witness his passage. *Source*: Wellcome Library, London.

3.1 Introduction

> . . . the last and greatest art is to limit and isolate oneself.
> Johann Wolfgang von Goethe 20 April 1825

Quarantine and isolation are the oldest methods used to try to prevent the geographical spread of communicable diseases between humans (**Figure 3.1**). The principle is simple and obvious – prevent spatial interaction between an infective or a fomite and a susceptible and the spread of infection is inhibited. Indeed, before the germ theory of diseases was available and antibiotics and vaccines developed, quarantine and isolation were the only methods by which the geographical spread of infectious diseases could be checked. And so our substantive discussion of methods of control in the next four chapters begins here with this most ancient of approaches, still used in certain circumstances today. We begin by defining what we mean by quarantine and isolation, and then consider each in turn.

Quarantine

The fifteenth edition of the American Public Health Association's bible, *Control of Communicable Diseases of Man* (Benenson, 1990, pp. 502–6), specifies very strict definitions for the terms, *quarantine* and *isolation*. *Quarantine* is used to denote restrictions upon the activities of **well** persons or animals (susceptibles, S in Figure 1.19) who have been exposed to a case of a communicable disease during its period of communicability. This is to prevent disease transmission ($I \rightarrow S$ in Figure 1.19) going beyond S if S should fall ill as a result of the contact with I. Failure to intercede would potentially allow the chains of infection to be maintained. Geographically, defensive isolation is employed as described in Section 1.4 and Figure 1.20. Quarantine may be *absolute* so that the S population has its freedom of movement curtailed for a period of time up to the longest usual incubation period of the disease in question. *Modified quarantine* is a selective, partial limitation upon the movements of those S who have come into contact with an I. It is designed to meet particular situations such as the exclusion of children from school, or the exemption of immunes (e.g. by vaccination) or recovereds, R, from the provisions applied to S. For modified quarantine to be successful, personal surveillance is essential so that if infection occurs, the person is removed from circulation, as well as segregation – the separation of some part of S from the herd for control or observation to protect uninfected from infected portions of a population. Examples of segregation include the removal of susceptible children to the homes of immunes, or the establishment of a sanitary boundary (*cordon sanitaire*) between susceptibles and infectives (cf. Sections 1.2–1.4).

Isolation

In contrast to quarantine, isolation refers to action taken with the **infected** rather than the susceptible population to prevent the transmission ($I \rightarrow S$). Isolation represents separation, for the period of communicability, of infectives from others in such a way as to prevent or limit the direct or indirect transmission of the infectious agent via the transmission ($I \rightarrow S$). This represents offensive containment in the terms of Figure 1.20. The US Centers for Disease Control and Prevention specifies seven grades of isolation. The general approach is *strict isolation* which is designed to prevent the transmission of highly contagious or virulent infections that may spread by both air and contact. The patient is isolated in a private room with, ideally, negative pressure to surrounding areas, and barrier nursed. The

other categories are less restrictive versions of strict isolation, i.e. *contact isolation* and *respiratory isolation* for less highly transmissible infections in which patients with the same pathogen may share a room; *tuberculosis isolation* with a special ventilated room and closed door but generally less severe barrier nursing; and *enteric*, *secretion* and *body fluid* precautions to prevent contamination of clothing and medical staff who then enter general circulation.

To some extent, these definitions look like splitting hairs. The end result will be the same – preventing the mixing of susceptible and infected persons in order to break the chains of infection from one person to another. In quarantine, the means used to prevent mixing focus on the suceptibles; in isolation, the focus is upon the infectives. In this book, we have followed the distinction drawn by Benenson. But we accept that much of the literature uses the term *quarantine* generically to refer to the separation of components of the S and I population. This is in line with both the spirit of the definition in the *Oxford English Dictionary* and common usage:

> Quarantine is a period of isolation (originally 40 days) imposed on an infected person or animal that might otherwise spread a contagious disease, especially on one who has just arrived from overseas or has been exposed to infection.

3.2 History of Quarantine

The large-scale practice of quarantine, as we know it today, began during the fourteenth century in an effort to protect coastal cities in Italy from plague epidemics (see Sections 1.2–1.4). The earliest attempts were made by Ragusa and Venice. Then, ships arriving at these cities from infected ports were required to sit at anchor for 40 days before landing. This practice, called quarantine, was derived from the Italian words *quaranta giorni* (40 days). As described in Section 2.5, the modern international development of ideas of quarantine is founded in the International Sanitary Conferences which took place from 1851, and whose primary purpose was to develop protocols to protect the world's peoples from the cholera pandemics which swept the world in regular waves from the early 1830s. Between the late nineteenth century and the inter-war period, the International Sanitary Conventions evolved to include an increasing number of so-called 'quarantine diseases' (cholera, plague, yellow fever, smallpox and louse-borne typhus fever; see Figure 2.22). From 1907, the Office International d'Hygiène Publique (Section 2.5) was charged with overseeing the international codification of procedures for quarantine and its associated surveillance and, in the aftermath of the First World War, the Paris Office continued its work in a formal collaboration with the League of Nations Health Organisation.

International Sanitary and Health Regulations

When the newly-created World Health Organization assumed responsibility for the international quarantine regulations in 1948, quarantine practice and procedure varied considerably from one country to another and the general situation was confused (World Health Organization, 1958). The International Sanitary Conventions then in force had been drawn up at different times, each with a specific objective in view. None completely replaced its predecessors because different countries adhered to different conventions or groups of conventions. Furthermore, since the adoption of the conventions, conditions had changed; hence they did not take account of the new methods available for the control of several of the diseases they covered, nor were they framed to deal adequately with the greatly increased volume and speed of international traffic (see Section 3.4).

It fell to the First World Health Assembly (1948) to replace this multiplicity of conventions by a single code based on modern epidemiological principles, and to provide an international instrument which could be adapted to changing conditions without the delays imposed by the formalities at each modification of signature and ratification. Provision for such an instrument existed in the Constitution of the World Health Organization, which, in Article 21, states that the World Health Assembly shall have the authority to adopt regulations concerning sanitary and quarantine requirements and, in Article 22, that regulations so adopted shall come into force for all Member States after due notice has been given of their adoption by the Health Assembly, except for such Members as may notify the Director-General of rejection or reservations within the period stated in the notice.

The International Sanitary Regulations (1951)

In the event, it was not until the Fourth World Health Assembly that final agreement was reached although preliminary studies had already been undertaken, 1946–48, on the possibility of drawing up a single set of regulations to replace the sanitary conventions. The regulations were signed off as WHO Regulations No. 2, on 25 May 1951. These regulations covered and still cover all forms of international transport – ships, aircraft, trains and road vehicles. They deal with the sanitary conditions to be maintained and measures to be taken against diseases at seaports and airports open to international traffic, including measures on arrival and departure, sanitary documents and sanitary charges. The Regulations represent "the maximum measures applicable to international traffic which a State may require for the protection of its territory against the quarantinable diseases . . .". The same principle – a minimum of interference with traffic and of inconvenience to passengers – is expressed in the stipulation that sanitary measures and health formalities "shall be initiated forthwith, completed without delay and applied without discrimination".

In the 1951 Regulations, there were special provisions relating to each of the (then) quarantine diseases (cholera, plague, yellow fever, smallpox, louse-borne typhus fever and louse-borne relapsing fever). These indicate the conditions under which vaccination may be required as a condition of entry into a country (**Figure 3.2**); conditions entailing the de-insecting of passengers, their isolation or surveillance; conditions entailing the de-ratting of vessels; and the measures to be taken in the case of "suspect" or "infected" ships and aircraft.

The Regulations, as they were first adopted, followed the example of the former international sanitary conventions and included provisions relating to the Mecca Pilgrimage. More than once in the nineteenth century the Pilgrimage had resulted in the catastrophic international spread of diseases, and it was to meet such dangers that an international sanitary convention for the Pilgrimage had been drawn up at the 1892 International Sanitary Conference in Venice, to give effect to conclusions reached at previous conferences in 1866 and 1874. Even in 1951, when the International Sanitary Regulations were adopted, it was considered that the Mecca Pilgrimage still needed special international sanitary controls.

The International Health Regulations (1969 and 2005)

The International Sanitary Regulations were revised and adopted by the WHO under the new title of the International Health Regulations in 1969. The number of diseases covered by the regulations reduced from six to four (cholera, plague, yellow fever and smallpox; see Figure 2.22). Smallpox was subsequently excluded by a regulatory amendment (1981) following its global eradication. Faced with the global health challenges posed by new and resurging infectious diseases in the late twentieth and early twenty-first centuries, WHO issued a fully revised set of International Health Regulations in 2005. As noted in Section 2.7, rather than focusing on a small and prescribed set of diseases, the 2005 regulations ushered in a new global public health surveillance regime that requires member states to notify WHO of *all events which may constitute a public health emergency of international concern* (Article 6.1) – whether naturally occurring, intentionally created or unintentionally caused. The regulations came into force on Friday 15 June 2007 and are a legally binding international instrument to "prevent, protect against, control and provide a public health response to the international spread of disease in ways that are commensurate with and restricted to public health risks and which avoid unnecessary interference with international trade and traffic" (World Health Organization, 2008b, p. 1).

The manner in which quarantine procedures and the associated reporting machinery described in Sections 2.5–2.7 have worked out in practice over time is most easily understood if we follow a single country example, here as in Chapter 2, the United States, and it is to this that we now turn.

Quarantine: The United States, 1878–2010

Early American Quarantine

For much of the early history of the North American colonies, the populations were too sparse to hold many infectious diseases in endemic form. Diseases such as smallpox and yellow fever would occasionally be introduced into southern ports by ships sailing from Latin America and the Caribbean, but the epidemics would rarely be sustained. The epidemiological isolation of the Colonies in these early years was bolstered by long sea journeys in small sailing ships, shipboard epidemics usually having run their course well before the Colonies were reached. But this situation changed in the nineteenth century as the epidemiological isolation of the United States was eroded by expanding international trade, immigration and the ever-increasing size and speed of ocean-going ships (Section 3.4). By the latter decades of the nineteenth century, major ports on the eastern seaboard were within epidemiological reach of many African, European and Latin American ports with which the United States had links. These, in turn, were potential sources of cholera, plague, yellow fever and many other infectious diseases.

The systematic development of quarantine procedures in the United States begins in the last quarter of the nineteenth century with the US Marine Hospital Service (USMHS), the forerunner of the US Public Health Service, which was established in July 1798 to provide healthcare and hospitals for ailing sailors (Williams, 1951; Furman, 1973; Bordley and Harvey, 1976; Greene, 1977; Bienia, *et al.*, 1983). In 1871, as a remedial response to the decimation of the health system wrought by the Civil War, the post of Supervising Surgeon of the Marine Hospital Service was created. The first person to occupy this position was John M. Woodworth (**Figure 3.3**) who was to play a pivotal role in the subsequent development of international disease surveillance by the United States.

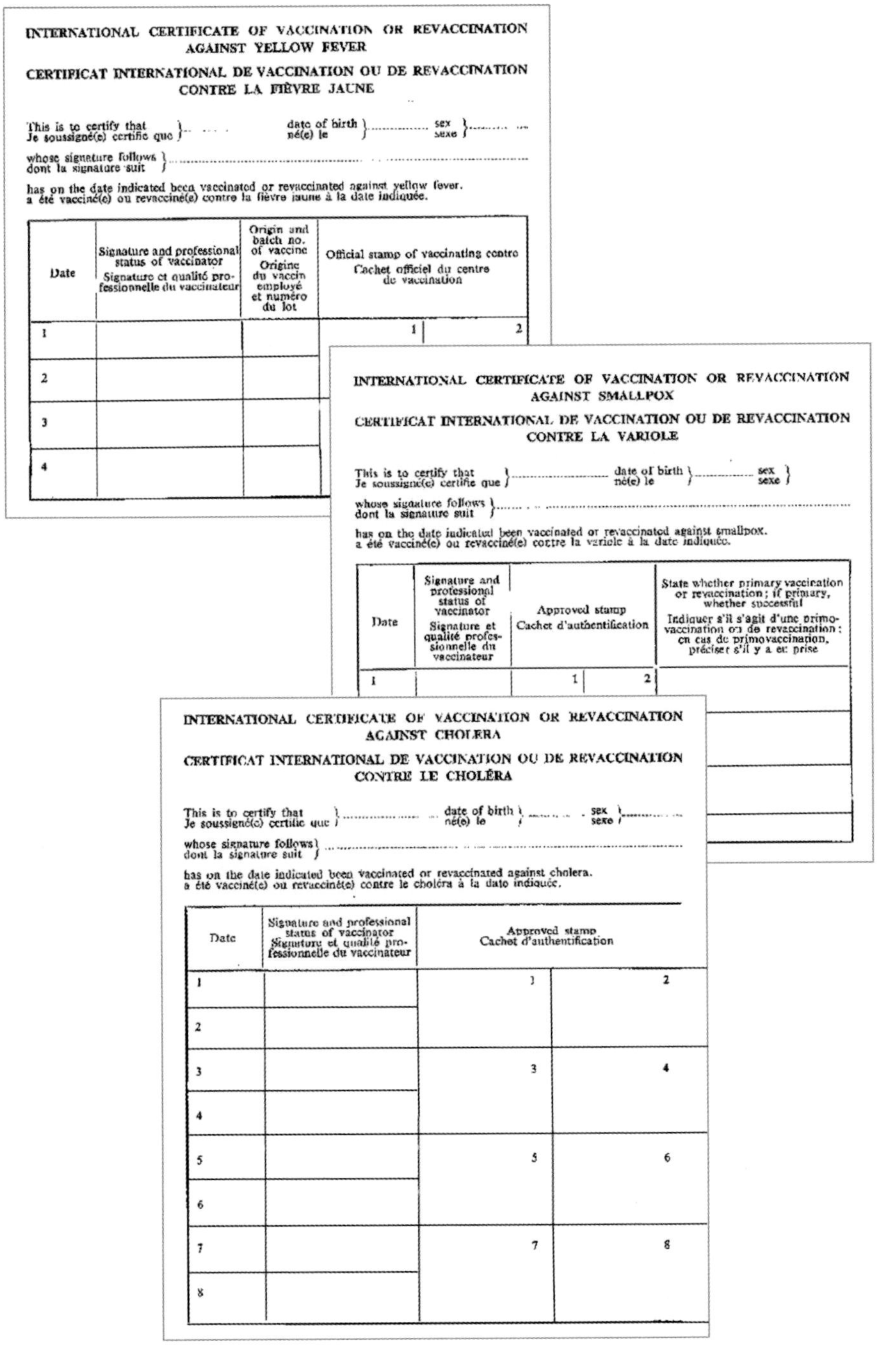

INTERNATIONAL CERTIFICATE OF VACCINATION OR REVACCINATION AGAINST YELLOW FEVER

CERTIFICAT INTERNATIONAL DE VACCINATION OU DE REVACCINATION CONTRE LA FIÈVRE JAUNE

This is to certify that / Je soussigné(e) certifie que .... date of birth / né(e) le .... sex / sexe ....

whose signature follows / dont la signature suit ....

has on the date indicated been vaccinated or revaccinated against yellow fever. / a été vacciné(e) ou revacciné(e) contre la fièvre jaune à la date indiquée.

Date	Signature and professional status of vaccinator / Signature et qualité professionnelle du vaccinateur	Origin and batch no. of vaccine / Origine du vaccin employé et numéro du lot	Official stamp of vaccinating centre / Cachet officiel du centre de vaccination
1			1 2
2			
3			
4			

INTERNATIONAL CERTIFICATE OF VACCINATION OR REVACCINATION AGAINST SMALLPOX

CERTIFICAT INTERNATIONAL DE VACCINATION OU DE REVACCINATION CONTRE LA VARIOLE

This is to certify that / Je soussigné(e) certifie que .... date of birth / né(e) le .... sex / sexe

whose signature follows / dont la signature suit ....

has on the date indicated been vaccinated or revaccinated against smallpox. / a été vacciné(e) ou revacciné(e) contre la variole à la date indiquée.

Date	Signature and professional status of vaccinator / Signature et qualité professionnelle du vaccinateur	Approved stamp / Cachet d'authentification	State whether primary vaccination or revaccination; if primary, whether successful / Indiquer s'il s'agit d'une primo-vaccination ou de revaccination; en cas de primovaccination, préciser s'il y a eu prise
1		1 2	

INTERNATIONAL CERTIFICATE OF VACCINATION OR REVACCINATION AGAINST CHOLERA

CERTIFICAT INTERNATIONAL DE VACCINATION OU DE REVACCINATION CONTRE LE CHOLÉRA

This is to certify that / Je soussigné(e) certifie que .... date of birth / né(e) le .... sex / sexe ....

whose signature follows / dont la signature suit ....

has on the date indicated been vaccinated or revaccinated against cholera. / a été vacciné(e) ou revacciné(e) contre le choléra à la date indiquée.

Date	Signature and professional status of vaccinator / Signature et qualité professionnelle du vaccinateur	Approved stamp / Cachet d'authentification	
1		1	2
2			
3		3	4
4			
5		5	6
6			
7		7	8
8			

Figure 3.2 Vaccination certificates. The International Sanitary Regulations (1951) laid out certain conditions under which the possession of a valid certificate of vaccination against yellow fever (*upper*), smallpox (*centre*) and cholera (*lower*) was a requirement for entry of an international passenger into a particular territory. Failure to produce a valid certificate could result in the placing of the passenger under a period of isolation or surveillance that reflected the incubation period of the disease.

The 1878 and 1893 Quarantine Acts

Woodworth contended that the most effective way to halt the spread of epidemic disease in the United States was to prevent it from entering the country. His first move was to revive the Quarantine Law of 1799 by ordering USMHS personnel to familiarise themselves with local quarantine regulations (**Figure 3.4**). Probably more significant, however, was his contribution to the report on the *Cholera Epidemic of 1873 in the United States* commissioned by Congress in 1874 (US Department of the Treasury, 1875). His 25-page preface, *The Introduction of Epidemic Cholera Through the Agency of the Mercantile Marine: Suggestions of Measures of Prevention*, argued that infectious diseases were permitted to break out in the United States because insufficient information was to be had of disease activity in foreign locations. To address the problem, Woodworth urged the President of the United States to instruct consular officials to inform the State Department of infectious diseases prevailing in their jurisdictions:

> A circular letter from his Excellency the President, through the Department of State, instructing consular officers to place themselves in communication with the health authorities of their respective localities; to advise promptly, by cable if necessary, of the outbreak of cholera (or other epidemic disease) at the ports or in any section in communication therewith; to inspect all vessels clearing for United States ports with reference to the original and intermediate as well

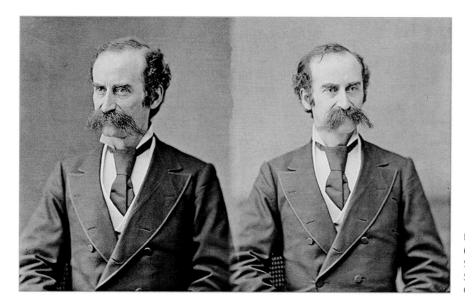

Figure 3.3 Dr John Maynard Woodworth (1837–1879). Supervising Surgeon and Supervising Surgeon General, US Marine Hospital Service, 1871–79. *Source*: Brady-Handy Photograph Collection, Library of Congress.

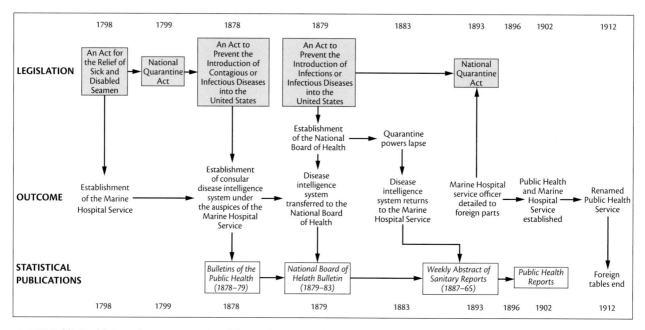

Figure 3.4 US Public Health Records, 1798–1912. Critical dates in disease surveillance in the United States. *Source*: Cliff, *et al.* (1998, Figure 2.6, p. 51).

as the final port of departure of emigrants thereon; and to report, always by cable, the sailing and destination of any such vessel carrying infected or suspected passengers or goods – this would be the first step (US Department of the Treasury, 1875, p. 13).

The resulting information, Woodworth proposed, should be collated and circulated to port health officers and other concerned parties. He concluded that:

> International sanitary action is too remote, and the steps toward it have been too vacillating in the past to admit of much hope from it in the near future. But the acquisition and diffusion of general sanitary knowledge is a matter in which each nation for itself may engage . . . Let the General Government do its share in collection and publishing the information – a work which it alone can do . . . (Woodworth, in US Department of the Treasury, 1875, p. 13).

The 1878 Quarantine Act

Woodworth's call for an international disease surveillance system materialised on 29 April 1878 with the passage of the National Quarantine Act: *An Act To Prevent The Introduction of Contagious Or Infectious Diseases Into The United States* (**Figure 3.4**). Not only did the Act grant the USMHS powers of detention over vessels originating from areas infected with epidemic disease. It also directed consular officers in foreign ports to forward weekly reports of sanitary conditions prevailing in their jurisdictions to the USMHS. This information was to be collated by the Supervising Surgeon General, and circulated in the form of a weekly abstract to USMHS officers and other interested parties; the first number was issued on 13 July 1878 under the title *Bulletins of the Public Health*.

The 1893 Quarantine Act

The National Quarantine Act of 1893 was to extend further the international powers of the USMHS. This Act provided that all ships headed from foreign ports to the United States must be issued with a bill of health signed by the US consul prior to departure. To assist in the process, officers of the USMHS could be detailed to foreign ports to serve in the office of the consul. Because of outbreaks of cholera in Europe, a number of medical officers were immediately assigned to consulates there (Furman, 1973).

The US Consular System and International Disease Surveillance

The idea of an international disease surveillance system which operated through consular officials was by no means new. Indeed, similar systems had been implemented in the city states of the Mediterranean as early as the fourteenth century (see Chapter 1). What was new, however, was the global scale of the operation mandated under the 1878 Quarantine Act. By the latter decades of the nineteenth century the US consular system had assumed a global pattern and included much of the Caribbean Basin and Latin America, northern, central and southern Europe, the St Lawrence Seaway and parts of Africa and Asia (**Figure 3.5**). Many consulates were located in the major urban centres of the most powerful

trading nations, in cities such as London, Paris and Rome. But other consulates were situated in small settlements, rarely heard of then as now (Mattox, 1989).

The 1878 Quarantine Act required all consuls in the jurisdictions plotted in Figure 3.5 to submit weekly reports of the sanitary conditions prevailing in their jurisdictions. This requirement fell within the jurisdication of a well-developed commercial intelligence system as evidenced by consular reports in the form of *Reports on the Commercial Relations of the United States* (House of Representatives, 1856–1902) and *Reports from the Consuls* (Department of State, 1880–1901). The sanitary information was usually drawn from local disease surveillance reports although other sources (including local gravediggers) were not unknown. Most of the sanitary reports reached the USMHS via the State Department in the form of consular dispatches. Examples of consular dispatches are reproduced in **Figure 3.6**. Sanitary dispatches rarely exceeded more than a few lines when favourable health conditions prevailed. But severe epidemics and poor sanitary conditions usually warranted much more information. Under these circumstances, dispatches frequently stretched to several handwritten pages and provided detailed qualitative and quantitative information pertinent to the health of the consular city. Under other conditions, dispatches simply served to refute popular rumours, to report the medical research of local luminaries, or as

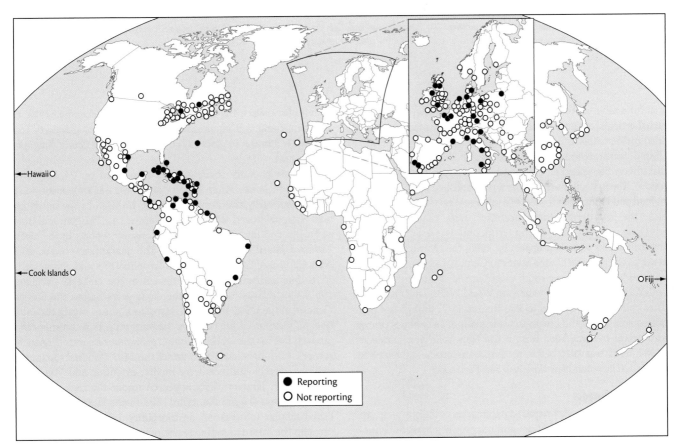

Figure 3.5 Location of US consulates and commercial agencies in 1888. The United States operated 277 consulates and 39 commercial agencies worldwide (circles), with major concentrations in Central America and the Caribbean Basin, along the St Lawrence waterway and the Canadian Great Lakes, Northern and Central Europe and in the Mediterranean Basin. Small clusters are also to be seen in the Southern cone of South America and along the coast of China. Elsewhere, in Africa and Asia, consulates and commercial agencies were restricted to the ports of a few major cities. Offices submitting mortality reports in 1888, towards the beginning of systematic surveillance, are indicated by black circles. *Source*: Cliff, *et al.* (1998, Figure 2.10, p. 66), drawn from information in US Department of State (1889).

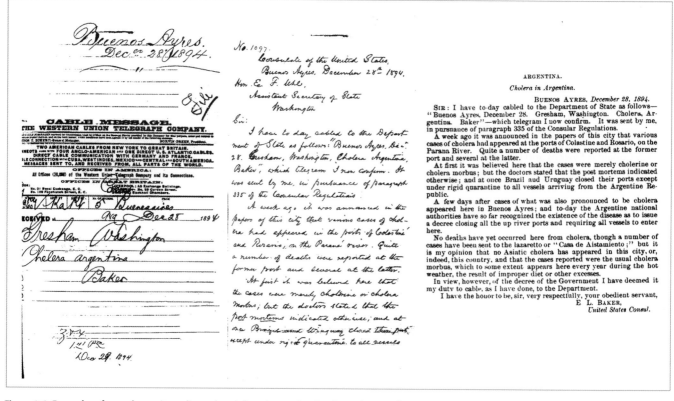

Figure 3.6 Examples of consular sanitary dispatches. *Left*, a telegram dated 28 December 1894 from Eugene Baker, Consul to Buenos Aires, Argentina, informing the State Department of the presence of cholera. *Centre*, a letter to confirm the telegram. *Right*, reproduction of the letter in the *Weekly Abstract*. *Source*: Cliff, *et al.* (1998, Plate 2.2, p. 56).

a call for action on the part of the USMHS. Newspaper clippings, journal articles, commissional reports and sundry other enclosures added further substance to the dispatches.

Rapid transmission of weekly consular dispatches depended critically on the telegraph (**Figure 3.7**, located in the colour plate section). The first submarine cable was established in 1850 between England and France, but it was 1866 (after several abortive schemes) before the first permanently successful trans-Atlantic cable was laid. Once complex cable-laying technology was established, new submarine links were laid apace. By 1890, the international cable network ran from the United States to Central and South America, and from Western Europe south to Africa and east to India, China, South Asia and Australia. By the First World War, most US consular offices could send telegrams to Washington D.C., though not without frequent delays and breaks in transmission. Telephone communication was to come later. Boston and New York were connected in 1884, but it was 1915 before the first transcontinental telephone line opened between New York and San Francisco.

The *Weekly Abstract*

The 1878 Quarantine Act required publication of the consular sanitary reports as a weekly abstract and this was begun as *Bulletins of the Public Health* on 13th July of that year (**Figure 3.8, left**). Issue No. 1 consisted of just 23 lines of text and detailed the sanitary conditions prevailing in Cuban ports, the occurrence of yellow fever in Florida and cholera on British troop ships in the Mediterranean. However, the *Bulletins* soon expanded to include reports of disease

activity in major cities around the world; by December 1878, the *Bulletins* contained summaries of morbidity and mortality from infectious diseases in places as far-flung as Brazil, China, Singapore and Ireland.

Publication of the *Bulletins* was suspended on 24 May 1879, after just 46 issues, when powers under the 1878 Quarantine Act were temporarily transferred from the USMHS to the newly created National Board of Health (see Figure 3.4). The National Board of Health continued to publish the consular reports in the weekly *National Board of Health Bulletin*. The quarantine powers of the National Board of Health were to lapse in 1883 and charge of the 1878 Quarantine Law again returned to the USMHS (Williams, 1951). But, it was to be a further four years before the Surgeon General of the USMHS, John B. Hamilton, was to regain the initiative; publication of the consular sanitary reports recommenced in January 1887 as the *Weekly Abstract of Sanitary Reports* (Figure 3.8, centre). With new legislation under the 1893 National Quarantine Act, the *Weekly Abstracts* were further extended and Volume XI, published in January 1896, appeared under the new title *Public Health Reports* (Figure 3.8, right). The *Public Health Reports* published tabular information on morbidity and mortality gathered through the international network of consuls and USMHS officers until 1912, although entries for cholera, yellow fever, plague and smallpox (the 'quarantine' diseases) continued in later years.

Although the *Weekly Abstract* and its successor publication, the *Public Health Reports*, was a vehicle for the dissemination of international sanitary information, it also assumed the role of

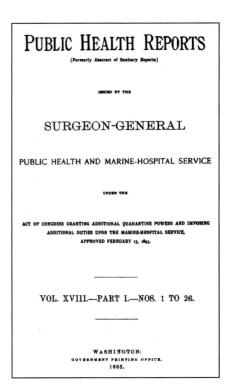

Figure 3.8 **Front covers of the *Weekly Abstract* under its various aliases.** (*Left*) Volume I appeared in 1878 as the *Bulletins of the Public Health*. (*Centre*) After a gap of nine years, Volume II emerged in 1887 as the *Weekly Abstract of Sanitary Reports*. (*Right*) The *Weekly Abstract* was renamed *Public Health Reports* in 1896. *Source*: Cliff, *et al.* (1998, Plate 2.3, p. 58).

the domestic disease surveillance report of the United States. The early editions restricted domestic information to brief statements, largely for port cities and quarantine stations. But, in June 1888, the *Weekly Abstract* began to tabulate disease reports for major US cities. This initiative continues today in the form of the US Centers for Disease Control and Prevention's *Morbidity and Mortality Weekly Report*.

Ellis Island

Once federal legislation had been passed in the shape of the 1878 Quarantine Act, which was reinterpreted in the early 1890s to provide the federal government more authority in imposing quarantine requirements following a series of cholera outbreaks from passenger ships arriving from Europe, the practical face of US quarantine emerged in the form of one of the world's great quarantine stations, Ellis Island (**Figure 3.9**). Located off New York City, Ellis Island operated for 62 years from 1892 to 1954. Over this period, more than 12 million immigrants – as many as 5,000 a day, with a record of nearly 13,000 – underwent immigration processing at Ellis Island. This total represents more than 66 percent of immigrants who came to America, and it is estimated that today more than 100 million Americans can trace their roots to an ancestor who came through Ellis Island. As described in Coan (1997, p. xiii), the Federal Immigration and Naturalization Service (INS), which operated the station, enforced a number of Acts to exclude mentally disabled persons, paupers and those who might become public charges. The INS also excluded those suffering from "a loathsome or contagious disease", or convicted of various crimes. Over the life of the station, 82,199 potential immigrants were rejected as mental or physical defectives. Screening for disease was carried out by Ellis Island doctors in a set of 15 medical buildings until 1932 when this

task was transferred to American consulates in originating countries. Thereafter, the role of Ellis Island declined until final closure in 1954.

Twentieth-century Quarantine Organization

In 1893, Congress passed legislation that further clarified the federal role in quarantine activities. As local authorities came to realise the benefits of federal involvement, local quarantine stations were gradually turned over to the US government. Additional federal facilities were built and the number of staff was increased to provide better coverage. The quarantine system was fully nationalised by 1921 within the Treasury Department when administration of the last quarantine station was transferred to the US government. Quarantine and the Public Health Service (PHS), its parent organisation, became part of the Federal Security Agency in 1939. The 1944 Public Health Service Act clearly established the federal government's quarantine authority for the first time. The Act gave the PHS responsibility for preventing the introduction, transmission, and spread of communicable diseases from foreign countries into the United States (**Figure 3.10**). Another transfer occurred in 1953 when quarantine and the PHS joined the Department of Health, Education, and Welfare (HEW). Quarantine was then transferred to the agency now known as the Centers for Disease Control and Prevention (CDC) in 1967. CDC remained part of HEW until 1980 when the department was reorganised into the Department of Health and Human Services.

When CDC assumed responsibility for quarantine, it was a large organisation with 55 quarantine stations and more than 500 staff members. Quarantine stations were located at every port, international airport and major border crossing. After evaluating the quarantine programme and its role in preventing disease transmission,

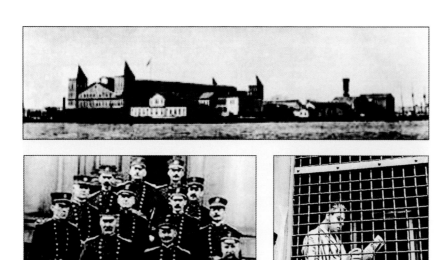

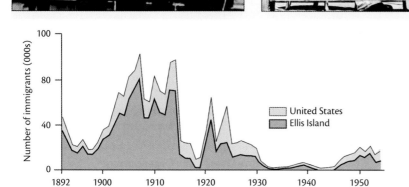

Figure 3.9 **Ellis Island quarantine station.** (*Upper*) Ellis Island Quarantine Station, New York City. The original Georgia-pine main building at Ellis Island, opened 1 January 1892. It was destroyed by fire in 1897 and then rebuilt. (*Centre left*) US Quarantine inspectors in Public Health Service uniforms c. 1912. (*Centre right*) Quarantine detention at the immigration station, Ellis Island c. 1930. Those suspected of having a communicable disease were segregated at once and, after confirmation of the diagnosis, admitted to the communicable disease hospital for care and treatment. (*Lower*) Number of immigrants passing through the Ellis Island station annually and the total number of arrivals in the USA, 1892–1954. *Sources*: (*Upper*) US National Park Service, Statue of Liberty National Monument website, reproduced in Cliff, *et al.* (2000, Plate 5.6, p. 200). (*Centre left*) Centers for Disease Control and Prevention website (http://www.cdc.gov/quarantine/HistoryQuarantine.html). (*Centre right*) National Library of Medicine, US Department of Health and Human Services, images of the history of the Public Health Service, p. 21 (http://www.nlm.nih.gov/exhibition/phs_history/images.dir/21.gif). (*Lower*) Cliff, *et al.* (2000, Figure 5.10, p. 199).

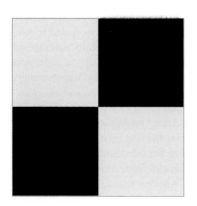

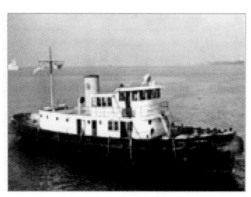

Figure 3.10 **US quarantine inspection of ships, mid-twentieth century.** (*Left*) The internationally-recognised yellow jack quarantine flag (the yellow squares of the flag are here shown in grey) flown by ships if they suspected they had quarantinable infection on board. (*Right*) US Public Health Service cutter used to transport quarantine inspectors to board ships flying the yellow quarantine flag. The flag was flown until quarantine and customs personnel inspected and cleared the ship to dock at the port. *Source*: Centers for Disease Control and Prevention website (http://www.cdc.gov/quarantine/HistoryQuarantine.html).

CDC trimmed the programme in the 1970s and changed its focus from routine inspection to programme management and intervention. The new focus included an enhanced surveillance system to monitor the onset of epidemics abroad and a modernised inspection process to meet the changing needs of international traffic (cf. Sections 2.6–2.8 and 3.4). The cutbacks are unsurprising given the long twentieth-century decline in the communicable diseases which made quarantine and isolation necessary; see Smallman-Raynor and Cliff (2012) for examples of this decline in the UK.

By 1995, all US ports of entry were covered by only seven quarantine stations. But the emergence of new and the re-emergence of old infections in the last quarter of the twentieth century posed new disease threats which led to an expansion of the US quarantine station network. A station was added in 1996 in Atlanta, Georgia, just before the city hosted the 1996 Summer Olympic Games. Following the severe acute respiratory syndrome (SARS) epidemic of 2003, CDC reorganised the quarantine station system, expanding to 18 stations with more than 90 field employees. The reorganisation led to the creation within CDC of a Division of Global Migration and Quarantine as part of CDC's National Center for Emerging and Zoonotic Infectious Diseases in Atlanta (**Figure 3.11**). The location of quarantine stations, currently 20, is mapped in **Figure 3.12** and covers all the ports (sea and air) of entry and land-border crossings where international travellers arrive in the US.

Under its delegated authority, the Division of Global Migration and Quarantine is empowered to detain, medically examine, or conditionally release individuals and wildlife suspected of carrying a communicable disease. The current list of quarantinable diseases is contained in an Executive Order of the President and includes both old and newly-emerging infections: cholera; diphtheria; infectious tuberculosis; plague; smallpox; yellow fever; viral haemorrhagic fevers such as Marburg, Ebola, and Crimean–Congo, and SARS. Influenza was added to the list in 2005 because of its pandemic potential. As noted, and reflecting the impact of mass vaccination upon the spectrum of vaccine-controllable diseases, many other illnesses of public health significance, such as measles, mumps, rubella, and chickenpox, are not contained in the list of quarantinable illnesses, although they continue to pose a health risk to the public.

Quarantine Islands

While Ellis Island is the most famous quarantine station of all, island settings have been favoured across the globe and throughout history for quarantine stations against a spectrum of diseases including cholera, leprosy, smallpox, yellow fever and measles (**Figure 3.13**).

Measles Invasions of Fiji (1879–1920)

One of the clearest examples of the yoking of changes in transport technology to the introduction of communicable diseases and the associated island quarantine response is provided by the history of the use of indentured labour on the Fiji sugar plantations, 1879–1920. The history of the first importation of measles into Fiji in January 1875 and the devastating impact on the native population over the ensuing six months is one of the classic cases of a 'virgin soil' outbreak and has been widely studied (McArthur, 1967; Cliff and Haggett, 1985). In the anxious years that followed, the islands provided what was essentially a test case in the use of quarantine to prevent further invasions of the measles virus.

Between 1879 and 1920, Indian immigrant ships made 87 voyages to Fiji carrying nearly 61,000 indentured emigrants. The main routes followed are mapped in **Figure 3.14A**. This illustrates an important distinction between voyages by sailing ships (used between 1879 and 1904) and steamships (used between 1884 and 1916). To take advantage of prevailing winds, sailing ships followed the route south of Australia and took about 70 days for the voyage. Steamships used the more direct Torres Strait north of Australia and halved the sailing ship times; they were also able to carry a larger number of immigrants. The health and welfare of the immigrants on board was the responsibility of the Surgeon-Superintendent who accompanied each ship and whose report was incorporated into the *Annual Reports on Indian Immigration* published regularly as Official Papers of Fiji's Legislative Council. These papers show how the transition from sail to steam dramatically altered the ways in which infectious diseases were transmitted between India and Fiji.

Since measles was an endemic disease in India, it is not surprising that cases were recorded on departure, although there were checks in the camps both at Calcutta and Madras (the two exit ports) before embarkation: the evidence in the Fijian annual reports shows a 1:3 probability of measles being detected on board on departure from India, and this proportion of infected voyages remained constant over the period. These are shown in Figure 3.14B in which each voyage is plotted in terms of the time taken and the passenger size of each vessel. For the smaller and slower sailing ships, around one-third of the vessels carrying labourers

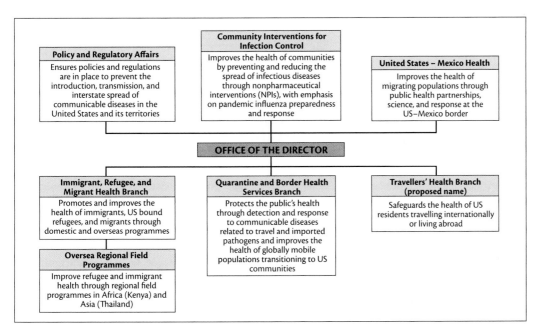

Figure 3.11 Centers for Disease Control and Prevention: Division of Global Migration and Quarantine. The organisational structure gives oversight over quarantinable diseases and travel and refugee entry into the US (http://www.cdc.gov/ncezid/pdf/ncezid-org-chart-july-2010.pdf; http://www.cdc.gov/ncezid/dgmq/index.html).

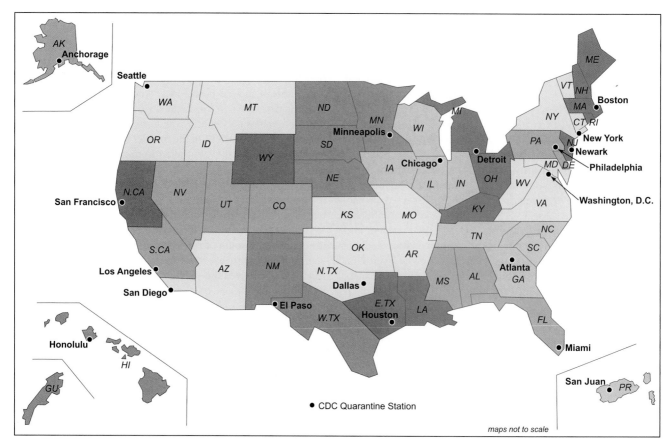

Figure 3.12 US quarantine stations. Location map of the 20 currently operating US quarantine stations with their geographical jurisdictions shaded. *Source*: CDC website (http://www.cdc.gov/quarantine/QuarantineStationContactListFull.html; http://www.cdc.gov/quarantine/HistoryQuarantine.html).

left India with infectives on board but the measles virus did not survive the journey. By the end of the voyage those infected had either recovered or died and the long chain of measles generations needed to maintain infection (up to six on slower voyages) was broken. But for the faster and larger steamships, Figure 3.14B shows the situation was different. Ships on one in three voyages still carried infectives on departure and, in 11 instances, the virus continued to thrive on arrival in Fiji. The larger susceptible population and shorter travel times (as few as two generations on the fastest voyages) ensured the virus persisted to pose a potential threat at the receiving end.

Intensive quarantine had been instituted on the smaller islands off Suva following the experience of the disastrous 1875 measles epidemic in Fiji which resulted in the loss of some 40,000 lives. As a result, during the period of indentured labour, quarantining of Indian passengers on immigrant boats was routine up to 1916. The first quarantine station was established on Yamuca Levu island between Ovalau and Moturiki islands and was used by the first immigrants from the *Leonidas* (**Figure 3.15**). With the shift of the Fijian capital to Suva, the quarantine station was moved to the island of Nukulau on the reef about 10 km east of Suva harbour. Immigrants were usually detained for a 14-day period before being delivered to the plantation areas.

Gillion (1962, p. 66) notes:

> All the ships, except the first, went to the port of Suva, where the Indians were transferred to barges and towed by steam launch or tug to the islet of Nukulau, which served as reception centre and quarantine station. There they were inspected by the Agent-General of Immigration and medically examined . . .

The ability to contain spread of disease by quarantine diminished rapidly during the steamship era. Nevertheless, quarantine was maintained by the first two chief medical officers for the next 30 years and then progressively abandoned in the face of changing transport technology. The threat of speeding the introduction of measles into Fiji by using the faster and larger steamships was considered by the medical officers on the ships but, by the early twentieth century, they did not rate the risk as critical:

> So far as can be judged as yet the introduction of immigrants by steamers has not had a prejudicial effect on their health, though it increases the chance of introducing diseases of a severe type into the colony and renders more likely the necessity of imposing quarantine (Fiji Legislative Council, 1903, p. 2).

The changing views of the value of quarantine were reflected by Fiji's chief medical officer, A. Montague, in 1921. While noting the catastrophic epidemic of 1875, he observed that:

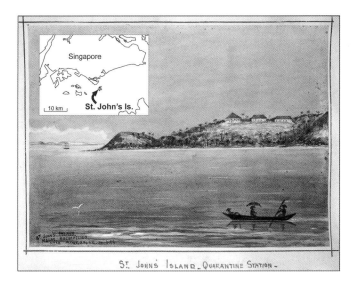

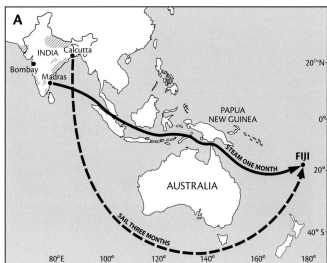

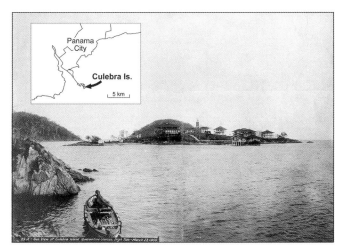

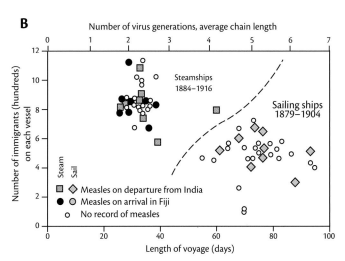

Figure 3.13 Island quarantine. (*Upper*) St John's Island, Malaysia, near Singapore. Watercolour by J. Taylor, 1879. In 1874, St John's Island became a quarantine station for cholera-stricken Chinese immigrants, and it became the world's biggest quarantine station in the 1930s, screening both Asian immigrants and Malay pilgrims from Mecca returning to Singapore. From 1901, victims of beri-beri, smallpox and leprosy were also brought here. Like Ellis Island, its quarantine function was abandoned in the 1950s when mass immigration into Singapore ceased. Gilbert Brooke (Figure 2.25) had oversight of St John's Island when he was Chief Health Officer for Singapore. (*Lower*) Culebra Island quarantine station, Panama, 1909. From the early years of the twentieth century, Culebra became the quarantine station to keep communicable diseases, especially malaria and yellow fever, from getting into the local population of the Panama isthmus – especially likely given its location on the Panama Canal and the fact that Culebra served the US military in various capacities, 1903–75. *Source*: Wellcome Library, London.

Figure 3.14 Measles transfer from India to Fiji. (A) Routes from India to Fiji via sailing ships and steamships. (B) Vessels carrying indentured immigrants between India and Fiji, 1879–1916, categorised by length of voyage in days and in measles virus generations (14-day periods), type of vessel and measles status. *Source*: Cliff, Smallman-Raynor, Haggett, *et al.* (2009, Figure 6.7, p. 312).

As a result, careful quarantine was unfortunately maintained against the disease [measles] and it was kept out until 1903 . . . since then no special measures have been taken and several localised epidemics have occurred . . . but the death rate has been very low (Montague, 1922, p. 4).

He concluded from the impact of the 1903 epidemic, after 28 essentially virus-free years, that it would be unwise to attempt to exclude measles any longer, since this would produce an adult, non-immune, population.

3.3 Isolation

As described in Section 3.1, isolation as a means of communicable disease control is concerned with the separation, for the period of communicability, of infectives from others so as to prevent or limit the direct or indirect transmission of the infectious agent to susceptibles. In this section, we begin by discussing the general theory of isolation for this purpose, before examining case studies to illustrate the practice.

Isolation: Theory

Isolation in the strict medical sense was the front line response used since Old Testament times to prevent the spread of infection, given (then) no or limited knowledge of the aetiology of different

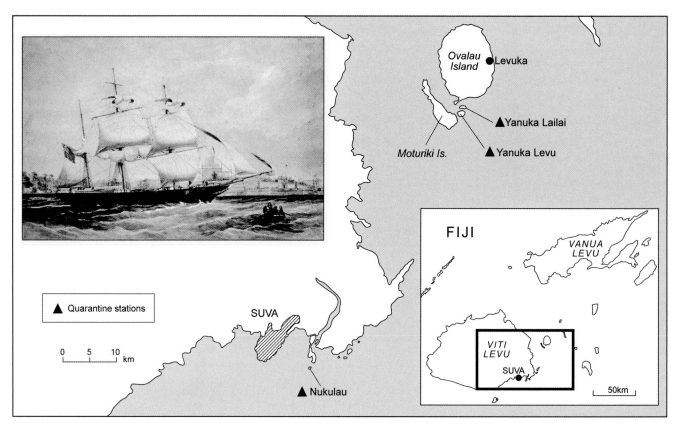

Figure 3.15 Quarantine in Fiji, 1879–1916. Locations of the quarantine stations in Fiji during the period of indentured labour. The inset shows the *Leonidas* from a watercolour probably by Frederick Garling, c. 1870. The *Leonidas* was a labour transport ship (schooner) that played an important role in the history of Fiji. Captained by McLachlan, the ship departed from Calcutta on 3 March 1879 and arrived at Levuka, Fiji, on 14 May. The indentured labourers who disembarked were the first of over 61,000 to arrive from the Indian subcontinent over the next 37 years, forming the nucleus of the Fiji Indian community that now comprises 40 percent of Fiji's population. A total of 498 passengers had embarked on the ship in Calcutta. While only three days out to sea there was an outbreak of cholera and smallpox on board. Despite efforts by the Surgeon Superintendent to isolate the infected passengers, 17 died before the ship arrived in Levuka, after a journey of 72 days. Since there was no quarantine facility in Levuka, it was decided to anchor the ship some distance from Levuka on the leeward side. To handle the crisis, Fiji's first (and temporary) quarantine station was established at Yanuca Lailai. Armed guards were placed in the narrow passage between Levuka and Yanuca Lailai, to prevent contact with the new arrivals. Fifteen more of the new arrivals died on the island from dysentery, diarrhoea and typhoid leaving only 463 survivors to be released into the general population on 9 August 1879. *Source*: *Leonidas*, State Library of New South Wales, image a353007.

communicable diseases and appropriate medication to control infection. It was believed, first with leprosy and second with plague, that it might be possible to avoid certain diseases by ensuring that no contact occurred between diseased and healthy persons. The practice of designating huts or villages in which severe infectious diseases such as plague or smallpox were present, as an indication that they were to be avoided, appears to have arisen independently among several different peoples in Africa, Asia and Europe (**Figure 3.16**). The isolation areas ranged in geographical size from camps down to individual houses. All had the same general idea of isolating patients externally from susceptibles living outside the isolation unit and internally within the unit from each other. It was difficult to achieve the efficient isolation of cases where diseases were endemic, but relatively easy when they were present on ships that approached disease-free ports. Thus the isolation of ships and their contents developed earlier and more successfully (cf. Venice in Section 1.2) than did effective isolation of infected patients on land.

The scientific underpinning of the concept of isolation had to await the enunciation of the germ theory of infectious diseases by Pasteur and Koch in the later nineteenth century but, long before this, a belief had developed that such diseases were spread by contagion. The best known early European exponent of this view, for smallpox and measles, was Girolamo Fracastoro of Verona (1478–1553). In a classic book, Fracastoro attributed these diseases to specific seeds, or *seminaria*, which were spread by direct contact from person to person by intermediate objects (fomites), or perhaps at a distance through the air (Fracastoro, 1546).

Historically, many infectious diseases were contained by isolation including, in addition to leprosy and plague, smallpox, tuberculosis, typhus, and typhoid (enteric fever) as well as general fevers like diphtheria and scarlet fever. In England and Wales, the Local Government Board (1882, 1912) discussed the utility of isolation in the control of infectious diseases and concluded (1912, pp. 59–60):

> Every populous district should be provided with hospital accommodation for the reception of cases of infectious disease, at least for such as are without proper lodging and accommodation or which occur under circumstances involving special danger to the public health. The proportion of cases which it may be desirable to isolate in hospital will vary to some extent with local circumstances. . . .

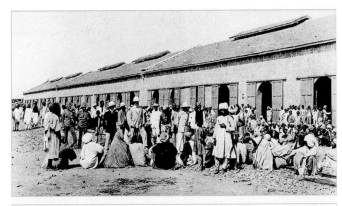

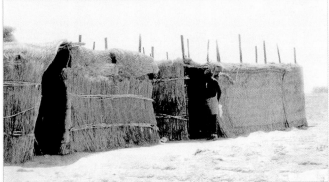

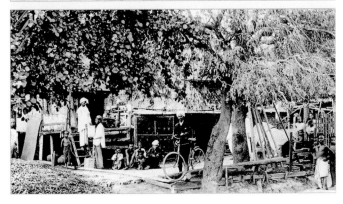

Figure 3.16 Disease control by isolation. (*Upper*) Isolation and quarantine area during a plague outbreak, Karachi, Pakistan, 1897. (*Middle*) Cerebrospinal meningitis camp outside a village near Zaris, Northern Nigeria, c. 1960. The graves of the dead comprise the drumlin-like ground in front of the camp. (*Lower*) Infected house in isolation/quarantine, India, 1906. Note the separate isolation units in the buildings in the upper and centre photographs. *Source*: Wellcome Library, London.

The diseases most commonly received into isolation hospitals are scarlet fever, diphtheria and enteric fever. It is undesirable that isolation hospitals should be reserved solely for scarlet fever, to the exclusion of diphtheria and enteric fever which are more formidable diseases. When not in use for the acute infectious diseases isolation hospitals may be used for the treatment of cases of pulmonary phthisis [tuberculosis].

As for the design of isolation hospitals, internal and external separation of patients was, if affordable, the order of the day (**Figure 3.17**).

Today, isolation is rarely recommended, but it does occur where the susceptibility of an immunosuppressed individual makes them high risk for infection – for example, in paediatrics – and with some

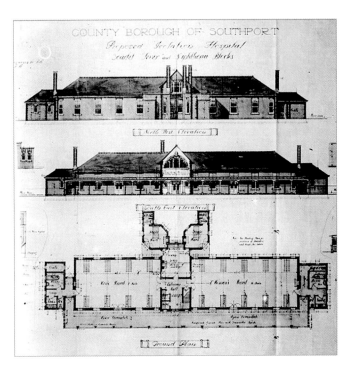

Figure 3.17 Southport's New Hall Isolation Hospital, 1927. Plan and elevation drawings for the scarlet fever and diphtheria isolation wings of the new hospital. The male ward is to the left of the central entrance and the female ward to the right. Note the principle of internal separation of patients achieved by the use of individual rooms and cubicles. There was an additional wing for the treatment of tuberculosis sufferers. *Source*: Wellcome Library, London.

extremely infectious diseases for which there is no cure – for example, haemorrhagic fevers like Ebola (**Figure 3.18**).

Isolation: Practice

Leprosy

The history of leprosy is well described by Carmichael (1993, 1997). Its origins are unknown, but lepers have been cast out into isolation from biblical times. In the Book of Leviticus, a disease called *zara'ath* was identified by the religious authorities. Those who suffered from it were cast 'outside the camp' and considered unclean. They were not exiled altogether from the community as were criminals but rather made to live apart as if the living dead. They were regarded as morally as well as physically tainted although not individually responsible for their disease. The opprobrium attached to leprosy affected attitudes in Western Europe for the next 2,000 years. During the high point of the Middle Ages (AD 1100–1300), lepers were identified by priests and ritually separated from the general community. Last rites might be said, sometimes as the lepers stood symbolically in an open grave. Once identified, the leper's ability to leave his or her city or village was severely limited. For example, Italian cities posted guards at the gates to identify lepers and to deny them entrance except under carefully controlled circumstances. Fears of contagion by lepers were much exaggerated as the disease is not particularly infectious. Local laws insisted that lepers had to be identifiable at a distance, leading to the creation of legendary symbols of the leper: a clapper or bell to warn those who might pass by too closely (**Figure 3.1**). Another symbol was the

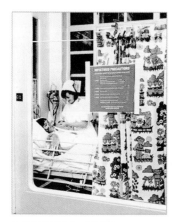
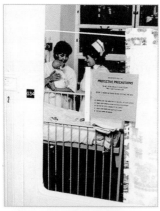
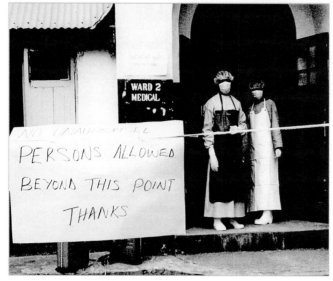

Figure 3.18 Spatial isolation at the patient level. (*Upper*) Isolation nursing to ensure infection control in paediatrics. (*Lower*) Warning notice outside Gulu hospital, Uganda, during the August 2000 outbreak of Ebola haemorrhagic fever. *Sources:* (*Upper*) Wellcome Library, London; (*lower*) World Health Organization (2000b, p. 3).

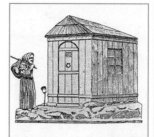
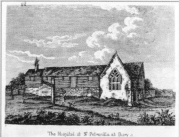
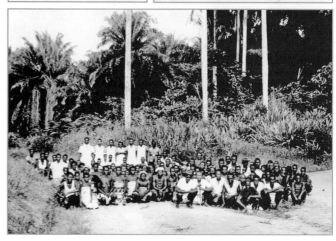

Figure 3.19 Isolation of lepers. (*Upper left*) A medieval leper's retreat in cast iron, fifteenth century. (*Upper right*) The medieval leprosarium at Bury St Edmunds, Suffolk, England. (*Lower*) Leprosy patients awaiting treatment cards, Bumba, Congo, 1955; photograph probably by Stanley Browne. *Source:* Wellcome Library, London.

long pole used to retrieve their alms cup or to point to items being purchased.

Lepers were also stigmatised outside Europe. In East Asia and in the Indian subcontinent, some legal rites were denied. For example, marriage to a leper or raising offspring with a leper was prohibited. Both western and eastern art depicted lepers as repulsive and sore covered. An exception to stigmatisation was Islamic society in which lepers were not exiled. Leprosaria, or isolation hospitals, to house lepers (usually with limited medical facilities) were constructed at church or communal expense. Outside the leprosaria, lepers had to depend upon begging or alms. **Figure 3.19** shows some of the isolation facilities provided.

Plague

Isolation hospitals, or lazarettos, for plague victims were widespread across Europe during the plague centuries. The examples from Venice, Genoa and Rome (Figures 1.12 and 1.13) illustrate the point, while John Howard's 1791 book (**Figure 3.20**) contains plans, prospects and commentary on the principal large hospitals. The operation of plague houses at the local scale has attracted a specialised literature (e.g. Henderson, 1994, on Florence).

Plague in Eyam, 1665–66

In the British Isles, the most famous geographical example of the use of isolation against plague is provided by Eyam, Derbyshire, in 1665–66. The story of the way in which the village decided to isolate itself from contact with the surrounding world in an attempt to prevent the spread of bubonic plague from the parish to the north of England, which was largely plague-free at the time, has been told and retold (Wood, 1865). It continues to fascinate and to attract the attention of demographers (Race, 1995), medical scientists (Massad, *et al.*, 2004) and mathematical modellers (Raggett, 1982a, b; Brauer, *et al.*, 2008, pp. 28–32) alike.

Sadly, Eyam's self-imposed isolation enhanced its own plague experience. At the time, Eyam parish consisted of three townships (Foolow, Woodlands and the larger village of Eyam). The parish population in 1664 has been estimated at c. 1,200–1,300 (Clifford and Clifford, 1993, p. v), and Eyam village at c. 350 persons. Eyam suffered by far the most serious outbreak of plague anywhere in the provinces during this plague visitation to the British Isles. By the time the plague expired in Eyam in November 1666, the village population had been reduced from c. 350 to c. 83, a decline of almost 75 percent (**Figure 3.21**).

Race (1995, p. 59) has assessed the severity of the outbreak on Eyam by calculating crisis mortality ratios (CMR). The CMR can be defined in a variety of ways; see, for example, Wrigley and Schofield (1981, pp. 646–49). But all consist of establishing the 'normal' or expected level of mortality in ordinary years, so that the ratio of actual:normal mortality is unity when nothing exceptional

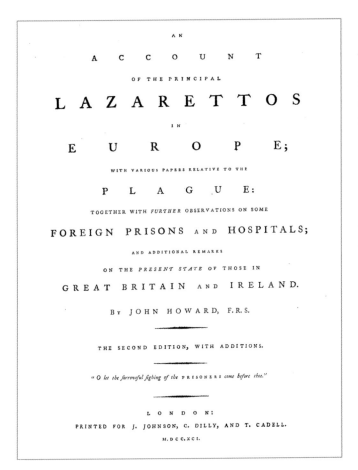

Figure 3.20 *The Lazarettos of Europe.* Title page of prison reformer John Howard's book on the condition and use of the principal plague lazarettos of Europe.

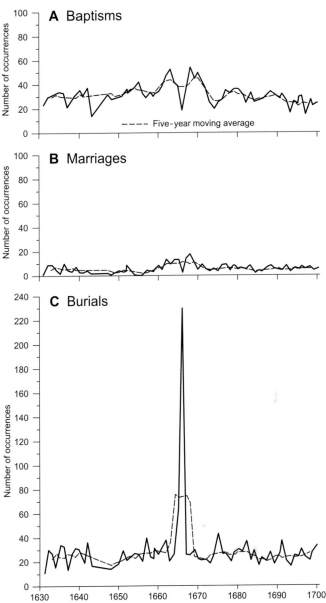

Figure 3.21 **Population of Eyam, Derbyshire, England, 1631–1700.** Annual baptisms (A), marriages (B) and burials (C), and associated five-year moving averages. The impact of the plague 1665–66 in reducing marriages (and therefore baptisms) is evident. Mortality rocketed. *Source*: based on Race (1995, Figures 1 and 2, p. 60).

is happening to mortality; values above one indicate higher than expected mortality and the converse. Race took 'normal' mortality as the average annual number of burials in the parish over the previous decade. The CMR in Eyam for the 12 highest epidemic months, 1665–66, was 10.2 compared with, for example, 5.9 for 47 London parishes in the Great Plague of the same period, and a value of 3.0 often taken by demographers to denote an exceptional crisis (Slack, 1985, p. 346, note 25).

It is generally accepted that the epidemic began in the bubonic form when the village tailor's assistant, George Vic[c]ars, who was lodging with the tailor, opened for drying in front of the cottage fire damp cloth which had arrived in a box from London at the beginning of September 1665. It probably also contained plague-carrying fleas which attacked Viccars as he unpacked the cloth. He rapidly sickened and died on 6 September 1665. After seeing that the epidemic was limited to the parish, the rector, William Mompesson, and a previous incumbent, Thomas Stanley, encouraged the villagers to agree to the unprecedented move of establishing a *cordon sanitaire* around the village to prevent catastrophic spread of the disease from Eyam to other localities. In doing so they made the apparent sacrifice of resigning themselves to death to save others. While the actual motives and reasoning of the inhabitants remain unclear, it now seems, with the benefit of modern medical science, that their actions contributed to an epidemic of almost unrivalled

severity for the village of Eyam (**Figure 3.22**). Massad, *et al.* (2004) have argued that, in the first 275 days of the outbreak, transmission was predominantly from infected fleas to susceptible humans. But from then on, mortality increased so sharply as to suggest a change in the transmission pattern caused by spatial confinement which facilitated the spread of the infection by direct transmission among humans rather than via the intermediate vector of rat fleas. This is also consistent with a switch from bubonic to pulmonary plague, a deadlier form of the disease.

Smallpox

One of the most momentous events in public health in the twentieth century was the global eradication of smallpox, declared in

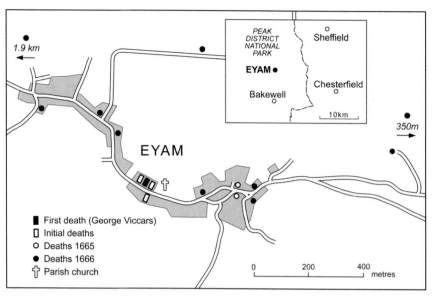

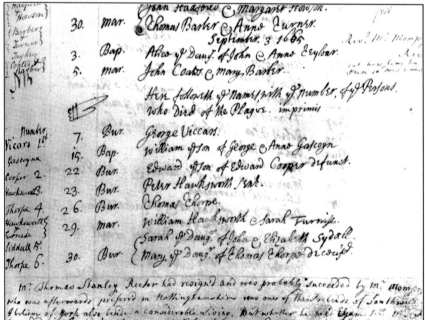

Figure 3.22 Geographical spread of plague in Eyam, 1665–66. The Eyam plague outbreak affected 76 out of 84 households in the village. On the map, the approximate settled area of the village is shown in grey with the principal roads marked. The plate shows the first entries in the Eyam plague register. The first death was of George Viccars on 6 September 1665 and yielded an early cluster of deaths in September in spatially contiguous households (square symbols). For those households whose geographical location is known, white and black dots are used to code the year of subsequent deaths. In 1665, the main focus of the epidemic was centred around the initial core of infection. When the epidemic resurged in the late spring of 1666, spread had reached the perimeter of the village and outlying cottages. Sources: drawn from parish data in Clifford and Clifford (1993, pp. 87–98) and publications of the Eyam Village Society, Eyam Museum.

1979 (Fenner, *et al.*, 1988). The last case in Britain occurred in 1978. All investigations illustrated that the practice of vaccination and revaccination, properly conducted, was a brilliant success, and Jenner's prediction in the early nineteenth century that smallpox could be eradicated by vaccination was correct (Section 4.2). However, before global eradication was achieved, practices additional to mass vaccination, which in an elementary form had antedated the concepts of variolation and vaccination, were invoked – namely, isolation and containment of smallpox patients and their contacts. So it was in 1881 when yet another smallpox epidemic badly affected London, the Metropolitan Asylums Board placed specially appointed hospital ships, moored at Long Reach in the Thames Estuary, for the treatment and care of smallpox patients (**Figure 3.23**). The smallpox hospital ships, in turn, were an alleged

source for the dissemination of the disease on both sides of the Thames in the epidemic of 1901–2, after which the use of the hulks was abandoned. On land, in the epidemic of 1881, the borough of St Pancras erected a temporary smallpox isolation hospital housed in a tented camp at Finchley which supplemented the permanent smallpox isolation hospital (**Figure 3.24**).

As described in Fenner, *et al.* (1988, pp. 274–6), the idea of isolation to control the spread of smallpox received a considerable stimulus with the popularisation of variolation, since it was soon recognised that one of the risks of this practice was the spread of smallpox to non-inoculated contacts. So it was, by the end of the eighteenth century, that some writers had already conceived the idea of controlling smallpox by a combination of variolation on a wide scale and the isolation of smallpox. By the middle of the nineteenth

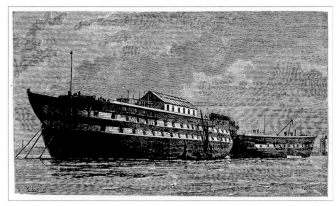

Figure 3.23 Smallpox hospital ships of the Metropolitan Asylums Board, London, 1881. Three vessels moored at Long Reach near Dartford, Thames Estuary, were used as hospitals for London's smallpox patients in the period 1881–1902. The wood engraving from the *London Illustrated News* (volume 79, 1881, p. 72) shows, from the left, *Atlas* (male patients) and *Endymion* (administration, stores and staff quarters). The hulk, *Castalia* (female patients), was moored further along the shore. *Source*: Wellcome Library, London.

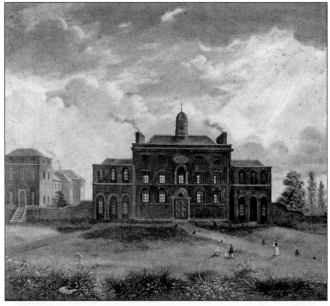

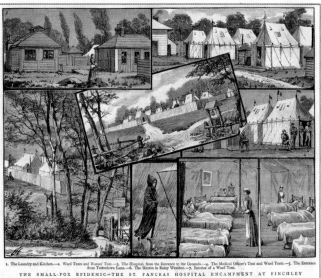

century, this approach had taken hold. An article by Sir James Simpson, famous for his introduction of chloroform for anaesthesia, aroused considerable interest and discussion (Simpson, 1868). In it he developed a proposal for eradicating smallpox and other infectious diseases, such as scarlet fever, measles and whooping-cough, by the isolation of cases. He recognised that his proposals could be most readily achieved with smallpox, because vaccination provided a means of protection for nurses and others who had to remain in contact with patients. His proposed *Regulations* were as follows (Fenner, *et al.*, 1988, p. 275):

1st. The earliest possible notification of the disease after it has broken out upon any individual or individuals.
2nd. The seclusion, at home or in hospital, of those affected, during the whole progress of the disease, as well as during the convalescence from it, or until all power of infecting others is past.
3rd. The surrounding of the sick with nurses and attendants who are themselves non-conductors or incapable of being affected, inasmuch as they are known to be protected against the disease by having already passed through cow-pox or small-pox.
4th. The due purification, during and after the disease, by water, chlorine, carbolic acid, sulphurous acid, etc., of the rooms, beds, clothes, etc., used by the sick and their attendants, and the disinfection of their own persons.

The most vigorous advocacy of isolation as a method of controlling smallpox was developed in Leicester, England, largely as a result of the local anti-vaccination movement (Fraser, 1980). The system (the so-called *Leicester Method*) developed during the 1870s and achieved notoriety in the 1890s. It depended critically on high-grade surveillance to recognise, report and isolate cases in the town's Fever and Smallpox Hospital (**Figure 3.25**). All immediate contacts were quarantined and compensated for loss of time from work. Vaccination was not mentioned – a reflection of the strong local disapproval of compulsory vaccination. Subsequently, the

Figure 3.24 Smallpox hospitals, St Pancras. (*Upper*) The St Pancras Smallpox Hospital on the King's Cross site, c. 1800. During the large smallpox epidemic of 1881, the hospital overflowed with victims and was supplemented (*lower*) by a temporary tented hospital at Finchley. The original hospital was founded on Windmill Street, Tottenham Court Road, in 1746, and was later moved to the parish of St Pancras on the site of the present King's Cross Station. The institution was rebuilt in c. 1793–94 when it received patients from the Cold Bath Fields Hospital in Clerkenwell, a foundation originating in Islington in 1740. Subsequent moves took the hospital to Highgate Hill in c. 1846, and Clare Hall, South Mimms c. 1895–99. It was acquired by the Middlesex Districts Joint Small Pox Hospital Board c. 1900–10. In May 1911, the Local Government Board made an order permitting the admission of patients with pulmonary tuberculosis. It was not unusual for the tuberculosis and smallpox isolation functions to be combined as indigenous smallpox waned and tuberculosis waxed in Great Britain. In 1949, its isolation role was supplemented when non-tuberculosis patients were admitted for treatment. The hospital was closed in 1975. Source: (*Upper*) Wellcome Library, London (oil painting, artist unknown); (*lower*) montage from the weekly newspaper, *The Graphic*, 1881, from a series of watercolour images of aspects of the camp hospital at Finchley by F. Collins.

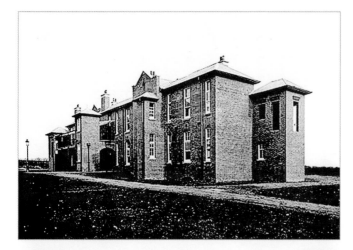

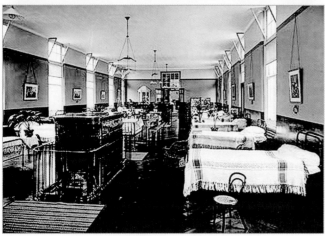

Figure 3.25 Leicester smallpox isolation hospital, 1901. The two-storey isolation block and a ward at Leicester Isolation Hospital at Gilroes. The new hospital was opened in 1900–1 and separated smallpox and tuberculosis isolation from fever isolation (scarlet fever, enteric fever, diphtheria and so on). Historically, all had been treated on a single site in a small combined fever and smallpox hospital built in 1871 on Freaks Ground in northwest Leicester. The buildings there were of corrugated iron and covered 2 acres. Despite enlargement in 1893, it proved inadequate to meet the demands placed upon it by the application of the Leicester Method to control infectious diseases, and this led to the building of the new hospital (McKinley, 1958, pp. 447–56). The old hospital then treated fevers only. *Source*: English Heritage Archives.

vaccination or revaccination of contacts was added to the routine procedure (Millard, 1914). In Fenner's view, the Leicester Method plus vaccination anticipated the surveillance and containment strategy of the World Health Organization's Intensified Smallpox Eradication Programme.

The Establishment of Smallpox Isolation Hospitals in Great Britain

The success of the Leicester Method led to its widespread adoption elsewhere in Great Britain during the first half of the twentieth century as the notion took hold that a special infectious diseases or smallpox hospital or ward should be an integral part of the control of smallpox. See Dixon (1962) who devotes a chapter of his book to the history of smallpox hospitals in Great Britain. Prior to 1900, hospitals were sometimes established in response to epidemics, often of smallpox, as in Quebec in 1639, and on frequent occasions

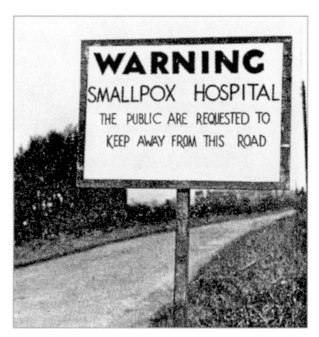

Figure 3.26 Smallpox isolation. A smallpox hospital sign in Yorkshire, England, associated with a 1953 outbreak. *Source*: Fenner, *et al.* (1988, Plate 23.2, p. 1078).

in towns in Great Britain. But, in general, smallpox patients were not admitted to hospitals. In England, one of the earliest smallpox isolation hospitals was the London Small-Pox and Inoculation Hospital, founded in 1746, initially for the treatment of poor persons with smallpox but soon afterwards mainly as a hospital for subjects undergoing variolation. An Inoculation Institute was established in Brno (Bohemia) at about the same time. Subsequently small private 'inoculation hospitals' were set up in most places in which variolation was practised extensively, to prevent the spread of smallpox to susceptible contacts.

As noted, the use of infectious disease hospitals as part of the machinery for controlling smallpox required an efficient system of notification which was easier for smallpox than for most other diseases. Notification formed the core of the Leicester Method and Fenner, *et al.* (1988, p. 276) regard it as a most important factor in limiting the spread of smallpox after importations into Europe and North America during the twentieth century. However, national notification of cases of infectious diseases was not introduced into Great Britain, for example, until 1899, and even an imperfect system of notification required a public health service far more effective than anything that existed during the nineteenth century in Great Britain or, for that matter, elsewhere. And so, even in the industrial countries of Europe, smallpox elimination was not achieved until well into the twentieth century and signs like **Figure 3.26**, along with the isolation use of their associated hospitals, passed into history.

Tuberculosis

Mortality from tuberculosis has been historically associated with population growth in cities. It was during the eighteenth century that the world's big epidemics of tuberculosis began. They were especially intense in those countries (England, United States, Italy and France) that experienced the greatest urbanisation and industrialisation (Johnston, 1993, p. 1059). Tuberculosis was so rampant that autopsies showed that close to 100 percent of some urban populations, such as those of London and Paris had, at some point in their lives, developed the disease although they had died from some other cause. By the early nineteenth century, rates of mortality from tuberculosis in most major American cities ranged from 400 to 500 per 100,000 population.

Early treatment of tuberculosis involved a wide range of quackeries. But, by the mid-nineteenth century and in the absence of antibiotics, therapies with fresh air and sunshine became increasingly popular in specialist isolation hospitals so that, in the 1880s, luxury sanatoria for the wealthy began to proliferate on both sides of the Atlantic and in Japan. One of the leading countries providing these treatments was Switzerland, with its 'healthy' mountain air, and four settlements specialised in this work – Davos, Leysin, Arosa and Montana. The village of Leysin had already become internationally known in 1798 when Thomas Malthus included six pages about it in his classic book, *An Essay on the Principle of Population*. Malthus quoted work by Muret the Elder (1764) who reported the average life

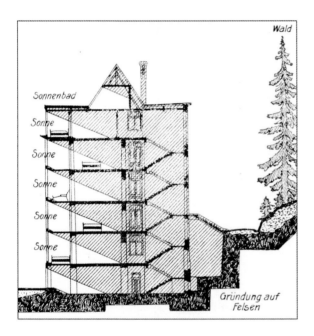

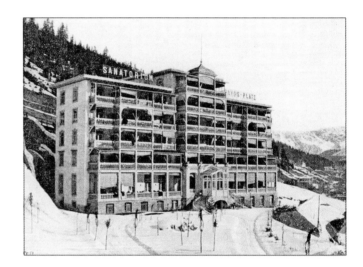

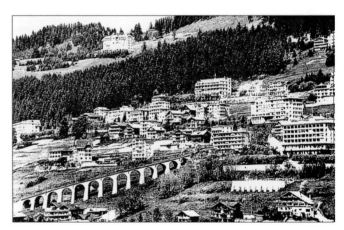

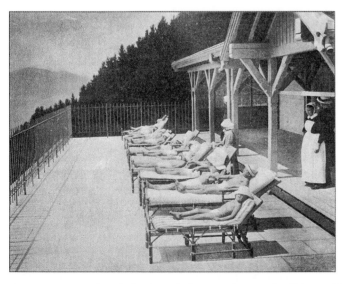

Figure 3.27 Sanatorium design in Leysin (1,263 m above sea level). (*Upper left*) Sanatoria were designed to make the best use of sunshine exposure for patients. The general design looked to exploit favourable geographical positions on south and southwest facing slopes of valleys, altitude, clear air and maximal insolation to treat tubercular patients. (*Lower left*) Wide balconies allowed patients to be wheeled out in their beds into the sun. (*Upper right*) The *Sanatorium Davos-Platz* shows the realisation of this design for a specific sanatorium in Davos. (*Lower right*) This view of Leysin in the 1930s shows that this basic design was repeated across the village producing a very characteristic townscape. Leysin's sanatoria varied greatly in size from small pavilions (the foreground chalets) to major structures (on the hillside). The viaduct carries a rack and pinion railway opened from Aigle in the valley below in 1900 to facilitate access by patients. *Sources*: (*upper left*) Commission Centrale Suisse pour la Lutte Antituberculeuse (Schweizerische Zentralkommission zur Bekämpfung der Tuberkulose), 1917, p. 323; (*remainder*) Photo Nicca, Leysin.

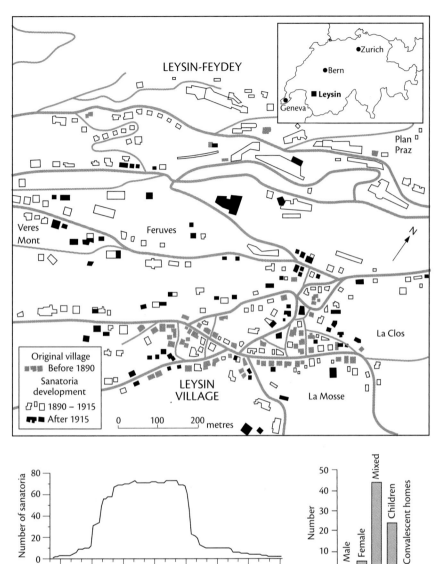

Figure 3.28 Sanatoria in Leysin. The map shows the original core of the village (grey) in 1890. Subsequent periods of development linked to Rollier's work providing tuberculosis treatments are shown by white and black boxes. The largest sanatoria on the highest south facing slopes north of the village were built first (white boxes, 1890–1915), with later sanatoria (black boxes) generally backfilling downslope to the original village core. The graphs show the number and demographic composition of sanatoria in Leysin, 1891–2001. The rapid growth after Rollier's arrival in 1903 is evident. The largest sanatoria were built in the period 1895–1910. At its height for tuberculosis care (1930), Leysin had 5,698 inhabitants. Of these, 3,000 were tuberculosis patients. Antibiotic treatment regimes for tuberculosis were developed after the Second World War, leading to closure of many of the sanatoria in the early 1950s (preceded by the Grand Hotel in 1942). By 1969, there were only eight clinics and convalescent homes left with fewer than 500 beds. *Source*: redrawn from a sketch map deposited in the Leysin Public Archives with the authorization of the Rollier family and data in Andrew (2002, pp. 252–69) also found in Cliff, *et al.* (2004, Figures 4.7 and 4.8, p. 58).

expectancy of inhabitants in Leysin was 61 years, as compared to 41 in Vaud (Switzerland) and 30.5 in London. The long life expectancy in Leysin was believed to be the result of both its sunny high altitude climate and the low incidence of infectious diseases.

Figures 3.27 and **3.28** illustrate sanatoria in Leysin. The first winter patient arrived in Leysin in 1873 and, in 1878, the first *pension* for foreigners was opened. In 1890, the Climatic Society of Leysin was founded, and its promotion of the climate of the village led to several early clinics being built. The first and grandest was the Grand Hotel for 120 patients, opened in 1892, emphasising the importance of international movements of monied patients. The development of Leysin as a centre specialising in the treatment of non-pulmonary tuberculosis awaited the arrival in the village of Dr August Rollier (1874–1954), 'The Sun Doctor', in 1903. Rollier's sun-treatment therapy involved a controlled regime of exposure of different parts of the body to sun for varying lengths of time. Tubercular patients flocked from

all over the world to Leysin to be treated. Rollier constructed 37 clinics with 1,150 beds. The design of the sanatoria broadly followed Figure 3.27. The clinics had wide doors and balconies so that bedridden patients could be wheeled into the sun. Rollier's theories are outlined in de Kruif's book, *Men Against Death*, while Mann (1932) in *The Magic Mountain* and Ellis (1958) in *The Rack* describe life inside one of the sanatoria.

By about 1900, state-sponsored sanatoria also began to be created in many parts of the world, and their use continued for the next half-century. **Figure 3.29** uses proportional circles to map the 1912 geographical distribution of isolation hospitals for tuberculosis by county in England and Wales. This function was often added to pre-existing isolation hospitals for smallpox. By mid-century, practically every borough had an isolation hospital for fevers, while hospitals for smallpox and tuberculosis were fewer and served larger catchment areas than the general fever hospitals. All changed with the advent of antibiotics, antivirals and a National Health Service to deliver mass vaccination programmes (see Chapter 4 and

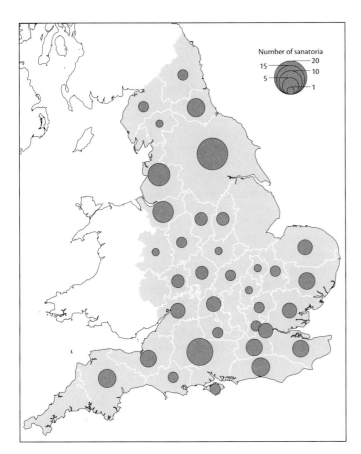

Figure 3.29 Tuberculosis isolation hospitals in England and Wales, 1912. The county level geographical distribution of TB hospitals is shown by proportional circles.

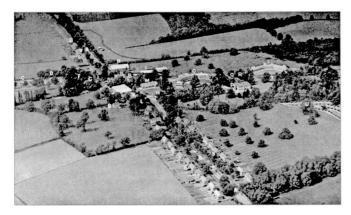

Figure 3.30 Papworth Village Settlement, near Cambridge. Aerial view of the Settlement. The Settlement was a tuberculosis treatment centre, established by Dr Pendrill Varrier-Jones in 1918 as an experiment in the holistic treatment of the disease. It consisted of a hospital and sanatorium (O and S) for the treatment of patients centred around the original Papworth Hall (P), along with a 'settlement' where former patients and their families ('colonists') could reside and work in a rural environment (A–N). Papworth became the model for other institutions involved in the treatment of tuberculosis in the 1920s and 1930s, including Preston Hall (Kent) and, on a smaller scale, Barrowmore Hall (East Lancashire), Wrenbury Hall (Cheshire) and Sherwood Forest Settlement (Nottinghamshire). The hospital was inherited by the newly formed National Health Service in 1948, and subsequently developed as a pioneering site for cardiology and cardiac surgery. *Source*: Department of Geography, University of Cambridge.

Smallman-Raynor and Cliff, 2012). Generalised population immunity meant cases and mortality from these infections ceased to be a significant public health problem. The isolation hospitals became redundant and were either closed or converted.

The holistic treatment of tuberculosis made its appearance in Great Britain as in Switzerland. The geographically isolated Papworth Village Settlement (**Figure 3.30**) near Cambridge was established by Dr Pendrill Varrier-Jones in 1918 as just such an experiment; see Varrier-Jones (1935), Trail (1961) and Bryder (1984). Initially based around Papworth Hall (P in Figure 3.30), the Settlement expanded in the Hall's grounds to include some 270 houses and flats. There were some 800 residents (settlers and their families), along with a further 175 colonists in hostels, and with around 500 people employed on-site in printing and bookbinding, woodworking, leather and metalworking industries by the early 1960s (Trail, 1961).

Typhus

Louse-borne typhus used to be a seemingly inevitable companion of war and other forms of social disruption. Louse-borne (epidemic) typhus fever appears to have first manifested as a pestilence of

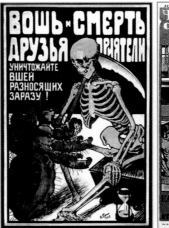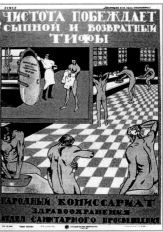

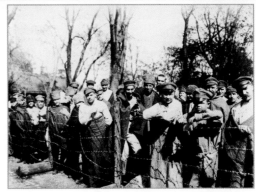

Figure 3.31 Typhus isolation in the First World War. (*Upper left*) The 1919 Russian lithograph by O. Grin illustrates the typhus louse shaking hands with Death. (*Upper right*) This lithograph by V.S. and Russian S.F.S.R. dates from 1921 and shows men washing themselves in a public or factory bathroom to prevent typhus while their clothes are cleaned in an industrial cleaner. (*Lower*) Typhus victims being kept in isolation during the First World War in Estonia. In Eastern Europe, Serbia was badly hit by major typhus epidemics in 1914 as were Poland and Russia in 1918. *Sources*: (*Upper*) Wellcome Library London, (*lower*) © Bettman/Corbis.

European wars in the latter part of the fifteenth century, spreading widely in the Spanish Army during the War of Granada (1482–92). From thereon, observes Prinzing (1916), the disease became the "Nemesis of belligerent armies" (p. 330), appearing in "almost every war that was waged between the beginning of the sixteenth century and the middle of the nineteenth century" and acquiring the appellation *war-plague* (p. 328). The notoriety continued into the twentieth century, with major epidemics of typhus fever spreading across Eastern Europe as a consequence of the First World War and its aftermath (Zinsser, 1935; Smallman-Raynor and Cliff, 2004, pp. 657–64), so that controlling the spread of typhus in its aftermath was an early focus of health-related work of the League of Nations (**Figure 3.31**). Until vaccination became available, isolation was a first line defence. In the Second World War, although there were some important outbreaks, typhus never got out of hand. Outside war zones, typhus struck particularly at major port cities – hence its other popular name of *shipboard fever*.

Typhoid

Typhoid and the carrier state

At the turn of the twentieth century, little was known or understood of the carrier state for typhoid, whereby an individual can be infected with typhoid bacilli, be asymptomatic themselves, and yet pass on the infection to others. The type example is "Typhoid Mary" (Mary Mallon, 1869–1938). Mary emigrated from Ireland to the United States in 1884 (Leavitt, 1996). Her trail of devastation began in 1900 when she commenced work as a cook in the New York City area. In 1900, she had been employed in a house in Mamaroneck, New York, for less than two weeks when the residents developed typhoid. She moved to Manhattan in 1901, and members of the family for whom she cooked developed fevers and diarrhoea, while the laundress died. She then went to work for a lawyer until seven of the eight household members developed typhoid. In 1906, she took a position in Oyster Bay, Long Island. Within two weeks, ten of eleven family members were hospitalised with typhoid. She changed employment again, and similar occurrences happened in three more households.

Mary was first identified as the source of these outbreaks in 1907 by a typhoid researcher, Dr George Soper (Soper, 1907, 1919, 1939). She was subsequently arrested and held in isolation after the New York City health inspector determined her to be a carrier. Under sections 1169 and 1170 of the Greater New York Charter, Mary was held in isolation for three years at a clinic located on North Brother Island (**Figure 3.32**). Mary came back into circulation when the then New York State Commissioner of Health decided that disease carriers would no longer be held in isolation. Her release in 1910

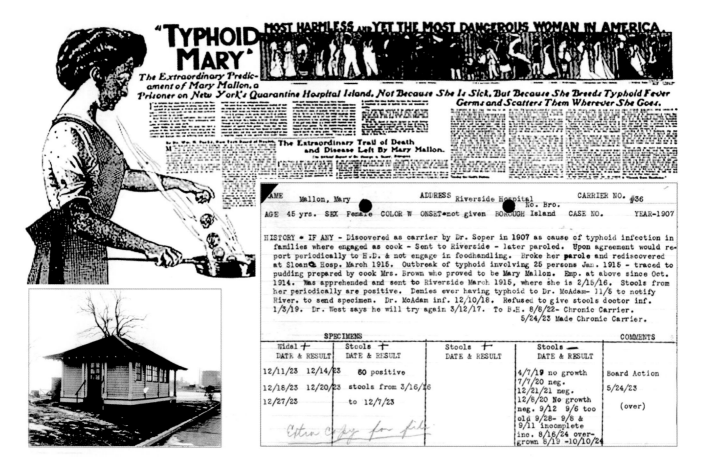

Figure 3.32 Mary Mallon ("Typhoid Mary") and the typhoid carrier state. When Mary Mallon was identified as a typhoid carrier, a lurid press developed around her. An article from the *New York American*, 20 June, 1909, portrays Mary breaking skulls, not eggs, into a frying pan. The inset images show a card in Mary's medical records detailing test results for typhoid, and the isolation cottage on North Brother Island where she was committed, 1907–10. *Sources*: Mary Mallon: Mary Evans Picture Library; medical card: New York County Clerk Archives; Brother Island cottage: World Health Organization Archives.

was conditional on her agreement to cease work as a cook and to take reasonable steps to prevent transmitting typhoid to others. After her release, Mary returned to the mainland and took a job as a laundress. The low wages paid to laundresses compared with cooks led Mary to disappear again, changing her name to Mary Brown to disguise her identity. She returned to her former occupation as a cook and, in 1915, was believed to have infected 25 people, one of whom died, while working as a cook at New York's Sloane Hospital for Women. Public-health authorities again found and arrested her. She was returned to North Brother Island isolation hospital for the remainder of her life. When she died, a post-mortem found evidence

of live typhoid bacteria in her gallbladder, although throughout her life she was in denial about her carrier state and regarded herself as persecuted by society.

Typhoid and the milk supply

As with Mary Mallon, the danger of an unknown typhoid carrier in the community is that they are likely to cause serial outbreaks of the disease prior to their identification. Such a situation occurred in Folkestone Urban District (1901 population 30,379), southern England, between 1896 and 1909 (Johnstone, 1910); see **Figure 3.33**.

In Folkestone, an investigation of enteric fever in the period 1896–1900 identified that a certain milker had worked upon three different farms that were associated with the dissemination of the disease in 1896, 1897 and 1899. At the time of this finding, pre-Mary Mallon, the existence of symptomless carriers was unknown. In succeeding years, 1901–9, inquiries revealed that this same milker was connected with milk farms again associated with the dissemination of enteric fever. Bacteriological studies in 1909 established that this milker was a typhoid carrier. The milker, N, was a man of about 60 years and had, to his knowledge, never suffered from enteric fever and had begun to work regularly as a milker in April 1893 at a farm in Elham Rural District, close to Folkestone. From thereon, he was employed as a cowman and milker on farms near Folkestone, working at four different farms in the years to 1909. Of the 323 indigenous (non-imported) cases of enteric fever identified in Folkestone in the period 1896–1909, 207 (64 percent) are known to have received milk from a farm at which N was then acting as a milker. Johnstone (1910) concluded that enteric fever in the Folkestone Rural District in this period has been spread mainly by milk, and that the milk was infected by a single typhoid carrier.

3.4 Quarantine and Isolation Today

In this section, we look at the impact of population movements, associated with technological changes in transport, upon the feasibility of quarantine and isolation as control strategies today. We then attempt to assess quantitatively their effectiveness using examples for twentieth-century influenza pandemics.

The Role of Movement

Quarantine and isolation are generally only effective control strategies if the surveillance and reporting systems which give early warning of the approach of infection are adequate; and it has always been simpler to control the arrival of infection by sea than overland. This was writ large in Chapter 1 in the early attempts by the states and principalities of Italy to control the spread of plague – compare, for example, Prato (Section 1.3) with the Venetian approach (Section 1.2), and Tatham's comments (Section 1.1) on disease surveillance in England and Wales.

In the twentieth century, the impact of the breakdown of surveillance and cross-border controls upon the spread of disease was nowhere more graphically illustrated than among the refugee and indigenous populations of Russia and Eastern Europe in the years after the end of the First World War in 1918. Aggravated by the population turbulence caused by the Russian Revolution, millions of displaced persons ranged across western Russia from the Black Sea to the Baltic, carrying with them all manner of infectious diseases – typhus, plague, relapsing fever, and cholera among them. Cholera was an especial concern. **Figure 3.34A** (Figure 3.34 located

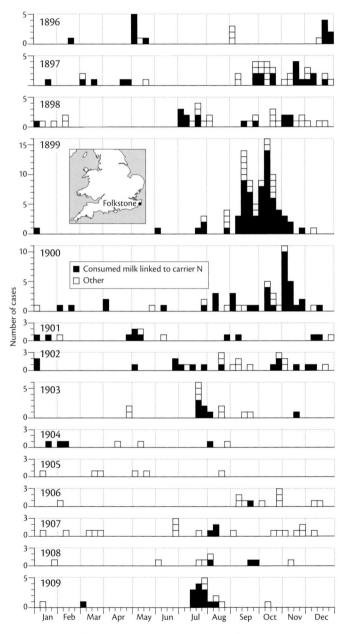

Figure 3.33 Weekly series of enteric fever cases in Folkestone Urban District, 1896–1909. Cases are classified according to whether the patients had consumed milk from one of four milk farms that employed the typhoid carrier, N, or not in the month prior to onset of illness. *Source*: redrawn from Johnstone (1910, unnumbered chart, between pp. 6–7).

in the colour plate section) shows the reported number of chol-era cases, other than on the railways, in western Russia in the first six months of 1922. Such was the role of travel in disseminating cholera from the Black Sea and the Ukraine that cholera cases on the railway were recorded separately (Figure 3.34B) while, for this water-borne disease, sanitary stations were established at regular intervals along the principal rivers (Figure 3.34C).

As we have noted, implementing quarantine and isolation has always been easiest for ships and when traffic volumes are low. In the twenty-first century, a radically different situation exists. Aircraft now provide the principal means of movement and international traf-fic volumes are vast. Figures from the World Tourism Organization show that international arrivals worldwide in 2009 for business, lei-sure and other purposes, amounted to 880 million. Travel for leisure, recreation and holidays accounted for just over half of this flux (51 percent). Some 15 percent of international travellers reported travel-ling for business and professional purposes and another 27 percent for specific purposes such as visiting friends and relatives, religious reasons and pilgrimages, and for health treatment. Slightly over half of travellers arrived at their destination by air transport (53 percent) in 2009, while the remainder travelled by surface (47 percent) – whether by road (39 percent), rail (3 percent) or sea (5 percent). Over time, the share for air transport arrivals has gradually increased so that international arrivals are expected to reach 1.6 billion by 2020.

Whether by land (**Figure 3.35**), sea (**Figure 3.36**) or air (**Figure 3.37**), the temporal story of transport for the last c. 250 years has been one of exponentially increasing carrying capacity and expo-nentially diminishing journey times.

If the shift from sail to steamships accelerated global interaction in the second half of the nineteenth century, aircraft did the same again in the second half of the twentieth century. Spurred on by the technological advances that accompanied the Second World War, notably the development of high-precision navigational aids and the gas turbine (jet) engine, passenger aircraft increasingly replaced ships as the international carrying medium. **Figure 3.37** charts the decline in passenger flight times at two geographical scales. Graph (A) shows the change in transcontinental flight times across the United States (approximately 3,000 miles). A crossing which took two full days in the late 1920s had been reduced to half a day by 1960. Graph (B) shows even more striking changes in the 12,000 mile England–Australia run since 1925. In both cases the exponen-tial decline in travel times is shown by a solid line, comparable in shape to the distance-decay curves for land and sea transport.

If we map the world in time–space using a technique like multi-dimensional scaling (MDS) (Cliff, *et al.*, 2000, pp. 219–29), rather than using a conventional geographical metric, a consequence of the collapse in travel times is that the world's countries have been rapidly moving closer together. **Figure 3.38** shows this effect for part of the Pacific Basin. Here MDS been used to construct a time accessibility map of 25 islands and island groups. Figure 3.38A is a conventional map of the locations of these islands. Figure 3.38B is the MDS representation of (A). Islands and island groups with sim-ilar levels of accessibility as measured by travel times are mapped together, irrespective of their geographical locations. The vectors show the way in which relatively inaccessible Papua New Guinea (PNG), the Trust Territories of the Pacific Islands (TTP) and Latin

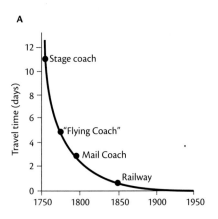

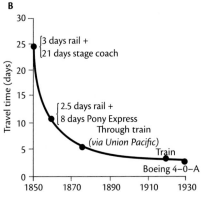

Figure 3.35 Historical time changes in land transport at two geographical scales. (A) London to Scotland, 1750–1950. (B) Transcontinental eastbound across the United States from New York to California, 1850–1930. The solid lines show the exponential decline in travel times. *Source*: based partly on Davies (1964, Figure 91, pp. 508–9).

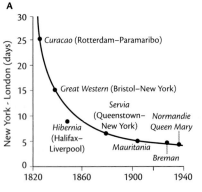

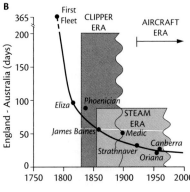

Figure 3.36 Time changes in intercontinental travel by sea transport. (A) Transatlantic travel times between Europe and North America, 1820–1940. (B) Travel times between England and Australia, 1788–2000. Names of vessels are in italic. The solid lines show the exponential decline in travel times. *Sources*: Davies (1964, Figure 91, pp. 508–9); Cliff and Haggett (2004, Figure 1A, p. 89).

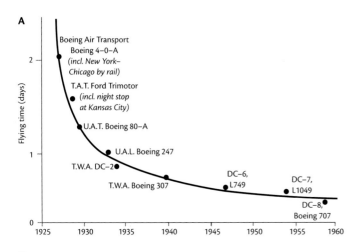

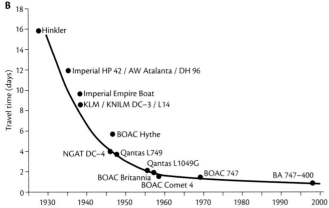

Figure 3.37 **Historic changes in travel times by air transport.** (A) Transcontinental in the United States eastbound New York–California, 1925–60. (B) Intercontinental between Europe and Australia, 1925–2000. Plane types are named. The solid lines show the exponential decline in travel times. *Sources*: adapted from Davies (1964, Figure 91, pp. 508–9) and Cliff and Haggett (2004, Figure 1B, p. 89).

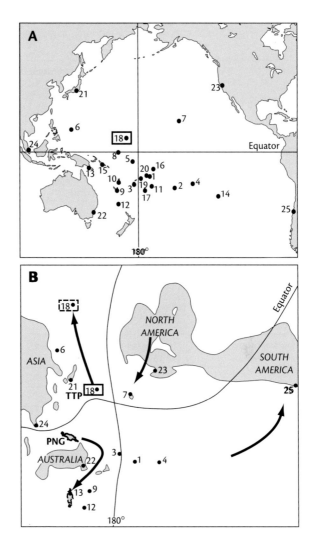

Figure 3.38 **A collapsing world: travel-time maps.** (A) Conventional map of the Pacific Basin with 25 islands, island groups and continental cities marked. (B) Time accessibility map of Pacific islands and Pacific Rim countries by scheduled airline carriers in the last quarter of the twentieth century, constructed by multidimensional scaling. Centres with similar levels of accessibility are mapped together irrespective of their geographical locations. 1 American Samoa; 2 Cook Islands; 3 Fiji; 4 French Polynesia; 5 Kiribati and Tuvalu; 6 Guam; 7 Hawaii; 8 Nauru; 9 New Caledonia; 10 Vanuatu; 11 Niue; 12 Norfolk Island; 13 Papua New Guinea; 14 Pitcairn; 15 Solomon Islands; 16 Tokelau; 17 Tonga; 18 US Trust Territories of the Pacific Islands; 19 Wallis and Futuna; 20 Western Samoa; 21 Tokyo; 22 Sydney; 23 San Francisco; 24 Singapore; 25 Santiago. *Source*: (B) is based upon unpublished work by P. Forer, Department of Geography, University of Canterbury, Christchurch, New Zealand.

America are moved from the centre of the time space, whereas the more accessible Pacific seaboard of the United States migrates in towards the centre of the time space.

Communicable Disease Consequences of Change

It was difficult to foresee in the two decades after the end of the First World War the long-term consequences of the collapse of geographical space for communicable disease diffusion and its control. Occasionally, a prescient view would be taken. Thus Massey (1933, p. v) in the preface to his book on *Epidemiology in Relation to Air Travel* remarks:

> Speedier transport is equivalent to a reduction of distance. This was shown when steamships superseded sailing vessels. It is demonstrated more forcibly today by the events of civil aviation. Among the momentous advantages, fraternal and commercial, born of this development, there is the disadvantage that countries affected by certain major infectious diseases are brought nearer to countries which ordinarily enjoy freedom therefrom.

Table 3.1, taken from Massey, goes to the heart of the matter by summarising the (then) relationship between ship and air travel

times to the UK, and the maximum incubation periods for four infectious diseases. It shows how the switch from steamship to air travel potentially opened up the UK to four of the quarantine diseases endemic in other parts of the world. Passenger aircraft reduced travel times to somewhat less than a third of the journey time by sea – and, in all instances, to less than the incubation periods of the diseases so that it became possible for an infected individual unwittingly to transfer sickness into a disease-free area before becoming symptomatic – and accordingly greatly reducing the effectiveness of any early-warning surveillance systems with their associated quarantine and isolation control strategies.

Table 3.1 Disease diffusion consequences of reduced travel times. Travel times by ship and air in relation to the incubation period of selected communicable diseases in days, 1933

Disease	Incubation period (maximum)	Infected countries trafficking with UK	Journey time to UK by sea	Journey time to UK by air
Plague	6	India	20	6
		Iraq	18	5
		Egypt	10	3
		East Africa	20	5
		West Africa	10	3
		South America	17	5
Cholera	5	India, Iraq	As above	As above
Yellow fever	6	W Africa, S America	As above	As above
Smallpox	14	India, Iraq, Egypt, W Africa, S America	As above	As above

All figures are in days.
Source: Massey (1933, p. 6).

Table 3.2 Putative spread of yellow fever. Travel time in days from regions with endemic yellow fever in 1933 to countries with no yellow fever experience

Destination country	Infected countries trafficking therewith	Travel time by sea	Travel time by air
UK	West Africa[1]	10	3
	Central America	17	5
	South America	17	6
	Caribbean islands[2]	14	5
France	West Africa[2]	8	2
	South America[2]	16	4
Belgium	Belgian Congo[1]	18	6
USA	Panama[2]	8 (to New York)	3 (to New York)
	Colombia[2]	8	3
	Caribbean islands[2]	7	2
South Africa	West Africa[1]	10	3
British East Africa	West Africa[1]	21	3
India	West Africa[1]	26	5

[1] Airlines likely to operate in the near future (1933)
[2] Airlines in operation (1933)
All figures are in days
Source: Massey (1933, p. 19)

Table 3.2 illustrates this problem in more detail for one of Massey's diseases, yellow fever. Massey was fearful that collapsing travel times within the incubation period of the disease would lead to a geographical diaspora of undetected yellow fever from endemic regions to new parts of the world. As noted in Section 2.5, the Office International d'Hygiène Publique took up the issue of quarantine regulations for air traffic in 1928; an International Sanitary Convention for Aerial Navigation was drawn up in 1932 and came into force in 1935. Part III (Chapter II) of the 1935 Convention was specifically aimed at the control of yellow fever, and this prompted the design of airports that incorporated elements of spatial isolation to lessen the risk of yellow fever virus transmission to passengers on stopovers in tropical locations (**Figure 3.39**).

The problem of spatially intercepting cases of communicable diseases and their contacts before they can spread infection to new areas has been exacerbated by the exponential increase in personal mobility in the last 50 years. **Figure 3.40** illustrates the point for 82 islands and island groups over the second half of the twentieth century for which UN data are available (1957–1992). The diagram shows on an annual basis the number of visitors per head of resident population. Representative islands from different geographical environments have been plotted with heavy lines. The pecked line is the sample median. Its gradient suggests that, over the sample, the visitor:resident population ratio has grown tenfold in 35 years. For 77 of the 82 islands, a simple linear regression of the visitor:population ratio against time produces positive slope coefficients; the log scale used for the vertical axis implies that the growth in the ratio has been exponential over the period.

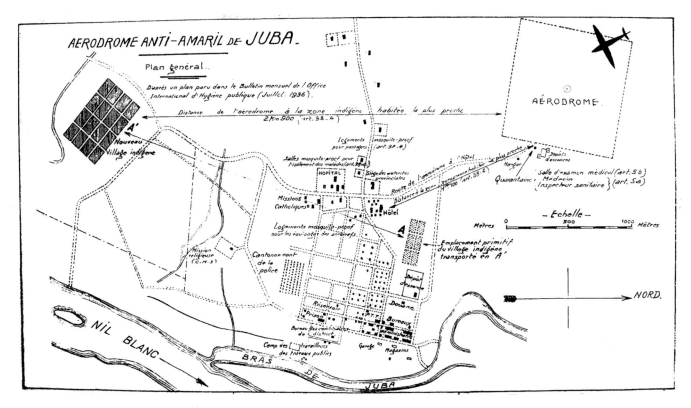

Figure 3.39 Inter-war plan of the anti-amaril aerodrome at Juba, Sudan. The putative identification of yellow fever virus (amaril) activity in southern Sudan in the mid-1930s necessitated remedial action if the aerodrome at Juba was to remain operative as a stopover on the Imperial Airways route between London and Cape Town. As implemented under Part III (Chapter II) of the International Sanitary Convention for Aerial Navigation (1935), 'Measures Applicable in Case of Yellow Fever', steps taken included the isolation of the airport from the indigenous population by relocating the village of Juba from site **A** (1.1 km to the southeast of the aerodrome) to site **A'** (2.9 km due south of the aerodrome), beyond the flight range of potentially infective mosquitoes. Other measures included the construction of mosquito-proof residences for air crew, isolation rooms for patients and a hotel for passengers, all located within approximately 1 km of the aerodrome. *Source*: Cliff, Smallman-Raynor, Haggett, *et al.* (2009, Plate 6.1, p. 351), originally from Pridie (1936, opposite p. 1296).

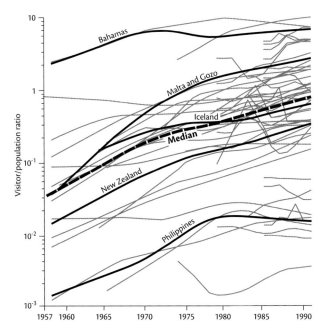

Figure 3.40 Population flux on 82 islands and island groups, 1957–1992. Line traces show number of visitors per head of resident population. Representative islands from different geographical environments are shown with heavy lines. The pecked line is the sample median. *Source*: Cliff, *et al.* (2000, Figure 5.12, p. 205).

Estimating the Impact of Quarantine and Isolation

Quarantine of the sort practised in Italy was a blunt instrument in that it attempted to limit the travel of people between communities (and often of goods as well) irrespective of their disease status. For humans, most quarantine efforts until the early years of the twentieth century focused upon controlling infection arising from maritime trade; Kilwein (1995a, b), Mafart and Perret (1998), Sattenspiel and Herring (2003) and Gensini, *et al.* (2004) provide reviews of the literature. The general experience with quarantine and isolation over this period was that it was more successful in reducing impact than in keeping areas disease-free – as in Italy with plague. But how successful was quarantine as an approach in the twentieth century as transport technology changed and the international flux of people multiplied exponentially year on year? And, recognising the possible adverse consequences that may follow from the implementation of large-scale quarantine action (Barbera, *et al.*, 2001), what are its prospects for the future? We consider these questions in this and the next subsection.

Canada, 1918–19

Sattenspiel and Herring (2003) used data from the Hudson's Bay Company records on the 1918–19 influenza pandemic among Aboriginal fur trappers in three northern communities (Norway House, Oxford House and God's Lake) in the Keewatin District of

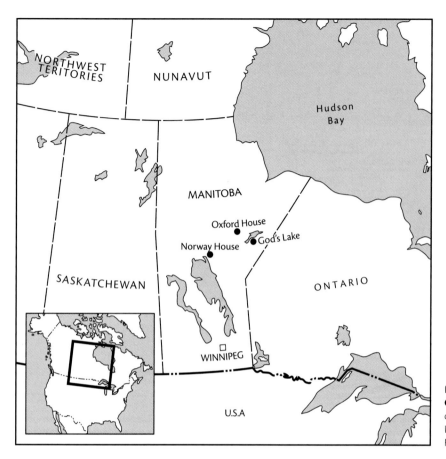

Figure 3.41 Keewatin District of central Manitoba, Canada. Location map showing positions of the trading communities of Norway House, Oxford House and God's Lake. *Source*: Cliff, Smallman-Raynor, Haggett, *et al.* (2009, Figure 11.12, p. 642).

Central Manitoba (**Figure 3.41**) to examine two topical questions relating to quarantine:

(i) What is the impact of varying the time during an epidemic at which intercommunity quarantine is implemented?

(ii) What is the effect of varying the duration of quarantine?

An *SIR* compartment model was used with a 30-day quarantine period which was applied only at Norway House. See Section 1.4 for the specification of an *SIR* model. The compartment model permits the mixing parameter, β, to vary spatially, thus allowing inhomogeneous mixing of susceptibles and infectives. In their version of the model, Sattenspiel and Herring (2003) replaced β with two parameters: σ, the rate of travel out of communities and ρ, the rate of return into communities. For a theoretical discussion of quarantine in infectious disease models, see Hethcote, *et al.* (2002).

Figure 3.42A shows the impact upon case levels at Oxford House of varying the time on the epidemic curve at which quarantine measures were introduced at Norway House (question (i) earlier), with epidemic starts at Norway House and God's Lake. Case load at the epidemic peak was minimised when quarantine was introduced well before the epidemic peaked, but not right at the beginning of an epidemic. The maximum effect was felt when quarantine was started about half way to the peak. Introduction of quarantine at this point on the epidemic curve also had the maximum delaying effect upon the epidemic peak. This is shown for God's Lake in Figure 3.42B. Such delay can buy public health authorities time to devise other control strategies.

Figure 3.42C shows the impact of quarantine periods of different lengths at Norway House upon the total number of cases estimated to occur at God's Lake. For quarantines of up to 30 days, the case total dropped sharply. There is no further benefit gained by quarantines of greater duration – although this will, of course, be affected by the serial interval of the disease (about 4–8 days for influenza), so that we might expect the optimal quarantine duration to be positively correlated with the serial interval of the disease.

The duration of quarantine will also be affected by its effectiveness. Figure 3.42D explores this for Oxford House. The curves show the time in days to the epidemic peak at Oxford House (vertical axis), against quarantine completeness at Norway House on the horizontal axis. The traces show that, once mobility goes above about 10 percent (i.e. the quarantine is less than 90 percent effective), quarantine did not delay the onset of the epidemic peak at Oxford House. Up to this threshold, the epidemic peak was delayed by several days. Sattenspiel and Herring also found a similar 10 percent threshold for the ultimate size of the epidemic.

United States, 1918–19 and 1957

Two studies, by Markel, *et al.* (2007) and by Haber, *et al.* (2007), have investigated the impact of various non-prophylactic techniques such as school closures as an approach to epidemic mitigation. Markel, *et al.* used data from 43 cities in the continental United States for the 24-week period from 8 September 1918 to 22 February 1919, to determine whether city-to-city variations in mortality were associated with the timing, duration, and combination of various non-pharmaceutical interventions (school closures;

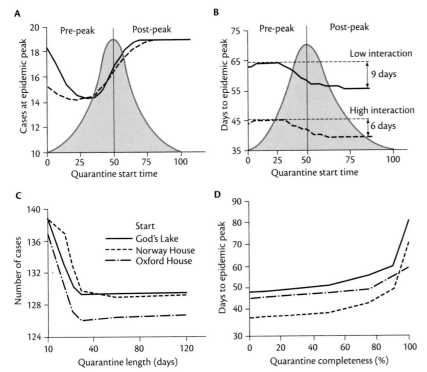

Figure 3.42 Quarantine in Canada, 1918–19. Estimated impact of inter-community quarantine upon the Spanish influenza pandemic in the Keewatin District of central Manitoba, Canada. (A) Oxford House (OH): Estimated cases at epidemic peak as a function of the time on the epidemic curve at which quarantine was started at Norway House (NH). Maximum case reduction occurred for quarantine start times about a quarter of the way through the epidemic. There was no effect after the epidemic peak. Curves for epidemics starting in NH and God's Lake (GL) are shown. The hypothesised epidemic curve is shaded. (B) God's Lake: Estimated delay in timing of the epidemic peak (in days) for different quarantine start times at NH and epidemics starting at NH and GL. Consistent with (A), maximum delay is delivered by starting quarantine about a quarter of the way through the epidemic. Curves are shown for high and low rates of inter-community travel. (C) God's Lake: Estimated size of epidemic (in cases) as a function of the quarantine period at NH and epidemic starts at NH, OH and GL. No appreciable effect is felt with quarantines > 30 days. (D) Oxford House: Days to epidemic peak as function of quarantine completeness at NH on a scale from 0–100 percent (no–complete quarantine), and epidemic starts at NH, OH and GL. *Source*: based upon graphs in Sattenspiel and Herring (2003, Figures 4–7, pp. 18–20).

cancellation of public gatherings; and isolation and quarantine); allowance was made for confounding variables like city size and population density. In a similar vein, but using simulation to evaluate different scenarios, Haber, *et al.* (2007) estimated the impact upon the ultimate size of an influenza epidemic of reducing contact rates among specified classes of citizens in a hypothetical small urban community in the United States. The community was assumed to have a distribution of household sizes and ages that followed the 2000 US Census. The interventions they investigated were school closures, confinement of ill persons and their household contacts to their homes, and reduction in contact rates among residents of long-term care facilities. Interventions were implemented at the start of the outbreak. Data from the 1957–58 Asian influenza pandemic were used to test the model. A mixing matrix was devised with the following age categories and mixing groups: < 1–4, 5–18, 19–64, ≥ 65 at home, ≥ 65 in long-term care; households, day-care centres, schools, workplaces, long-term care facilities and the community.

Markel, *et al.* took the weekly excess death rate per 100,000 population (*EDR*) as a measure of the success of different interventions. Over the 24-week study period, there were 115,340 excess pneumonia and influenza deaths (*EDR* = 500) in the 43 cities analysed. Every city adopted at least one of the three non-pharmaceutical interventions: school closure; cancellation of public gatherings; and isolation/quarantine. School closure and public gathering bans was the most common intervention combination, implemented in 34 cities (79 percent), with a median duration of 4 weeks (range, 1–10 weeks). The longer the period of non-pharmaceutical intervention, the lower was the *EDR*. This is illustrated in **Figure 3.43A** by, comparing St Louis (143 days of non-pharmaceutical intervention) and New York City (73 days). The cities which implemented non-pharmaceutical

interventions earlier also had greater delays in reaching peak mortality (Spearman $r = -0.74$, $p < 0.001$) and lower peak mortality rates (Spearman $r = 0.31$, $p = 0.02$); see Figure 3.43. There was a statistically significant inverse correlation between duration of non-pharmaceutical interventions and total mortality (Spearman $r = -0.39$, $p = 0.005$) and, as noted, cities experienced lower total mortality when intervention started early (Spearman $r = 0.37$, $p = 0.008$); see Figure 3.43C.

Haber, *et al.* used a different measure of the success of non-prophylactic interventions in their study, namely *effectiveness*, defined as:

$$effectiveness = (baseline\ influenza\ rate - rate\ with\ intervention)/\ baseline\ rate.$$

Figures 3.43D and E show the estimated impact upon outbreak size of (D) school closures and (E) confinement of sick people to home. For schools, closure at around 10 percent sick and for 14 days was the most effective compromise in the trade off between reducing infection and increasing societal disruption. By striking early, children incubating the disease are taken out of circulation, while 14-day closure exceeds the serial interval of influenza. As graph (D) shows, delay (as measured by percent illness required to trigger closure) allows incubators and infectives to produce secondary downstream cases, thus greatly reducing effectiveness. Within the family, chart 3.43E shows that the same principles apply. By confining sick individuals and their contacts to home with high isolation compliance greatly reduces the chances of community-wide contacts between infectives and susceptibles; it is a highly effective intervention. Haber, *et al.* also found that, for long-term care facilities (LTCF), reducing contacts of the healthy residents with sick co-residents has a significant impact upon illness levels. This is an

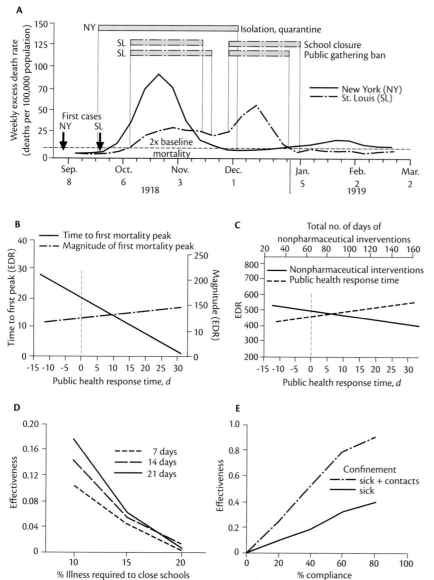

Figure 3.43 United States: estimated impact of non-prophylactic interventions upon rates of illness and mortality in the influenza pandemics of 1918 and 1957. (A) Weekly excess death rate (*EDR*) in New York City and St Louis, September 1918–February 1919 in relation to the duration of non-pharmaceutical interventions. The lower excess mortality in St Louis may be attributed to the longer duration of intervention. (B) and (C), regression lines showing (B) the relationship between public health response time (PHRT) and the timing and magnitude of the first influenza peak in 43 cities and (C) Weekly *EDR* in relation to timing and duration of non-prophylactic interventions. The vertical line indicates the day on which the pandemic accelerated in each city. An intervention introduced on this day was given a PHRT of zero; interventions introduced on days before acceleration have negative PHRTs and, on days after, positive PHRTs. (D) Impact of school closures for varying levels of sickness and closure periods. (E) Impact of home confinement of sick individuals and their contacts for varying levels of quarantine compliance. In (D) and (E), *effectiveness* is defined as: *effectiveness* = (baseline rate − rate with intervention)/baseline rate, where the baseline rate is that for illness during the 1957–58 pandemic in the United States. *Source*: Cliff, Smallman-Raynor, Haggett, *et al.* (2009, Figure 11.14, p. 646).

important finding since LTCF residents respond poorly to vaccination and often escape vaccination entirely in the US.

The findings of the Markel and Haber studies are consistent with that of Sattenspiel – the application of non-pharmaceutical interventions which reduce mixing between infectives and susceptibles early in an epidemic has the capability of reducing both the ultimate size of an epidemic and delaying the peak of infection. It suggests, as do the recent studies by Davey and Glass (2008) and Meltzer (2008), that in planning for future severe influenza pandemics, non-pharmaceutical interventions should be considered for inclusion as companion measures to developing effective vaccines and medications for prophylaxis and treatment (cf. Barbera, *et al.*, 2001). Haber, *et al.* estimate that, by combining these interventions, rates of illness and death in a community might be reduced by as much as 50 percent. Such non-prophylactic interventions are included in the current US Department of Health and Human Services Influenza Pandemic Plan (US Department of Health and Human Services, 2005, 2007).

Similar findings have also been found for international travel. On a global scale, Cooper, *et al.* (2006) used simulation models hypothetically to track how the 1968–69 Hong Kong influenza pandemic would have spread globally if it had been injected into the world's passenger airline network as it existed in 2000. They examined two scenarios: (i) with intervention to suspend 99.9 percent of air travel from affected cities and (ii) for comparison, no intervention, at two dates – August 1968 and February 1969 – two and eight months respectively after the first cases on 1 June 1968; see **Figure 3.44** (located in the colour plate section). In the simulation, intervention was made after 100 cases occurred in a city (or 1,000 cases for Hong Kong, the city of origin). As the airline links dropped out so the speed of spread of the epidemic was reduced by up to three weeks as compared with the no intervention scenario – sufficient time to consider local interventions including vaccination provided a suitable vaccine was predistributed to doctors (as was the case in the UK during the influenza A/H1N1/09 pandemic of 2009). The highly connected nature of the air travel network prevents minor delays between pairs of cities combining into substantial delays over the whole network.

These ideas were tested further by Epstein, *et al.* (2007) who used a stochastic epidemic model to study global transmission of pandemic influenza, including the effects of travel restrictions and vaccination. They found that the distribution of first passage times to the United States and the numbers of infected persons in metropolitan areas worldwide could be slightly delayed by international air travel restrictions alone. When other local containment measures were applied at the source of infection, in conjunction with travel restrictions, delays could be much longer and case load reduced.

Plague in India, 1994

Beginning on 26 August 1994, outbreaks of bubonic and pneumonic plague began to be reported in south-central, southwestern and northern India (Dutt, *et al.*, 2006). The outbreak probably resulted in some 5,150 pneumonic or bubonic plague cases and 53 deaths in eight Indian states, with the majority from south-central and southwestern regions. Of the 5,150 cases, the majority (2,793) were reported from Maharashtra state (including Bombay), with much of the balance from Gujarat state (1,391 cases) and Delhi (749 cases); the remaining 169 cases were from Andhar Pradesh, Haryana, Madhya Pradesh, Rajasthan, Uttar Pradesh and West Bengal (Centers for Disease Control and Prevention, 1994a, b). By 19 October, the outbreak was under control.

As Madan (1995) and Fritz, *et al.* (1996) observe, the initial reports of the 1994 outbreak caused considerable international concern, especially among countries which were uncertain of the effectiveness of their own public healthcare systems, over the possible importation of pneumonic plague from India by air travel. The

response from the World Health Organization was benign, so that a number of countries adopted their own ad hoc procedures. These ranged from increased surveillance and checking of passengers (e.g. France, Germany and the United States) at airports, through to border closure (offensive containment in terms of Figure 1.20B) in others (six of the Gulf States). Many countries, particularly in Asia, banned flights to and from India. For example, Saudi Arabian authorities refused a scheduled Air India flight from Bombay permission to land in Jeddah (Madan, 1995). Air India aircraft were fumigated on arrival at airports in Rome and Milan and passengers were subjected to special health checks. In Moscow, authorities ordered six-day quarantines for passengers from India and banned travel to India. The response reflected recognition of the risk of transmission in the modern global community, and India was de facto in pseudo-isolation/quarantine for a period with a ring of nations around its borders implementing restrictions on travel and trade to try to prevent cross-border transfer of infection (**Figure 3.45**). Together, these countries effectively comprised an isolation *cordon sanitaire* around India. The economic impact on India was enormous and it took the country months to recover. In addition, some 300,000 Indians fled the infected regions, creating an internal migration problem.

Severe Acute Respiratory Syndrome (SARS), 2003

SARS was the first new emerging infectious disease to hit the world in the twenty-first century with the potential to become a global epidemic. It was caused by a previously unknown coronavirus subtype (SARS-CoV), which crossed the species barrier with subsequent human-to-human transmission. As a result of this transmission, from November 2002–July 2003, 8,096 SARS

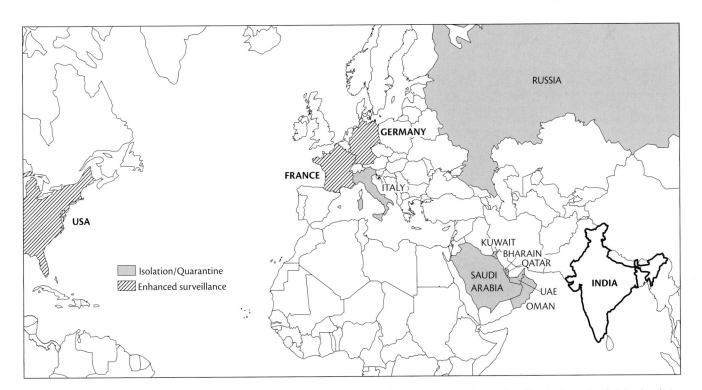

Figure 3.45 Containing plague in India, 1994. Countries are identified if they adopted defensive measures to prevent plague from India crossing their borders during the Surat outbreak, August–October 1994. Measures used ranged from banning trade and travel (isolation and quarantine, grey shading) at one extreme through to enhanced surveillance and vaccination at the other (diagonal shading).

cases and 774 deaths were reported from 29 countries and areas. More than 95 percent of cases occurred in 12 countries of the Western Pacific Region. Mainland China was the worst affected with 5,327 cases. A fifth of the world-wide SARS cases occurred among healthcare workers. The average global case fatality ratio was estimated at around 15 percent, increasing to more than 55 percent for people above 60 years of age (Ahmad and Andraghetti, 2007).

During the outbreak, and dealing with a novel disease agent about which little was initially known, contact tracing, quarantine and isolation were used globally as the principal tools to limit disease spread. Such traditional intervention methods had not been used on this scale for several decades. In many countries, legislative changes were required to facilitate the approach (Rothstein, *et al.*, 2003). WHO was strongly interventionist in leading the global response. Over the longer run, as the characteristics of the causative coronavirus were established, it became clear that it had low transmissibility between humans (basic reproductive number R_0 about 3 compared with c. 7 or more for influenza A and c. 15–18 for measles prior to widespread immunisation) and that peak infectiousness followed the onset of clinical symptoms. These characteristics conspired to make the simple public health measures used initially, such as isolating patients and quarantining their contacts, very effective in the control of the epidemic (Anderson, *et al.*, 2004).

Figures 3.46 and **3.47** show the geographical diffusion process. The index case was a 72-year-old man who was taken ill while returning on 15 March 2003 from a trip to Hong Kong to his home in Beijing on China Airways flight CA112. On the flight he transmitted SARS virus to a number of fellow travellers seated near him (Figure 3.46A; Olsen, *et al.*, 2003, and Whaley, 2006). The aircraft was a Boeing 737-300 which can typically carry up to 126 passengers; on this flight there were 112 with eight crew members. The index case had stayed at the Metropole Hotel in Hong Kong. Subsequent tracking confirmed that 22 fellow passengers and two crew members were infected by this index case, four of whom eventually died. WHO studies of other flights with SARS cases on board showed within-plane virus spread on only four of 35 flights, so CA112 looks like an extreme event on the virus spreading scale.

Rapid onward spread of the virus occurred because many of the man's fellow travellers, now infected, flew on to Taipei, Singapore, Bangkok and Inner Mongolia. As Figure 3.46C shows, this onwards geographical spread continued so that, by May 2003, cases of SARS were occurring worldwide, driven by international air travel. The temporal sequence of cases and deaths at the global scale by July 2003 is mapped in **Figure 3.47**.

In the absence of a vaccine or effective therapies, the options for intervention within a country were limited to public health

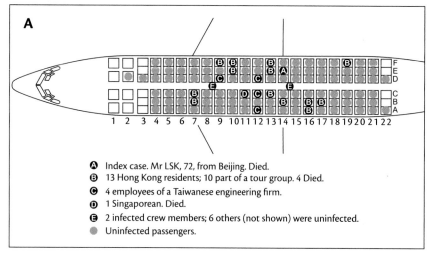

A

A   Index case. Mr LSK, 72, from Beijing. Died.
B   13 Hong Kong residents; 10 part of a tour group. 4 Died.
C   4 employees of a Taiwanese engineering firm.
D   1 Singaporean. Died.
E   2 infected crew members; 6 others (not shown) were uninfected.
●   Uninfected passengers.

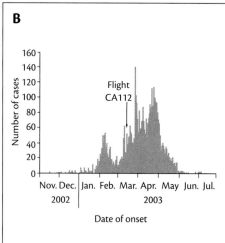

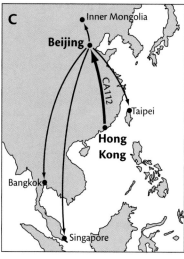

Figure 3.46   Pattern of SARS spread, 2003, by aircraft.
(A) Contacts within an aircraft cabin. SARS infections on Flight CA112 from Hong Kong to Beijing, 15 March 2003. (B) SARS epidemic curve, November 2002–July 2003 showing fuelling of the curve by flight CA112 and its *sequelae*. (C) Subsequent movement of infected passengers. *Source:* Whaley (2006, Figure 15.1, p. 150).

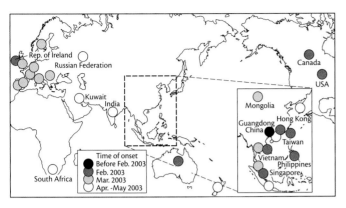

Figure 3.47 Global spread of severe acute respiratory syndrome (SARS), November 2002–May 2003. Sequence of appearance of probable SARS cases in 29 countries and major administrative regions, November 2002–May 2003. Timings are based on the date of onset of the first recorded case in a given geographical area. *Source*: based on information in World Health Organization (2005f).

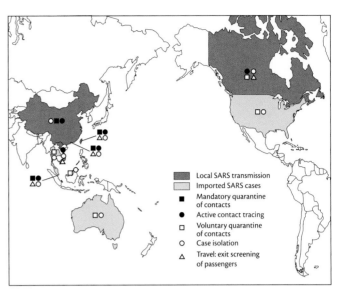

Figure 3.48 SARS control measures, 2002–3. Symbols and shading are used to indicate the main public health control measures adopted in each of the 10 countries principally affected. There is a clear difference between countries with local SARS transmission, where mandatory quarantine and vigorous contact tracing were undertaken to try to break the chains of infection, and the more permissive approach in countries with solely imported cases. *Source*: drawn from data in Ahmad and Andraghetti (2007, Tables 1–7, pp. 13, 15, 17, 20–1, 23, 25, 27).

measures. There are essentially six intervention categories, namely: (i) restrictions on entry to the country and screening at the point of arrival for fever; (ii) isolation of suspect cases; (iii) the encouragement of rapid reporting to a healthcare setting following the onset of defined clinical symptoms, with subsequent isolation; (iv) rigorous infection control measures in healthcare settings; (v) restrictions on movements within a country (restricting travel, limiting congregations such as attendance at school); and (vi) contact tracing and isolation of contacts (Ahmad and Andraghetti, 2007; Anderson, *et al.*, 2004). **Figure 3.48** uses symbols and shading to indicate which interventions were used in each of the countries chiefly affected.

Affected countries fell into two distinct categories: *Category 1*, countries with local SARS transmission (Singapore, Hong Kong, mainland China, Taiwan, Vietnam and Canada) and *Category 2*, countries with imported SARS cases (United States, Thailand, Malaysia and Australia). The Category 1 countries experienced 98 percent of the world's cases (Ahmad and Andraghetti, 2007, p. 7). Once the presence of SARS was realised, all countries set up SARS task forces and committees at central and regional level for coordinating surveillance, response, and communication activities. They were generally supervised by the national Ministry or Department of Health. All countries made legislative amendments in their infectious disease acts making SARS a notifiable disease. Apart from Vietnam and Canada, all the Category 1 countries implemented mandatory quarantining of contacts; no Category 2 countries went that far. All countries implemented intensified surveillance and reporting. Those in Category 1 instituted active tracing of close contacts. Mandatory home quarantining of contacts of cases, actual and suspected, was commenced in Category 1 except for Vietnam and Canada. Voluntary home quarantining occurred in Canada and Category 2. Vietnam implemented institutional quarantine at affected sites. Eventually, the various public health measures used were sufficient to cause the epidemic to die out in the middle of 2003.

Summary

The burden of evidence of the studies described in this section is that, since the turn of the twentieth century, non-prophylactic

interventions have had diminishing impact in preventing the geographical spread of communicable diseases. However, they are still used in certain circumstances. The decline in their general utility as control interventions has been precipitated by changes in the speed and volume of international travel brought about by developments in the internal combustion and jet engines. Now no parts of the populated globe are more than 24–48 hours apart, well within the incubation period of most communicable diseases. This can allow inter-area disease spread to occur asymptomatically and thus undetected, perpetuating chains of infection. The main value of quarantine and isolation today is that careful use (having regard as to when and for how long to implement the measures) will delay rather than prevent inter-community propagation of infection. They may also reduce the ultimate caseload. These interventions may thus buy precious time to deploy other control methods.

3.5 Conclusion

The public health responses of quarantine, isolation, closure of public facilities and the cessation of community events to contain the geographical spread of communicable diseases were widely used until the end of the first quarter of the twentieth century. Indeed, without the availability of appropriate vaccines and antibiotics, they were the only realistic measures which could be deployed for disease containment. But, as we have seen, both quarantine and isolation became progressively less sustainable as stand-alone control strategies as the century unfolded. The main value of quarantine and isolation when used in the modern era has been to slow the geographical spread of infection. Fortunately, medical advances in vaccines and antibiotics have enabled other defensive strategies to be developed, and it is these which we consider in the next chapter.

CHAPTER 4

Vaccination: Interrupting Spatial Disease Transmission

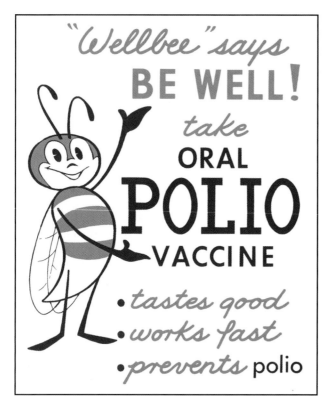

Figure 4.1 Poster to encourage the uptake of oral poliovirus vaccine (OPV) in the United States, 1963. The "Wellbee" character was first used in US public health promotion campaigns to promote the uptake of Sabin Type-II poliovirus vaccine. It was later incorporated into campaigns for the promotion of diphtheria and tetanus immunisation, hand washing, physical fitness and injury prevention. *Source*: CDC/Mary Hilpertshauser (CDC Public Health Image Library ID #7224).

4.1 Introduction

> The impact of vaccination on the health of the world's peoples is hard to exaggerate. With the exception of safe water, no other modality, not even antibiotics, has had such a major effect on mortality reduction and population growth.
>
> Susan and Stanley Plotkin (2008, p. 1)

Vaccines are broadly defined by Parish (1968, p. 2) as "preparations of *any* antigen which induces a specific active immunity to the corresponding infective agent". The term 'vaccine' stems from the Latin word *vacc(a)* (cow) and was originally applied to the material used by Edward Jenner to infect humans with cowpox, the antibodies to which provided protection against smallpox. Vaccination – the process of conferring immunity to diseases through the administration of a vaccine – is now considered to be among the safest and most effective of health interventions, and has been used as a means of controlling an expanding list of infectious diseases since the late eighteenth century. In this chapter, we briefly review the history of vaccination (Section 4.2) and the principles that underpin the use of vaccination as a disease control strategy (Section 4.3). We then examine the vaccine control of common childhood and other infections at the global level through the World Health Organization's Expanded Programme on Immunization (WHO-EPI) (Section 4.4) and at the national level through US strategies to eliminate the sustained indigenous transmission of poliomyelitis (**Figure 4.1**) and measles (Section 4.5). Finally, we look at the risks posed by faulty vaccines, vaccine scares and the spatially heterogeneous uptake of vaccines (Section 4.6). The chapter is concluded in Section 4.7.

4.2 History of Vaccination

Historical summaries of vaccination are provided by Parish (1965, 1968) and Plotkin and Plotkin (2008). Practices analogous to the process of conferring increased resistance to infection ('immunisation') can be traced to antiquity. Parish (1968), for example, cites Mithridates VI of Pontus (134–63 BC) who, in an endeavour to protect himself against assassination by poisoning, experimented with sub-lethal doses of toxins to engender a tolerance to their effects. The first recorded evidence of the artificial induction of immunity to an infectious disease agent dates to the late sixth century AD and Chinese descriptions of the process of variolation in which immunity to smallpox was induced by exposure to smallpox pus or scabs derived from mild cases of the disease. The practice of variolation, which may have developed independently in India, spread westwards in later centuries, reaching North Africa by the thirteenth century and Europe by the eighteenth century. As early as 1714, a letter to the *Philosophical Transactions* of the Royal Society described inoculations conducted in Turkey, while Lady Mary Wortley Montagu, wife of the English Ambassador to Constantinople, introduced the practice to the British court in the same decade. By the 1720s, variolation had become accepted as a medical practice in Britain, if not so in some other European countries. Elsewhere, in North America, the Reverend Cotton Mather (1663–1728) learnt of the practice of variolation in West Africa from his slaves. Mather persuaded a medical colleague (Dr Zabdiel Boylston) to introduce the practice and 280 patients were inoculated with a fatality rate well below the 15 percent in the control population (Parish, 1968; Fenner, *et al.*, 1988).

Early Vaccine Developments to 1900

The modern history of vaccines dates to the late eighteenth century and local knowledge from the southwest of England that dairy-farm workers who contracted cowpox were immune to smallpox. In 1774, Benjamin Jesty, a farmer in Dorset, drew on this knowledge to immunise experimentally his wife and sons against smallpox by exposing them to pustular material from a cow with cowpox. But it was the English physician, Edward Jenner (**Figure 4.2**), who studied and promoted the prophylactic powers of cowpox. On 14 May 1796, Jenner vaccinated James Phipps with material obtained from a pustule on the hand of a milkmaid. Six weeks later he attempted, without success, to infect Phipps with pus from a smallpox patient. After twelve more successful vaccinations, he privately published a report of his findings (**Figure 4.3**). Jenner's ideas were triumphant. It was as if " … an angel's trumpet had sounded over the earth" (Winslow, 1974; cited in Kiple, 1993, p. 1012). More than 100,000 were vaccinated in England in 1801 alone (cf. Figure 1.1). Within three years, Jenner's *Inquiry* had been translated into six languages. Between 1804 and 1814, two million were vaccinated in Russia, and so on across the industrialising world.

Jenner's ideas were taken up enthusiastically in the New World by Dr Benjamin Waterhouse of Boston. In 1800 he vaccinated four of his children and placed them in the smallpox hospital, a highly contaminated environment. Their successful survival provided a boost for the practice, despite the offsetting of uncontrolled vaccination by charlatans and sharks. As the nineteenth century progressed, so standardisation of vaccination practice began to show very positive results. Its benign effect on death rates was everywhere evident and, in disciplined countries like England, Sweden and Prussia, smallpox deaths towards the end of the century were moving towards zero (Fenner, *et al.*, 1988).

The Development of 'Scientific Immunisation'

While the early work on smallpox vaccine was empirical and undertaken with no knowledge of the aetiology of the disease, the development of what Parish (1968, p. 21) terms 'scientific immunisation' awaited advances on several fronts. Lancaster (1990) has tabulated the dates on which the 'modern' causes of 50 major diseases were established (see **Table 4.1**). Beginning with the identification of the intestinal worm *Trichinella spiralis* as the cause of trichniosis in 1835, the rate of detection of disease agents increased decade by decade from the 1830s until the 1880s when, in the golden age of bacteriology, the causes of nearly half the diseases listed were determined in a single decade. These advances, in turn, reflected the tools available for clinical examination and laboratory analysis. The compound microscope was not developed commercially until 1840; versions of the electron microscope to allow virus recognition did not appear until 1932, and entered general scientific use only from c. 1940. Examination of human tissues through the freezing, supporting and paraffin imbedding of samples was developed in 1843, 1853 and 1869 respectively. Stains for the study of cell structures began to be used from 1847.

Theory also played a critical role. Rokitansky's great text on systematic pathology was published between 1842 and 1846, while Virchow announced the cell theory in 1855. By the middle of the century, a small number of diseases had been shown to be caused by living organisms (Table 4.1) and Henle had given his closely-reasoned account of the hypothesis that infectious diseases were not the result of unspecified 'miasmas' but transmitted by living

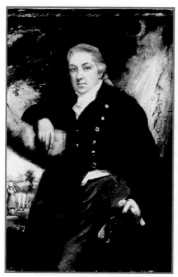
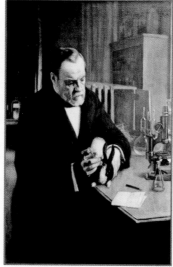
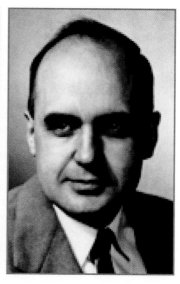

Figure 4.2 Three pioneers in the development of human vaccines. (*Left*) Edward Jenner (1749–1823), a Gloucestershire physician and one of the discoverers of smallpox vaccination. In 1775 he began to examine the truth of the traditions that cowpox provided some protection against smallpox. In 1796 he confirmed his hypotheses by successfully inoculating an eight-year-old patient. Artist: John Raphael Smith (pastel, 423 mm × 332 mm). (*Centre*) Louis Pasteur (1822–95), a French chemist and the first scientist to attenuate viruses artificially for use in vaccines. He created several veterinary vaccines (including a vaccine for chicken cholera, the first vaccine to be developed in a laboratory) before successfully administering his human rabies vaccine in 1885. (*Right*) Maurice Hilleman (1919–2005), pictured c. 1958. Hilleman was an American microbiologist who worked on the development of over 40 vaccines in the post-war years, including mumps, measles, rubella, hepatitis A and hepatitis B. *Sources*: (*left*) and (*centre*) Wellcome Library, London; (*right*) National Library of Medicine and the Walter Reed Army Medical Centre (Wikimedia Commons).

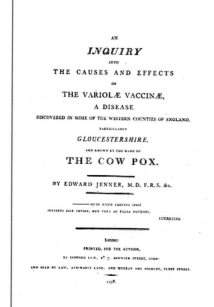
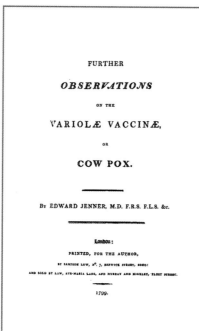

Figure 4.3 Jenner's treatise on smallpox vaccination. In 1798 Edward Jenner proposed inoculation without contagion, using cowpox pustules instead of smallpox pustules as the source of inoculation material. Title page of Jenner's self-published treatise on the subject from 1798 (*left*) and two subsequent publications offering further facts and observations from 1799 (*centre*) and 1800 (*right*).

Table 4.1 Discovery of the causes of 50 major human diseases, 1835–1935

Year	Disease	Modern name of organism	Discoverer
1835	Trichinosis	*Trichinella spiralis*	Paget, Owen
1843	Hookworm disease	*Ancylostoma duodenale*	Dubini
1849, 1876	Anthrax	*Bacillus anthracis*	Pollender, Koch
1853	Schistosomiasis	*Schistosoma mansoni*	Bilharz
1860, 1875	Amoebic dysentery	*Entamoeba histolytica*	Lambl, Loesch
1868	Leprosy	*Mycobacterium leprae*	Hansen
1868	Filariasis	*Wuchereria bancrofti*	Wucherer
1873	Relapsing fever	*Treponema recurrentis*	Obermeier
1877–78	Actinomycosis	*Actinomyces israeli*	Bollinger, Israel
1878–79, 1881	Suppuration	*Staphylococcus aureus*	Koch, Pasteur, Ogston
1879	Childbed fever	*Streptococcus pyogenes*	Pasteur
1879,1885	Gonorrhoea	*Neisseria gonorrhoeae*	Neisser, Bumm
1880	Malaria	*Plasmodium falciparum*	Laveran
1880,1884	Typhoid fever	*Salmonella typhi*	Eberth, Gaffky, Klebs, Koch
1881	Suppuration	*Streptococcus pyogenes*	Ogston
1881	Rabies	*Rabies virus*	Pasteur
1882	Glanders	*Pseudomonas mallei*	Loeffler & Schutz
1882	Tuberculosis	*Mycobacterium tuberculosis*	Koch
1882	Pneumonia	*Klebsiella aerogenes*	Friedländer
1883	Erysipelas	*Streptococcus pyogenes*	Fehleisen
1883	Cholera	*Vibrio cholerae*	Koch
1883–84	Diphtheria	*Corynebacterium diphtheriae*	Klebs, Loeffler
1884–89	Tetanus	*Clostridium tetani*	Nicolaeir, Kitasato
1886	Pneumonia	*Streptococcus pneumoniae*	Fraenkel
1886	Poliomyelitis	*Poliovirus*	Medin
1886, 1892	Smallpox	*Smallpox virus*	Buist, Guarnieri
1887	Cerebrospinal meningitis	*Neisseria meningitidis*	Weichselbaum
1887	Scarlet fever	*Streptococcus pyogenes*	Klein
1887	Undulant fever	*Brucella melitensis*	Bruce
1888	Food poisoning	*Salmonella enteritidis*	Gaertner
1889	Soft chancre	*Haemophilus ducreyi*	Ducrey
1892	Gas gangrene	*Clostridium welchii*	Welch
1894	Bubonic plague	*Yersinia pestis*	Kitasato, Yersin
1896	Botulism	*Clostridium botulinum*	Ermengem
1896	Bacillary dysentery	*Shigella shigae*	Shiga
1900	Paratyphoid fever	*Salmonella paratyphi*	Schottmüller
1901, 1903	Sleeping sickness	*Trypanosoma gambiense*	Forde, Bruce, Castellani
1903	Kala azar	*Leishmania donovani*	Leishman, Donovan
1905	Tick-borne relapsing fever	*Borrelia duttoni*	Dutton & Todd
1905	Syphilis	*Treponema pallidum*	Schaudinn & Hoffmann
1906	Whooping cough	*Bordetella pertussis*	Bordet & Gengou
1909	American trypanosomiasis	*Trypanosoma cruzi*	Chagas
1909	Bartonellosis	*Bartonella bacilliformis*	Barton
1911, 1938	Measles	*Measles virus*	Anderson & Goldberger, Plotz
1912	Tularemia	*Francisella tularensis*	McCoy & Chapin
1915	Leptospirosis	*Leptospira icterohaemorrhagiae*	Inada
1916	Typhus	*Rickettsia prowazekii*	Rocha Lima
1916	Rocky Mountain spotted fever	*Rickettsia rickettsii*	Ricketts
1917	Chickenpox	*Varicella-zoster virus*	Paschen
1933	Influenza	*Influenza A virus*	Smith, Andrewes & Laidlaw

Source: Cliff, *et al.* (1998, Table 1.5, pp. 22–3), modified from Lancaster (1990, Tables 2.3.1 and 2.3.2, pp. 16, 17).

organisms. The second half of the nineteenth century saw the heyday of bacteriological theory and practice with Louis Pasteur (1822–95), Ferdinand Cohn (1828–98) and Robert Koch (1843–1910) using the new laboratory tools to establish hypotheses of infection and contagion, often against entrenched opposition.

The early laboratory vaccines

The successful development of laboratory vaccines began with the pioneering work of the nineteenth-century French chemist, Louis Pasteur (Figure 4.2). Initially concerned with the development of attenuated veterinary vaccines for fowl cholera (1879), anthrax (1881) and, somewhat less successfully, swine erysipelas (1883), Pasteur's rabies vaccine (1885) was the first laboratory vaccine to make an impact on human disease. Pasteur developed both the theory and the experimental practice for attenuating the (then unknown) rabies virus in the spinal chords of rabbits. Having initially demonstrated the protective effect of the vaccine on dogs, the first human test of the vaccine came in July 1885 when a nine-year-old boy who had been bitten by a rabid dog two days earlier was brought to Pasteur's laboratory.

The successful development of vaccines against a series of major human bacterial diseases followed in short order. By 1896, the German scientist Wilhelm Kolle – an assistant to Robert Koch – had developed a heat-inactivated cholera vaccine that would serve as a model for cholera vaccines in the next century. In the same year, the British bacteriologist Almroth E. Wright developed a killed vaccine against typhoid fever that would subsequently be used by the British Army during the Second Boer War (1899–1902), while Waldemar Haffkine's plague vaccine was developed and introduced in India in 1896–97 (Parish, 1968).

Post-1900 Developments

While antitoxins and vaccines were developed for a range of bacterial diseases (including anthrax, cholera, diphtheria, plague, tetanus, typhoid and tuberculosis) in the early decades of the twentieth century, the rapid development of virus vaccines awaited the advent of the electron microscope, from the 1930s, and methods for the laboratory culture of viruses. Vaccines for poliomyelitis and other common childhood diseases such as measles, mumps, and rubella followed in quick succession (**Table 4.2**). In the late twentieth and early twenty-first centuries, new methods and techniques have been adopted in vaccine development (notably recombinant DNA technology), while vaccine research has expanded to include cancers and non-infectious conditions such as addictions and allergies. To illustrate the pace and dimensions of these developments, Table 4.2 gives the year in which sample vaccines and antitoxins were licensed/approved in the USA from the implementation of the Biologics Control Act (1902) to the early twenty-first century, while Figure 4.4 gives a timeline for the introduction of sample vaccines in the United Kingdom.

In Appendix 4.1, we survey the development of vaccines against common infectious diseases that, today, form a central part of the routine childhood immunisation schedules of many countries and whose administration has been promoted since 1974 by the World Health Organization's Expanded Programme on Immunization (WHO-EPI) (Section 4.4). These vaccines include those against diphtheria, tetanus, pertussis, poliomyelitis, measles, mumps and rubella, tuberculosis, *Haemophilus influenzae* type b, hepatitis B, invasive meningococcal and pneumococcal diseases and rotavirus gastroenteritis.

4.3 Vaccination Strategies and Disease Control

In Section 1.4, we saw how natural breaks in chains of infection for a specific disease can occur depending upon the sizes of the communities in which the disease agent is circulating. This gave rise to the notion of critical community size (*CCS*) – the population size of a community above which a sufficiently large stock of susceptibles will exist to enable the disease to be endemic – and below which the stock of susceptibles will not be large enough to maintain continuous chains of infection. In studies of the *CCS*, total population of a community is generally used as a convenient correlate of the difficult-to-estimate true susceptible population. Many studies have attempted to estimate the *CCS* for a range of common infectious diseases, and the results of these are summarised in **Table 4.3**, while Cliff, *et al.* (2000, pp. 85–117) have shown how the *CCS* is affected by factors such as geographical isolation and population density.

The basic notion of a threshold population below which an infectious disease becomes naturally self-extinguishing is paramount in articulating spatial control strategies. It implies that vaccination may be employed to reduce the susceptible population below some critical mass so that the chains of infection are broken. Once the susceptible population size of an area falls below the threshold then, when the disease concerned is eventually eliminated, it can only recur by reintroduction from other reservoir areas.

Critical Community Size, Vaccination and Disease Elimination

As shown in Table 4.3, the *CCS* for measles in an unvaccinated population is generally estimated to be around 250,000, above which the continuous epidemic chains displayed by settlement **A** in Figure 1.18C occur. In general, Griffiths (1973) has shown that the effect of vaccination is to raise the *CCS* for a given disease by a factor of $1/x^2$, where x is the proportion of the population that is not immunised by vaccination. Thus 50 percent immunisation against measles increases the critical community size from 250,000 to one million, while 90 percent immunisation increases the threshold to 25 million. So, for all practical purposes, when the percentage of the population vaccinated reaches the mid-90s, *herd immunity* is established and major epidemics will not occur; 100 percent vaccination is impossible to achieve because there always exist subgroups in a population who are inaccessible for any number of reasons (for example, objection to vaccination on religious grounds and inaccurate demographic recording). For a further consideration of the concept of *CCS* in relation to disease elimination, see Gay (2004).

Vaccination Impact on Epidemic Cycles

Although obviously not ideal, levels of vaccination well below herd immunity still severely disrupt chains of infection. **Figure 4.5** shows the predicted effect of partial immunisation against measles, sustained over 15 years, at 80 percent of the one- to two-year-olds in a theoretical population. The slow damping of epidemic amplitude is evident as the cumulative impact of vaccination is felt. Eventually the endemic cycle is broken and whole epidemics are missed. Thus natural fadeout becomes very widespread, enhancing the possibility of local elimination and long-run global eradication of a disease.

Table 4.2 Year in which sample vaccines and antitoxins were licensed/approved in the USA, 1902–2010[1]

Year	Disease	Vaccine
1914	**Rabies**	**Rabies vaccine**
1914	**Typhoid fever**	**Typhoid vaccine**
1915	**Pertussis**	**Pertussis vaccine**
1923	**Diphtheria**	**Diphtheria toxoid**
1935	**Yellow fever**	**Live yellow fever vaccine (17D)**
1937	**Tetanus**	**Adsorbed form of tetanus toxoid**
1945	**Influenza**	**Inactivated influenza vaccine**
1947	Diphtheria, tetanus	Combination diphtheria & tetanus toxoids
1949	Diphtheria, tetanus, pertussis	Diphtheria & tetanus toxoids & pertussis (DTP) vaccine
1952	Typhoid fever	Heat-phenol inactivated typhoid vaccine
1953	Yellow fever	Yellow fever vaccine
1953	Tetanus, diphtheria	Tetanus & diphtheria toxoids (adult formulation)
1955	**Poliomyelitis**	**Inactivated poliovirus vaccine (IPV)**
1961	Poliomyelitis	Oral polio vaccine (OPV) types 1 & 2
1962	Poliomyelitis	Oral polio vaccine (OPV) type 3
1963	**Measles**	**Inactivated measles vaccine (Pfizer-vax Measles-K)**
1963	Measles	Live virus measles vaccine (Rubeovax)
1963	Poliomyelitis	Trivalent oral polio vaccine (OPV)
1965	Measles	Live, further attenuated measles virus vaccine (Lirugen)
1967	**Mumps**	**Mumps virus vaccine live (MumpsVax)**
1968	Measles	Measles virus vaccine live (Attenuvax)
1969	**Rubella**	**Rubella virus vaccines (Rubelogen; Meruvax; Cendevax)**
1971	Measles, mumps, rubella	Combined measles, mumps & rubella (MMR) and measles & rubella (M-R-Vax) vaccines
1973	Measles, mumps	Measles & mumps virus vaccine live (M-M-Vax)
1974	**Invasive meningococcal disease**	**Monovalent (group C) meningococcal polysaccharide vaccine**
1977	**Invasive pneumococcal disease**	**Pneumococcal vaccine**
1978	Invasive meningococcal disease	Monovalent group A (Menomune-A), group C (Menomune-C) and bivalent groups A & C (Menomune-A/C) vaccines
1978	Yellow fever	Yellow fever vaccine (YF-Vax)
1979	Rubella	Rubella virus vaccine live (Meruvax)
1980	Rabies	Rabies vaccines (Imovax Rabies & Wyvac)
1981	Invasive meningococcal disease	Meningococcal polysaccharide vaccine, groups A, C, Y & W-135 Combined (Menomune A/C/Y/W-135)
1981	**Hepatitis B**	**Hepatitis B viral vaccines**
1983	Invasive pneumococcal disease	Enhanced pneumococcal polysaccharide vaccines (Pneumovax & Pnu-Imune)
1985	**Invasive Hib disease**	***Haemophilus influenzae* type b (Hib) polysaccharide vaccines (b-CAPSA 1, Hib-VAX & Hib-IMUNE)**
1986	Hepatitis B	Hepatitis B vaccine (recombinant) (Recombivax)
1987	Invasive Hib disease	Protein-conjugated *Haemophilus influenzae* type b vaccine (ProHibit)
1988	Invasive Hib disease	Conjugated *Haemophilus influenzae* type b vaccine (HibTITER)
1989	Hepatitis B	Hepatitis B vaccine (recombinant) (Engerix-B)
1989	Typhoid fever	Typhoid vaccine live oral Ty21a (Vivotif)
1989	Invasive Hib disease	*Haemophilus* b conjugate vaccine (PedvaxHIB)
1990	Poliomyelitis	Poliovirus vaccine inactivated (Ipol)
1991	Diphtheria, tetanus, pertussis	Diphtheria & tetanus toxoids & acellular pertussis vaccine (Acel-Imune) for use as fourth & fifth doses
1992	Diphtheria, tetanus, pertussis	Diphtheria & tetanus toxoids & acellular pertussis vaccine adsorbed (Tripedia by Connaught) for use as fourth & fifth doses
1993	Invasive Hib disease, diphtheria, tetanus, pertussis	Combined Hib & whole cell DTP vaccine (Tetramune)
1993	Invasive Hib disease	*Haemophilus* b conjugate vaccines (ActHIB and OmniHib)
1994	Typhoid fever	Typhoid Vi polysaccharide vaccine (Typhim Vi)
1995	Varicella virus	Varicella virus vaccine live (Varivax)
1995	**Hepatitis A**	**Hepatitis A vaccine, inactivated (Havrix)**
1996	Hepatitis A	Hepatitis A vaccine, inactivated (Vaqta)

Table 4.2 (*Continued*)

Year	Disease	Vaccine
1996	Invasive Hib disease, Hepatitis B	*Haemophilus* b conjugate vaccine (meningococcal protein conjugate) & hepatitis B vaccine (recombinant) (Comvax)
1996	Diphtheria, tetanus, pertussis	Diphtheria & tetanus toxoids & acellular pertussis vaccine adsorbed (Tripedia by Aventis Pasteur)
1996	Diphtheria, tetanus, pertussis, invasive Hib disease	Combination diphtheria & tetanus toxoids & acellular pertussis & Hib vaccine (TriHIBit)
1996	Diphtheria, tetanus, pertussis	Diphtheria & tetanus toxoids & acellular pertussis vaccine (Acel-Imune)
1997	Diphtheria, tetanus, pertussis	Diphtheria & tetanus toxoids & acellular pertussis vaccine adsorbed (Infanrix)
1997	Rabies	Rabies vaccine (RabAvert)
1998	Diphtheria, tetanus, pertussis	Diphtheria & tetanus toxoids & acellular pertussis vaccine adsorbed (Certiva)
1998	**Rotavirus gastroenteritis**	**Rotavirus vaccine, live, oral, tetravalent (RotaShield)**
1998	**Lyme disease**	**Lyme disease vaccine (recombinant) (LYMErix)**
1999	Diphtheria, tetanus, pertussis	Diphtheria & tetanus toxoids & acellular pertussis vaccine adsorbed (Tripedia by Connaught)
2000	Invasive pneumococcal disease	Pneumococcal 7-valent conjugate vaccine (Prevnar)
2001	Hepatitis A, B	Hepatitis A inactivated & hepatitis B (recombinant) vaccine (Twinrix)
2002	Diphtheria, tetanus, pertussis	Diphtheria & tetanus toxoids & acellular pertussis vaccine adsorbed (Daptacel)
2002	Diphtheria, tetanus, pertussis, hepatitis B and poliomyelitis	Diphtheria & tetanus toxoids & acellular pertussis vaccine adsorbed, hepatitis B (recombinant) & inactivated poliovirus vaccine combined (Pediarix)
2003	Influenza A, B	Influenza vaccine, live, intranasal (FluMist)
2004	Tetanus, diphtheria	Tetanus & diphtheria toxoids adsorbed for adult use (Decavac)
2005	Invasive meningococcal disease	Meningococcal polysaccharide (serogroups A, C, Y & W-135) diphtheria toxoid conjugate vaccine (Menactra)
2005	Tetanus, diphtheria, pertussis	Tetanus toxoid, reduced diphtheria toxoid & acellular pertussis vaccines, adsorbed (Adacel, Boostrix)
2005	Influenza	Influenza virus vaccine, trivalent, types A & B (Fluarix)
2005	Measles, mumps, rubella, varicella virus	Measles, mumps, rubella & varicella virus vaccine live (Proquad)
2006	Rotavirus gastroenteritis	Rotavirus vaccine, live, oral, pentavalent (RotaTeq)
2006	**Cervical cancer, genital warts**	**Human papillomavirus quadrivalent (Types 6, 11, 16, 18) vaccine, recombinant (Gardasil)**
2007	Influenza A/H5N1	Influenza virus vaccine, H5N1
2007	Influenza A, B	Inactivated influenza virus vaccine (Afluria)
2008	Rotavirus gastroenteritis	Rotavirus vaccine, live, oral (Rotarix)
2008	Diphtheria, tetanus, pertussis, poliomyelitis	DTaP-IPV vaccine (Kinrix)
2009	Influenza	Influenza A (H1N1) 2009 monovalent vaccines
2009	Cervical cancer	Human papillomavirus bivalent (Types 16, 18) vaccine, recombinant (Cervarix)
2009	Influenza A, B	Inactivated influenza virus vaccine, trivalent, types A & B (Fluzone High-Dose)
2010	Invasive pneumococcal disease	Pneumococcal 13-valent conjugate vaccine (Prevnar 13)

Notes: [1] The earliest licensed vaccines for sample diseases are shown in bold.

Source: data from the U.S. Food and Drug Administration (FDA).

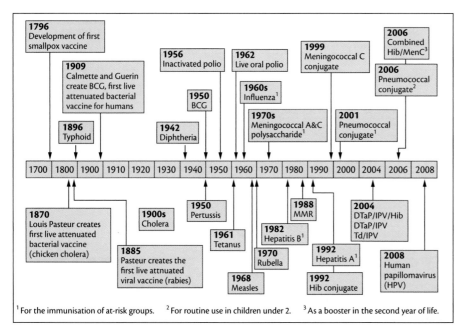

Figure 4.4 Timeline of vaccine developments and the introduction of vaccines in the United Kingdom, 1796–2008. BCG (Bacillus Calmette-Guérin) tuberculosis vaccine. Hib (*Haemophilus influenzae* type b) vaccine. MMR (measles, mumps and rubella) combined vaccine. DTaP (diphtheria and tetanus toxoids, and acellular pertussis) vaccine. IPV (inactivated poliovirus vaccine). Td (tetanus and diphtheria toxoids) vaccine for adults. DTaP/IPV, DTaP/IPV/Hib and Td/IPV are combined preparations. *Source*: adapted from National Health Service (NHS) website.

Table 4.3 Critical community size and disease properties: Icelandic evidence, 1888–1988

Disease	Transmission	Immunity	Critical community size (thousands)		Normal infectious period in days (rank, 1 = shortest)
			Quoted[1]	Estimated CCS: Iceland	
Scarlet fever	Intimate contact	Some repeat cases		48	15 (3)
Diphtheria	Normal contact	Usually lasting		67	21 (5)
Whooping cough	Airborne droplet	Lasting		106	18 (4)
Rubella	Airborne droplet	Lasting	132	151	7 (2=)
Measles	Airborne droplet	Lasting	250–500	259	7 (2=)
Influenza	Airborne droplet	Specific	1,000,000	102	5 (1)

Notes: [1] Ramsay and Emond (1978); Yorke, *et al.* (1979); Cliff, *et al.* (1986); and Cliff and Haggett (1990).

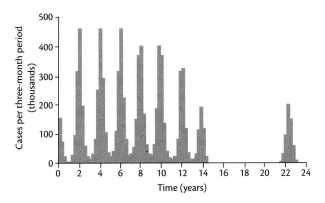

Figure 4.5 Predicted effects of widespread measles immunisation.
Application of the *SIR* model with the level of immunisation held constant for 15 years at 80 percent of one- to two-year-olds. *Source:* redrawn from Cliff, Smallman-Raynor, Haggett, *et al.* (2009, Figure 11.17, p. 654), adapted from Cutts (1990, Figure 10, p. 23).

Ring Vaccination Strategies

The use of vaccination to establish a containing 'ring of immunity' around outbreaks has been considered by a number of workers; see, for example, Greenhalgh (1986) and Cliff and Haggett (1989). While the approach has occasionally been invoked for infectious diseases in human populations (Kretzschmar, *et al.*, 2004; Lau, *et al.*, 2005), the principles involved are readily illustrated by disease outbreaks among farm animals and we draw here on Tinline's (1972) study of foot-and-mouth disease (FMD) in cattle.

Based on data relating to the 1967–68 epizootic of FMD in the United Kingdom, Tinline demonstrated that airborne spread of FMD virus downwind of an initially infected area was an important cause of additional disease outbreaks during the epizootic. To contain the disease, therefore, Tinline investigated the possibility of implementing vaccination in areas downwind of an initial outbreak in order to create a 'buffer zone' of immunity across which the virus could not easily pass. The principles involved are illustrated in **Figure 4.6A**. In the upper-left map of Figure 4.6A, the immediate ('blanket') vaccination of all herds downwind of the initial outbreak is called on confirmation of the outbreak. Recognising the manpower difficulties in the implementation of such a scheme, the remaining maps provide different schemes for the priority order (cell codes 1 and 2) of vaccine delivery. The results of simulations to test the efficacy of the different schemes are summarised in Figure 4.6B. With the exception of blanket vaccination, which would reduce the number of FMD cases to just 14 percent of the no vaccination scenario, Tinline identified ring vaccination scheme III as the most successful in reducing FMD transmission. The key feature of this scheme is the prioritisation of vaccination from the outside, in towards the initially infected area. Practical difficulties arise, however, in the implementation of such ring vaccination strategies, including the need for accurate 20-day wind forecasts from the date of the initial onset of the FMD outbreak; see Cliff and Haggett (1989) and Haggett (2000).

Applications: Equine Influenza in Eastern Australia

Perkins, *et al.* (2011) provide an example of the practical application of ring vaccination, in conjunction with blanket vaccination and predictive vaccination strategies, to contain an outbreak of equine influenza among horses in New South Wales and Queensland, Australia, in 2007 (**Figure 4.7**, located in the colour plate section). Ring vaccination of horses was implemented through the establishment of 'vaccination buffer zones' – strips or corridors of land that were typically ≥ 10 km wide and which were formed around infection foci with the view to limiting the lateral transmission of equine influenza by wind or other local spread mechanisms. Within the buffer zones, the objective was to vaccinate a sufficiently high proportion of horses to yield a barrier of immunity that would inhibit the spatial transmission of natural infection. The vaccination buffer zones in New South Wales were positioned sufficiently far away from areas of active infection to allow time for the development of immunity in vaccinated horses, and were formed in relation to natural geographical barriers, including lakes, escarpments and expanses of land in which horses were known to be absent. Within the buffer zones, vaccination was prioritised from the outside, in towards the infection foci (cf. Tinline's ring vaccination schemes II and III in Figure 4.6). Queensland adopted a broadly similar approach, with an initial outer vaccination buffer zone, supplemented by an inner buffer zone when it became apparent that the rate of expansion of the disease in the area had begun to slow. Although the control of the outbreak was ultimately attributable to a range of control strategies that included movement controls and the implementation of biosecurity measures, available evidence suggests that equine influenza breached the vaccination buffer zones on only two occasions (Perkins, *et al.*, 2011).

A

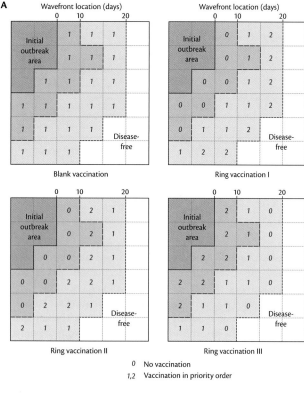

B

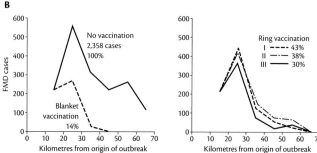

Figure 4.6 Ring vaccination schemes to control the spread of FMD virus. Tinline's simulations of alternative vaccination schemes to control the spread of the 1967–68 epizootic of FMD among cattle herds in central England. (A) Prioritisation of vaccination of herds downwind of an initial outbreak (grey shaded) area. Each cell represents a 10 km × 10 km area, with priority of vaccination indicated by codes 1 (first priority) and 2 (second priority); code 0 = no vaccination. (B) Results of simulations of the number of FMD cases with distance from the initial outbreak area for no vaccination and blanket vaccination schemes (left) and for ring vaccination schemes I–III (right). Percentage estimates of the number of FMD cases in a given vaccination scenario, relative to the no vaccination scenario (= 100 percent), are given. *Source*: redrawn from Haggett (2000, Figure 4.10, p. 118), from Tinline (1972).

4.4 Global Programmes: The Expanded Programme on Immunization (EPI)

In Section 5.2, we examine one of the outstanding achievements of the World Health Organization (WHO): the global eradication of smallpox. Although the final eradication of smallpox was not formally announced by the WHO until December 1979, confidence was growing by the early 1970s that this would eventually be achieved. At this time, therefore, policy advisors both within and outside the WHO looked for an initiative which could become a successor to the smallpox eradication campaign. Representatives from industrialised countries, particularly those from Europe, were now seeing the results from their own immunisation programmes against a variety of childhood diseases and urged that these diseases be made the new WHO target area. The resolution creating the Expanded Programme on Immunization (EPI) was adopted by the World Health Assembly in 1974, with the initial aim of targeting six vaccine-preventable diseases (diphtheria, measles, pertussis, poliomyelitis, tetanus and tuberculosis) for a substantial reduction in global incidence. The term 'expanded' was used to recognise the fact that immunisation services of some sort already existed in virtually all countries. It indicated that the WHO programme would work to increase them, both in terms of coverage of the susceptible population and in terms of the number of antigens being used.

Programme policies of the EPI were formalised by the World Health Assembly in 1977. It was at this time that the twin goals were set of: (i) providing immunisation services for all children of the world by 1990 and (ii) giving priority to developing countries. In the formal terms of the policy documents, the EPI is "a worldwide collaborative programme of Member States in the sense that it aims at total coverage of susceptible populations and age-groups throughout the world, irrespective of whether or not WHO is directly involved" (Keja and Henderson, 1984, p. 2).

When the EPI began, no global immunisation information system existed and best guesses were that vaccine coverage for the six EPI target diseases was < 10 percent in developing countries (excluding China). In light of knowledge subsequently obtained, it seems likely that the figure was actually < 5 percent. From this low baseline, immunisation services in developing countries were extended to almost 80 percent of children (aged < 1 year) by the mid-1990s (Bland and Clements, 1998). Nevertheless, some 34 million children were being born each year in areas of the world that lacked adequate immunisation programmes. In response, the Global Alliance for Vaccines and Immunization (GAVI) was established in 2000 with the specific aim of promoting the reach of the EPI in the world's poorest countries. The GAVI Alliance is formed as a coalition of UN agencies and institutions (WHO, UNICEF and the World Bank), the Bill and Melinda Gates Foundation, the Rockefeller Foundation, the vaccine industry, NGOs, and donor and implementing countries, among others. National governments of 72 countries with a gross national income (GNI) per capita of < US$1,000 in 2003 are eligible to apply for support from the GAVI Alliance for the supply of vaccines and the strengthening of health systems and immunisation services.

EPI and the Global Immunization Vision and Strategy (GIVS)

The operations of the EPI are currently set within the framework of the Global Immunization Vision and Strategy (GIVS). GIVS was launched as a collaborative initiative of the WHO and UNICEF in 2006 with the aim of providing a 10-year framework for controlling morbidity and mortality from vaccine-preventable diseases. As described in the GIVS framework document (World Health Organization, 2005a), the strategic areas of GIVS include: (i) the immunisation of more people against more diseases; (ii) the introduction of new vaccines and technologies; (iii) the integration of other critical health interventions with immunisation; and (iv) the management of vaccination programmes within the context of global interdependence. The specific goals of GIVS are summarised in **Table 4.4**. Set relative to the year 2000, these goals include a two-thirds (or greater) reduction in childhood morbidity and mortality due to vaccine-preventable diseases by 2015 – a contribution to achieving the United Nations' Millennium Development Goal 4 ('to reduce childhood mortality').

Additional EPI Target Diseases

Within the framework of GIVS, the EPI has been charged with continuing to promote the introduction of appropriate new vaccines into national immunisation programmes. The original six EPI target diseases were selected in 1974 on the basis of their high incidence in countries around the world and the availability of safe, effective and affordable vaccines. As new vaccines have been developed, so additional diseases have been added to the EPI list. Many countries have included *H. influenzae* type b (Hib) and hepatitis B vaccines in their routine infant immunisation schedules. A number of countries are also in the process of including pneumococcal conjugate vaccine, rotavirus vaccine and human papillomavirus vaccine, while yellow fever vaccine has been included in some at-risk countries.

Trends in Global Vaccine Coverage

Regional overviews of immunisation practices in the twenty-first century are provided in Plotkin, *et al.* (2008, pp. 1479–1571). **Figure 4.8** plots, as line traces, WHO/UNICEF estimates (broken line traces) and officially reported levels (full line traces) of annual global vaccine coverage for the six original EPI target diseases (graphs A–G) and three additional target diseases (graphs H–J) in the 30 years to 2009. The discrepancies between the two sets of coverage data arise from situations in which the official reports, supplied by WHO member states, are deemed by the WHO/UNICEF to be compromised and therefore potentially misleading (Burton, *et al.*, 2009; World Health Organization, 2010a). Global counts of the target diseases are plotted, where available, as the bar charts.

The Original EPI Target Diseases

A prominent feature of Figures 4.8A–G is the rapid increase during the 1980s in global vaccine coverage for the six original EPI target diseases. This development was driven by the push to achieve the WHO/UNICEF goals for Universal Childhood Immunization, with the specific aim of immunising 80 percent of all children by 1990 (**Figure 4.9**). The increase in global vaccine coverage at this time was attributable to both an increase in the number of WHO member states that had established immunisation services and to an increase in vaccine coverage in these member states, most notably in the WHO Regions of Africa, Eastern Mediterranean, South-East Asia and the Western Pacific. Thereafter, global vaccine coverage for the target diseases grew steadily, with WHO/UNICEF estimates ranging between 75 and 88 percent in 2009. Some impression of the associated reduction in disease activity is provided by the bar charts, and by **Table 4.5** which gives the global incidence of the EPI target diseases in 1980 and 2009. Over the 30-year interval, reported measles cases fell from > 4.21 million (1980) to < 0.23 million (2009), diphtheria from little under 100,000 cases (1980) to < 1,000 cases (2009), while pertussis fell from > 1.98 million cases to < 0.11 million cases (World Health Organization, 2010a).

Additional EPI Target Diseases

An increasing proportion of WHO member states have incorporated Hib (Figure 4.8H) and hepatitis B (Figure 4.8I) vaccines into routine immunisation services since the 1990s, with WHO/UNICEF estimates of global vaccine coverage rising to 38 percent (Hib) and 70 percent (hepatitis B) of the respective target populations by 2009. Of the 45 member states and territories of the WHO Africa (31), Americas (12) and Eastern Mediterranean (2) Regions that are deemed to be at risk for yellow fever, 35 had incorporated yellow fever into their routine immunisation schedules by 2009 and vaccine coverage approximated 50 percent (Figure 4.8J). Additional vaccines had also been incorporated into the routine immunisation schedules of WHO member states by 2009, including pneumococcal

Table 4.4 Key goals of the WHO-UNICEF Global Immunization Vision and Strategy (GIVS)

By 2010 or earlier
• **Increase coverage.** Countries will reach at least 90% national vaccination coverage and at least 80% vaccination coverage in every district or equivalent administrative unit.
• **Reduce measles mortality.** Globally, mortality due to measles will have been reduced by 90% compared to the 2000 level.
By 2015 or earlier
• **Sustain coverage**. The vaccination coverage goal reached in 2010 will have been sustained.
• **Reduce morbidity and mortality.** Global childhood morbidity and mortality due to vaccine-preventable diseases will have been reduced by at least two-thirds compared to 2000 levels.
• **Ensure access to vaccines of assured quality.** Every person eligible for immunisation included in national programmes will have been offered vaccination with vaccines of assured quality according to established national schedules.
• **Introduce new vaccines.** Immunisation with newly-introduced vaccines will have been offered to the entire eligible population within five years of the introduction of these new vaccines in national programmes.
• **Ensure capacity for surveillance and monitoring.** All countries will have developed the capacity at all levels to conduct case-based surveillance of vaccine-preventable diseases, supported by laboratory confirmation where necessary, in order to measure vaccine coverage accurately and use these data appropriately.
• **Strengthen systems.** All national immunisation plans will have been formulated as an integral component of sector-wide plans for human resources, financing and logistics.
• **Assure sustainability.** All national immunisation plans will have been formulated, costed and implemented so as to ensure that human resources, funding and supplies are adequate.

Source: World Health Organization (www.who.int).

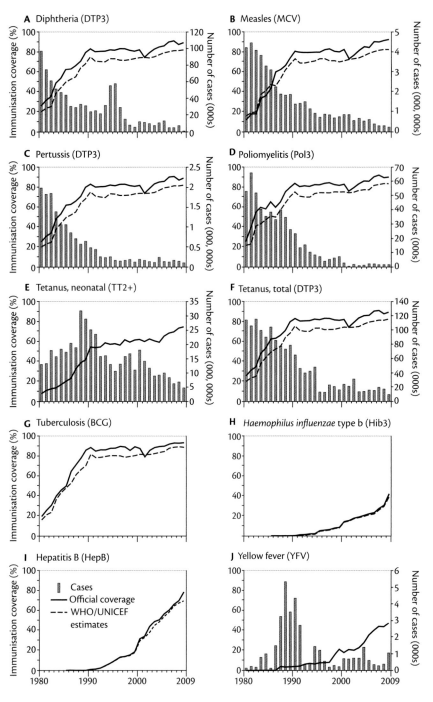

Figure 4.8 Trends in global vaccine coverage, 1980–2009. Official reports by WHO member states (full line traces) and WHO/UNICEF estimates (broken line traces) of annual global vaccine coverage for the original six EPI target diseases (graphs A–G) and for three additional target diseases (H–J). Vaccine coverage is expressed as a percentage of the target population for vaccination, most commonly formed as the number of infants surviving the first year of life. Bar charts plot the global count of reported cases of sample diseases. (A) Diphtheria, coverage with the third dose of diphtheria, tetanus and pertussis vaccine (DTP3) at < 1 year of age. (B) Measles, coverage with the first dose of measles-containing vaccine (MCV) at < 1 year of age. (C) Pertussis, coverage with the third dose of diphtheria, tetanus and pertussis vaccine (DTP3) at < 1 year of age. (D) Poliomyelitis, coverage with the third dose of oral or inactivated poliovirus vaccine (Pol3) at < 1 year of age. (E) Tetanus (neonatal), coverage with at least two doses of tetanus toxoid (TT2+) among pregnant women in priority countries for neonatal tetanus elimination and developing countries where tetanus is in the national immunisation schedule for women of childbearing-age. (F) Tetanus (total), coverage with the third dose of diphtheria, tetanus and pertussis vaccine (DTP3) at < 1 year of age. (G) Tuberculosis, coverage with BCG vaccine at < 1 year of age. (H) *H. influenzae* type b, coverage with the third dose of *H. influenzae* type b vaccine (Hib3) at < 1 year of age. (I) Hepatitis B, coverage with the third dose of hepatitis B vaccine (HepB) at < 1 year of age. (J) Yellow fever, coverage with yellow fever vaccine (YFV) at < 1 year of age in countries that are considered to be at risk for the disease. *Source*: redrawn from World Health Organization (2010a, pp. 8, 10, 12, 14, 16, 18, 20, 22, 24, 26).

conjugate (44 member states), rotavirus (22), rubella (130) and human papillomavirus (29) vaccines (World Health Organization, 2010a).

Regional Contexts: WHO Western Pacific Region

As Figure 2.31 shows, the WHO Western Pacific Region (WPR) encompasses a vast swathe of continental east Asia and the western Pacific Ocean. In 2010, the combined population of the region's 27 member states was 1,776 million, with China (1,336 million), Japan (128 million), Philippines (88 million) and Vietnam (87 million) as the most populous states and the remote south Pacific islands of Tuvalu (11,000), Nauru (10,000), and Niue (2,000) as the least populous.

In the 1970s and 1980s, the establishment of routine immunisation systems for the EPI target diseases formed the main focus of EPI activities in the region (**Figure 4.10**). With the 1988 resolution of the World Health Assembly to eradicate poliomyelitis globally (Section 5.3), the WPR-EPI entered a new phase that centred on disease eradication, elimination and accelerated control. Sustained interruption of wild poliovirus transmission was achieved within 10 years (Figure 4.10D); the last indigenous cases of the disease were recorded in 1997 and the Western Pacific Region was certified to be poliomyelitis-free on 29 October 2000 (**Figure 4.11**).

The poliomyelitis eradication initiative resulted in substantial investment in resources and had the effect of strengthening routine

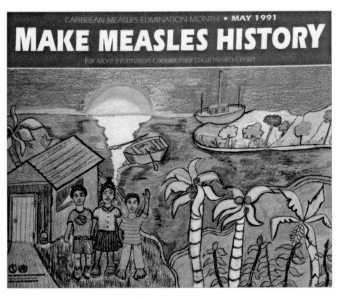

Figure 4.9 The Expanded Program on Immunization in the Americas. The 'Make Measles History' campaign was launched when the Caucus of Caribbean Community and Common Market (CARICOM) Ministers Responsible for Health resolved, in 1988, to eliminate the indigenous transmission of measles in the Caribbean by 1995. A primary strategy of the campaign was to immunise simultaneously all susceptible people in the region and, to these ends, May 1991 was declared 'Measles Elimination Month'. In this month, an attempt was made to immunise all people aged < 15 years against measles, regardless of vaccination status or measles history. *Source*: Castillo-Solórzano, *et al.* (2009, unnumbered plate, p. 5).

Table 4.5 Reported global incidence of WHO EPI target diseases, 1980 and 2009

Disease	Global incidence	
	1980	2009
Original EPI target diseases		
Diphtheria	97,511	857
Measles	4,211,431	222,408
Pertussis	1,982,355	106,207
Poliomyelitis	52,795	1,779
Tetanus		
neonatal	13,005	4,712
total	114,251	9,836
Tuberculosis	–	–
Additional EPI target diseases		
H. influenzae type b	–	–
Hepatitis B	–	–
Yellow fever	144	1,044

Source: data from World Health Organization (2010a).

immunisation services in WPR member states (Alward, *et al.*, 1997). This has contributed to a substantial decline in the incidence of diseases such as diphtheria (Figure 4.10A), pertussis (4.10C) and tetanus (4.10E), while new initiatives have followed. In 2003, the WPR Regional Committee Meeting established the twin goals of measles elimination (Figure 4.10B) and hepatitis B control (4.10H) by 2012. In addition, new and underutilised vaccines, including Hib (Figure 4.10G), pneumococcal, rotavirus and Japanese encephalitis vaccines, have been targeted for increased use (Clements, *et al.*, 2006; WHO Western Pacific Region, 2008).

Beyond the EPI: Towards Second-Generation Programmes?

John, *et al.* (2011) suggest that one of the original objectives of the EPI, namely the development of vaccination programmes and sustainable infrastructure for their delivery in low- and middle-income countries, has been achieved. But the higher objective of the control of the EPI target diseases requires a second-generation programme that builds upon and subsumes the achievements of the EPI; a programme that has clear objectives to control a cluster of childhood diseases, and one whose outcomes are measured in terms of disease reduction rather than vaccine coverage. John, *et al.* (2011) propose that this second-generation programme could be named Control of Childhood Communicable Diseases (CCCD). CCCD would provide a platform for the integration of vertical disease control programmes from which to establish a public health infrastructure for childhood disease control in lower and middle-income countries. In addition to immunisation, such a programme would include: (i) the systematic reporting of diseases; (ii) the analysis and monitoring

of diseases; (iii) the investigation of the occurrence of diseases that have been designated for control; and (iv) action to prevent, control and eliminate diseases and disease outbreaks.

4.5 National Programmes: Mass Vaccination and Disease Elimination in the United States

A review of immunisation in the United States is provided by Orenstein, *et al.* (2008). In this section, we examine how US programmes for the elimination of two major viral diseases of children, poliomyelitis and measles, have been articulated. Our account draws, in part, on Smallman-Raynor, *et al.* (2006, pp. 433–68) and Cliff, *et al.* (1993, pp. 217–44).

Poliomyelitis

The development and mass administration of safe and effective poliovirus vaccines has been one of the important public health achievements of the United States in the post-war era. The licensing of Salk's inactivated poliovirus vaccine (IPV) in April 1955 marked the first specific federal involvement in immunisation (Orenstein, *et al.*, 2008) and was accompanied by a dramatic reduction in disease incidence. But it was the introduction and mass administration of Sabin's live attenuated oral poliovirus vaccine (OPV) from the early 1960s (Figure 4.1) that finally broke the chain of wild poliovirus transmission. Some impression of the scale and timing of the US vaccination programme required to effect the control of indigenous wild poliovirus is provided by **Figure 4.12**. In the words of Schonberger, *et al.* (1984, p. S424),

The successful control ... involved the total net distribution of ~483 × 10⁶ doses of inactivated poliovirus vaccine (IPV), ~114 × 10⁶ doses of each of the three types of monovalent oral poliovirus vaccine (MOPV), and ~423 × 10⁶ doses of trivalent oral poliovirus vaccine

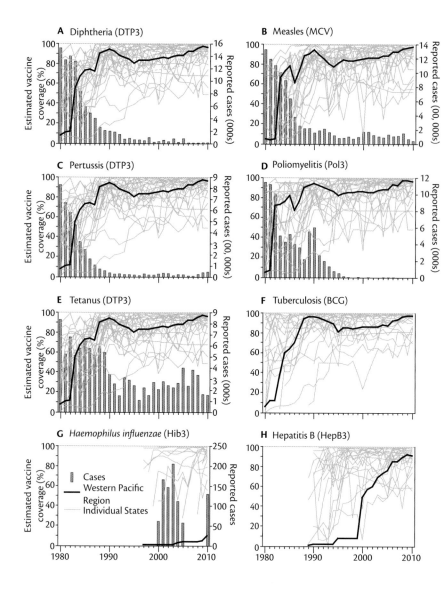

Figure 4.10 Trends in vaccine coverage in the WHO Western Pacific Region, 1980–2010. WHO/UNICEF estimates of annual vaccine coverage for the original six EPI target diseases (graphs A–F) and for two additional target diseases (G, H) for individual member states (fine line traces) and for the Western Pacific Region as a whole (heavy line trace). Vaccine coverage is expressed as a percentage of the target population for vaccination. Bar charts plot the regional count of reported cases for sample diseases. (A) Diphtheria, coverage with the third dose of diphtheria, tetanus and pertussis vaccine (DTP3). (B) Measles, coverage with the first dose of measles-containing vaccine (MCV). (C) Pertussis, coverage with the third dose of diphtheria, tetanus and pertussis vaccine (DTP3). (D) Poliomyelitis, coverage with the third dose of oral or inactivated poliovirus vaccine (Pol3). (E) Tetanus (total), coverage with the third dose of diphtheria, tetanus and pertussis vaccine (DTP3). (F) Tuberculosis, coverage with Bacille Calmette-Guérin (BCG) vaccine. (G) *H. influenzae* type b, coverage with the third dose of *H. influenzae* type b vaccine (Hib3). (H) Hepatitis B, coverage with the third dose of hepatitis B vaccine (HepB). *Source*: data from World Health Organization.

(TOPV). Almost 90% of the IPV was distributed between 1955 ... and 1962 but as many as 5.5×10^6 doses were distributed in 1966, 4.0×10^6 doses in 1967, and 2.7×10^6 doses in 1968. About 93 percent of the doses of MOPV were distributed during 1962–1964, a fact that reflects the emphasis given to vaccinating both children and adults in mass vaccination campaigns and community-wide programs. Since the switch in 1965 to the current practice of routine vaccination of infants with TOPV, the annual distribution of TOPV has remained relatively stable, averaging ~23×10^6 doses.

The massive uptake of both IPV and OPV had an immediate and dramatic impact on the US poliomyelitis curve (**Figure 4.13**). The first year of immunisation with Salk vaccine resulted in a 47 percent reduction in notified cases, with a further 64 percent reduction in the following year. A decade or so later, in 1967, only 41 cases of poliomyelitis were reported throughout the United States, representing a decrease of 99.7 percent in notified cases since vaccination began. By January 1972, the incidence of the disease was deemed too low to justify the routine reporting of notifications in the flagship US disease surveillance report, *Morbidity and Mortality*

Weekly Report (*MMWR*), while poliomyelitis associated with wild poliovirus – including importations – had fallen to near-zero levels by the early 1980s (Schonberger, *et al.*, 1984).

The Geography of Vaccine-Induced Poliomyelitis Retreat, 1955–71

Between the onset of poliovirus vaccination in April 1955 and December 1971, some 70,300 cases of the disease were notified in the conterminous United States – a case total that was underpinned by annual epidemic upswings of rapidly diminishing magnitude to virtual extinction in the late 1950s and early 1960s (Figure 4.13). **Figure 4.14** plots, as a monthly average, the state-level poliomyelitis notification rate per 100,000 population for April 1955–December 1971 (map D); the equivalent information for time intervals in the pre-vaccination phase (July 1910–March 1955, maps A–C) is shown for reference. From an established pattern of raised activity in the interval 1941–55, Figure 4.14D shows that the introduction of mass poliovirus vaccination was accompanied by a marked contraction in levels of poliomyelitis incidence. Average monthly case

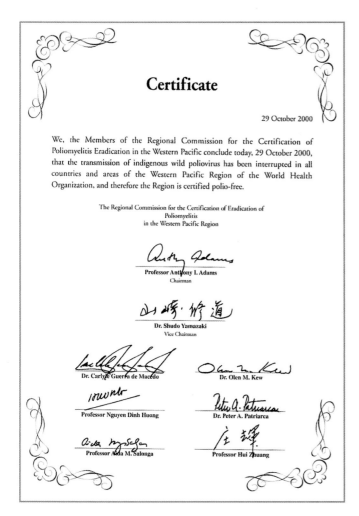

Figure 4.11 Certificate for the eradication of poliomyelitis in the WHO Western Pacific Region, 29 October 2000.

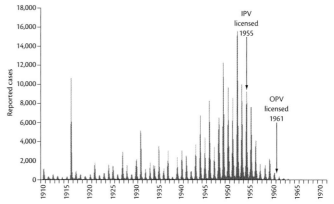

Figure 4.13 Monthly count of poliomyelitis notifications in the conterminous United States, 1910–71. The years in which Salk's inactivated poliovirus vaccine (IPV) and Sabin's oral poliovirus vaccine (OPV) were first licensed in the United States are indicated.

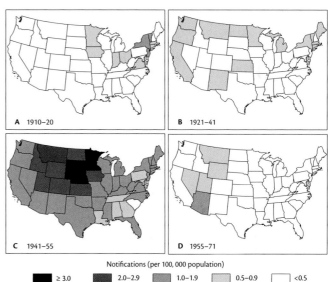

Notifications (per 100, 000 population)

≥ 3.0 ■ 2.0–2.9 1.0–1.9 0.5–0.9 <0.5

Figure 4.14 Average monthly rate of poliomyelitis notifications (per 100,000 population) by state, conterminous United States, 1910–71. Map (D) plots the average monthly rate of poliomyelitis notifications for the vaccination phase (April 1955–December 1971). As a benchmark, Maps (A)–(C) plot the equivalent information for time intervals in the pre-vaccination phase (July 1910–March 1955). *Source*: adapted from Smallman-Raynor, *et al.* (2006, Figures 7.3 and 10.6, pp. 270, 446).

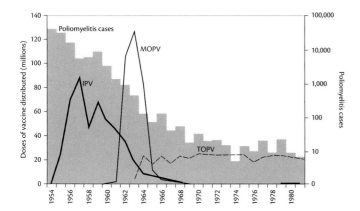

Figure 4.12 Annual number of doses of poliovirus vaccine distributed in the United States, 1954–81. Line traces plot the number of doses of inactivated poliovirus vaccine (IPV), monovalent oral poliovirus vaccine (MOPV) and trivalent oral poliovirus vaccine (TOPV). The annual count of poliomyelitis notifications is plotted as a bar chart. *Source*: redrawn from Smallman-Raynor, *et al.* (2006, Figure 10.5, p. 444), based on data in Communicable Disease Center (1964, p. 5) and Centers for Disease Control (1982, Tables 2 and 7, pp. 8, 19).

rates ≥ 0.5 per 100,000 population were limited to just a handful of states in the western United States (Arizona, Montana, Nevada, Utah and Wyoming).

Critical community size

In Section 4.3, we noted how the effect of vaccination is to raise the critical community size (*CCS*) required to maintain a target disease in endemic form. In the absence of vaccination, Eichner and colleagues (1994) have estimated the *CCS* for poliomyelitis to be of the order of 250,000 (range 50,000–500,000). Adopting a working estimate of 250,000, application of the computational procedure of Griffiths (1973) yields *CCS* estimates for poliomyelitis of 1 million (50 percent vaccination coverage; $x = 0.5$) and 25 million

(90 percent vaccination coverage; $x = 0.1$) – estimates that are identical to those given for measles in Section 4.3. On this basis, it is possible to estimate the level of vaccination required to force the *CCS* for poliomyelitis above the population size of a given US state.

Figure 4.15 plots, on the horizontal axis, the estimated (minimum) level of vaccination coverage required to raise the *CCS* for poliomyelitis above the population size of each US state against, on the vertical axis, the first calendar year of the state-level time series (1955–71) with zero poliomyelitis notifications. Subject to the complicating factor of sub-clinical infection, the latter measure provides an indication of the year in which vaccination had forced the *CCS* above the population of a given state. For reference, circle sizes in Figure 4.15 are drawn proportional to the mid-period estimates of state populations.

Inspection of Figure 4.15 reveals, as we would expect, that the more populous states, which require higher estimated levels of vaccination coverage to achieve virus extinction, cross the empirically defined *CCS* threshold at relatively later dates than the less populous states implying that, from the early 1960s, poliomyelitis was progressively pinned back into a limited number of reservoir states with relatively large populations.

Poliomyelitis in a Heavily Vaccinated Population: The Last Cases (1972–88)

Between 1972 and the 1988 resolution of the Forty-First World Health Assembly to eradicate poliomyelitis globally, only two outbreaks of poliomyelitis were recorded in the United States. Both were associated with the spread of wild type 1 poliovirus in minority religious communities, and both were the consequence of residual pockets of susceptibility in an otherwise heavily vaccinated population. The first occurred in October 1972. It was associated with 11 cases of poliomyelitis (including 8 cases of paralysis) and was centred on Daycroft private boarding school at Greenwich, Connecticut, whose faculty and 128 students were Christian Scientists (Centers for Disease Control, 1974). As a remedial

response to the demonstrably low vaccination coverage (46 percent) of the student population, vaccination of students, faculty members, and all other school employees was undertaken on 26–27 October. Other Christian Science families living in Greenwich, and whose children did not attend Daycroft School, were also contacted and administered trivalent OPV as required.

The second outbreak occurred in 1979 and was centred on members of a US Mennonite sect (Amish), some of whom reject immunisation on religious grounds. The outbreak first manifested in Pennsylvania (eight cases), with additional cases in Iowa (three cases), Wisconsin (three cases) and Missouri (one case); see **Figure 4.16**. The ultimate source of the virus was traced to a large epidemic of poliomyelitis among unvaccinated members of a Protestant sect of fundamentalist reformed churches (Netherlands Reformed Congregation) in the Netherlands in 1978, with the virus spreading to the United States via sect members in Canada (World Health Organization, 1978; Furesz, 1979; Centers for Disease Control, 1981). The outbreak illustrates how residual pockets of

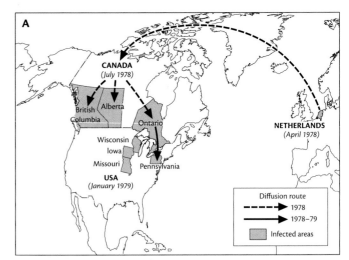

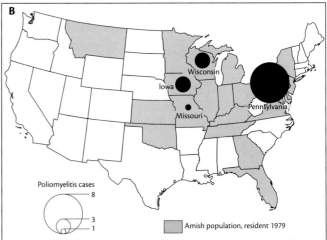

Figure 4.16 The 1979 outbreak of poliomyelitis among the Amish in the United States. (A) Vectors plot the diffusion of type 1 poliovirus in 1978 (Netherlands→Canada) and 1978–79 (Canada→USA). (B) Cases of poliomyelitis associated with the 1979 outbreak in the United States. Proportional circles show the number of poliomyelitis notifications by state. States in which Amish populations are resident have been shaded grey. *Source*: redrawn from Smallman-Raynor, *et al.* (2006, Figure 10.16, p. 465).

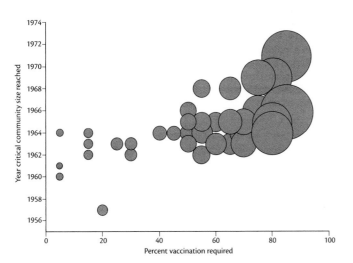

Figure 4.15 Critical community size (CCS) and poliomyelitis vaccination in the United States. The graph plots, on the vertical axis, the year in which states first reported no poliomyelitis cases against, on the horizontal axis, the percentage vaccination coverage of the population required to achieve this. Circles are drawn proportional to state populations. *Source*: redrawn from Smallman-Raynor, *et al.* (2006, Figure 10.8, p. 449), originally from Nettleton (2002, Figure 7.21(a), p. 307).

susceptibility can sustain chains of infection over long distances. We return to this theme in Section 4.6 with an analogous outbreak of measles among the Amish in 1987–88.

The last cases of wild-virus poliomyelitis

Since the 1979 outbreak, all reported cases of disease due to wild poliovirus have been associated with importations from abroad (see, for example: Strebel, *et al.*, 1992; Centers for Disease Control and Prevention, 1997b). During the period 1980–88, a total of five imported cases of wild-virus poliomyelitis were recorded in the United States – a rate of somewhat less than one case per year. Of the five cases, Mexico (two), Haiti (one), Nepal/Burma (one) and Zaire (one) were the presumed sources of infection, with the disease occurring in three travellers and two recent immigrants. No secondary cases of disease were attributed to the imported cases. The fifth and final case in the series, detected in 1986, was the last confirmed case of wild-virus poliomyelitis in the United States (Strebel, *et al.*, 1992; Centers for Disease Control and Prevention, 1995). On the basis of the five documented cases of wild-virus disease, and with an assumed infection-to-paralytic case ratio of 200:1, Strebel, *et al.* (1992, p. 575) estimate that the average number of wild poliovirus importations (clinical and sub-clinical) was of the order of 100 per year in the 1980s.

Vaccine-associated paralytic poliomyelitis (VAPP)

Poliomyelitis due to live vaccine strains of poliovirus, manifesting in vaccine recipients or through virus transmission to their contacts, may represent the predominant form of the disease when levels of wild-virus infection are low. In the United States, vaccine-associated paralytic poliomyelitis (VAPP) has been the principal form of the disease since 1973 and, with one possible exception, the only form since 1986 (Strebel, *et al.*, 1992). Between the mid-1960s and the late 1980s, the level of VAPP remained approximately constant at 3–4 cases per 10 million doses of OPV distributed. As **Table 4.6** shows, 83 cases of VAPP were recorded in the United States in the period 1980–88, with an approximately equal distribution between (i) vaccine recipients (43 cases) and (ii) contacts of vaccine recipients (40 cases).

Measles

In the early years of the twentieth century, thousands of deaths were caused by measles in the United States each year and, at mid-century, an annual average of more than 0.5 million cases and nearly 500 deaths were reported. It was against this background of

great need and vaccine availability that the US Centers for Disease Control (CDC) evolved in the United States a programme for the elimination of indigenous measles once a safe and effective vaccine was licensed for use in 1963 (Appendix 4.1). In 1966, CDC announced that the epidemiological basis existed for the elimination of indigenous measles from the United States. This was the first of three measles elimination drives to be implemented in the latter part of the twentieth century (**Figure 4.17**), each consisting of the basic strategies of high vaccination coverage among preschool and school-aged children, case surveillance and outbreak control.

The First Elimination Drive (1966–70)

Following the announcement of possible measles elimination in 1966, considerable effort was put into mass measles immunisation programmes throughout the United States. To achieve elimination, the immunisation of 90–95 percent of the childhood population was aimed for (i.e. herd immunity). Federal funds were appropriated

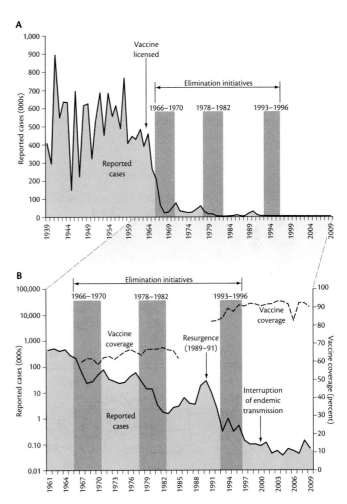

Figure 4.17 Measles reduction in the United States. (A) Annual reports of measles cases, 1939–2009. (B) Annual reports of measles cases 1961–2009 (solid line trace) and population coverage with measles-containing vaccines 1967–2009 (pecked line trace). Periods associated with elimination initiatives are identified by the grey shading. Note that pre-1993 immunisation data relate to children aged 24 months (National Immunization Survey), while later data relate to children aged 19–35 months (National Immunization Program and the National Center for Health Statistics, CDC). *Source*: data from Centers for Disease Control and Prevention (CDC).

Table 4.6 Number of cases of vaccine-associated paralytic poliomyelitis (VAPP) in the United States, 1980–88

Exposure category	Cases
Vaccine recipients	**43**
Immunologically normal	33
Immunologically compromised	10
Contacts of vaccine recipients	**40**
Immunologically normal	35
Immunologically compromised	5
Total	**83**

Source: information from Centers for Disease Control and Prevention (1997a, Table 1, p. 80).

and, over the next three years, an estimated 20 million doses of vaccine were administered. The discontinuity induced in the national time-series of reported cases is shown in Figure 4.17A. In 1962, the year before measles vaccine was introduced, there were over 481,500 cases of measles reported in the United States. Within four years, this figure had been halved and, within six years, the reported incidence had plummeted to only 22,000. In 1969, however, emphasis shifted to the administration of the newly-licensed rubella vaccine (Table 4.2) and, by the following year, federal funding for measles vaccination had ceased. One determining factor in the ultimate fate of the elimination drive was its failure to achieve and sustain high levels of immunisation in preschool-aged children. So, as Figure 4.17B shows, annual coverage of two-year-olds did not exceed 62 percent in the latter years of the 1960s. Moreover, less than 50 percent of states had school immunisation requirements which would ensure the objective of high immunisation coverage at school entry (Hinman, *et al.*, 2004).

The Second Elimination Drive (1978–88)

Measles soon began to rebound. To remedy the situation, a nationwide Childhood Immunisation Initiative was launched in April 1977, followed by the announcement of a programme to eliminate indigenous measles from the United States within five years (the 'Make Measles a Memory' campaign). The immunisation goal was again 90–95 percent of the childhood population. The geographical impact of this second push against the disease is seen in **Figure 4.18**. The maps show the distribution of counties in the United States

reporting measles cases at the start of the campaign (1978, Figure 4.18A) and five years later in 1983 (4.18B). The contraction of infection from most of the settled parts of the United States in 1978 to restricted areas of the Pacific Northwest, California, Florida, the northeastern seaboard and parts of the Midwest is pronounced. The persistence of indigenous measles in many of these regions may be explained by the importation of cases from Mexico and Canada. By 1983, 12 states and the District of Columbia reported no measles cases, and 26 states and the District of Columbia reported no indigenous cases.

The second elimination drive failed to achieve its goal by the target date of 1 October 1982 and measles incidence began to rise once again. This major resurgence was associated with 55,685 reported cases, 11,000 hospital admissions and 123 deaths in 1989–91 (Figure 4.17B). This resurgence was part of a more general upturn in disease activity in the Western Hemisphere which had resulted in the importation of hundreds of cases into the US. The principal causes of this epidemic were vaccine failure among a small proportion of school-aged children who had received one dose of measles vaccine, and low vaccine coverage among preschool-aged children (Hinman, *et al.*, 2004; Orenstein, *et al.*, 2004).

The Third Elimination Drive (1993–96)

Following the measles resurgence of 1989–91, a new childhood immunisation initiative was implemented in 1993 that included a call for the elimination of six vaccine-preventable diseases (including measles) by 1996. The geographical distribution of measles

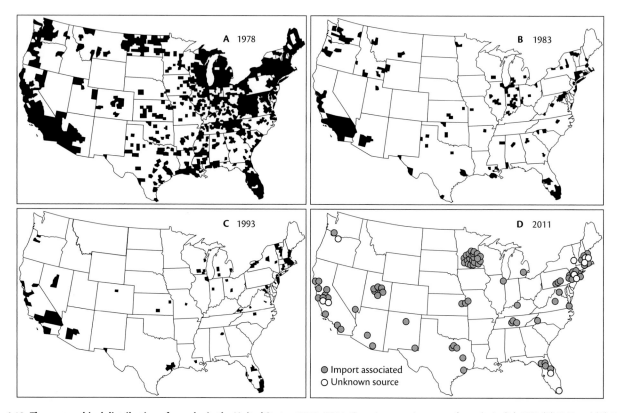

Figure 4.18 The geographical distribution of measles in the United States, 1978–2011. Counties reporting cases of measles in (A) 1978, (B) 1983 and (C) 1993. Map D plots the distribution and source (import associated or unknown) of reported measles cases, 1 January–20 May 2011. *Source*: maps (A) and (B) redrawn from Cliff and Haggett (1988, Figures 4.9(C) and (D), p. 165); map (C) redrawn from Centers for Disease Control and Prevention (1993a, p. 39); map (D) redrawn from Centers for Disease Control and Prevention (2011a, Figure 1, p. 666).

cases at the start of the third drive is shown in Figure 4.18C. The elimination strategy involved four elements: (i) to maximise population immunity through vaccination, including the timely immunisation of preschool-aged children and the delivery of a second dose of measles vaccine to school children; (ii) to ensure adequate surveillance; (iii) rapid outbreak response; and (iv) to work in partnership with other countries towards the achievement of global measles control. As Figure 4.17B shows, the annual count of notified measles cases had fallen to just 500 in 1996 and, by the end of the decade, to less than 100 (Hinman, *et al.*, 2004).

The interruption of endemic measles transmission

In March 2000, the National Immunization Program of CDC convened a meeting to assess whether measles was currently endemic in the United States. It was recognised that elimination of endemic disease does not require a total absence of indigenous cases; rather, it requires the absence of continuing indigenous transmission. The implication is that the disease can be eliminated as an indigenous condition even though recurrent outbreaks still occur. In the period 1997–99, a total of 338 measles cases (< 1 case per million population) were recorded. Of these, 34 percent were imported, 30 percent were epidemiologically linked to an imported case or were caused by an imported virus genotype, while the remaining 36 percent had an unknown source. The reproductive rate of measles, R, was estimated at < 0.8 in the period 1997–99, with molecular data supporting the proposition that endemic measles virus transmission had been interrupted in the country. R is defined in its basic form, R_0, in Section 6.2. Here, it is sufficient to note that, when $R > 1.0$, each measles case generates an average of more than one secondary case, thereby resulting in an increase in cases and sustained transmission of measles virus. Conversely, when $R < 1.0$, the measles transmission chain will be broken. On the basis of information available, the meeting concluded that measles was not currently endemic in the United States (Katz and Hinman, 2004).

The continuing problem of measles importation

Over a decade after the declaration of the interruption of sustained indigenous measles virus transmission in the United States, imported cases of the disease continue to occur. In the period 1 January–20 May 2011, for example, 118 measles cases were reported from 23 states and New York City – the highest reported number in the period since 1996 (Figure 4.18D). The majority of these (105 cases) were acquired directly or indirectly from abroad, and 9 outbreaks were recorded. The largest of the outbreaks (21 cases) was in Minnesota and occurred among children who were unvaccinated owing to concerns over the safety of the combined measles, mumps and rubella (MMR) vaccine (Centers for Disease Control and Prevention, 2011a). We return to the implications of declining immunity arising from the MMR vaccine scare, with special reference to the United Kingdom, in Section 4.6.

Economic Evaluations of Vaccination Programmes

Economic analyses of vaccine policies are reviewed by Miller and Hinman (2008). Over the years, decisions about the use of vaccines and their incorporation into routine immunisation schedules have been increasingly informed by economic evaluations of their relative costs (inputs) and benefits (outcomes) as public health interventions (Szucs, 2000). Costs are ordinarily assessed in terms of the monetary investment in vaccines and their delivery, manpower and programme administration, and the costs of the treatment of vaccine side effects. Benefits are typically measured in terms of the healthcare savings that accrue from morbidity and mortality averted. Here, we briefly summarise the results of sample cost–benefit studies in relation to the poliomyelitis and measles elimination campaigns in the United States.

Poliomyelitis elimination. Beginning with the onset of mass vaccination with IPV in 1955, and projected through to 2015, Thompson and Duintjer Tebbens (2006) estimate the investment of the United States in poliovirus vaccines at US$2002 36.4 billion. In the same 60-year interval, 1.7 billion doses of vaccine will have been delivered, resulting in the prevention of 1.1 million cases of paralytic poliomyelitis (including > 160,000 deaths) and yielding, net of treatment costs, economic benefits of almost US$2002 180 billion.

Measles elimination. Taking a hypothetical 2001 US birth cohort of approximately 3.8 million and following the cohort to age 40 years, Zhou, *et al.* (2004) estimate that the two-dose MMR vaccine strategy adopted as part of the 1990s elimination drive would avert 3.4 million measles cases, 2.1 million mumps cases and 1.8 million rubella cases, 616 cases of congenital rubella syndrome (CRS) and 2,888 deaths as compared to a no-vaccination scenario. The net savings of the two-dose programme from direct costs are estimated at US$2001 3.5 billion, with every US$ spent on the programme yielding savings of > US$14 in direct costs and > US$10 in additional costs to society. While the delivery of the second dose of MMR vaccine was not judged by Zhou and colleagues to yield net economic savings, this component of the two-dose strategy is acknowledged to have been pivotal to the interruption of indigenous measles.

4.6 Vaccination Risks

Faulty Vaccines

Vaccines are not risk-free (Offit, *et al.*, 2008). Ever since the early work on smallpox vaccination, adverse events have been shown to follow their administration. Sometimes manufacturing faults may result in the very diseases against which they are supposed to protect. Or the vaccines may unwittingly contain other pathogenic microorganisms that cause disease outbreaks (for example, Anonymous, 1942a, b on jaundice following yellow fever vaccination). Vaccines may also cause severe adverse events that are not associated with faulty production. Examples include poliovirus vaccine-associated paralytic poliomyelitis (Table 4.6) and Guillain–Barré syndrome following the receipt of swine influenza A vaccine (Offit, *et al.*, 2008). Here, we illustrate what may happen with faulty vaccine manufacture using the well-known Cutter incident which occurred in the early history of the US poliomyelitis vaccination campaigns (Section 4.5) and which were based upon Salk's inactivated poliovirus vaccine (IPV).

Poliomyelitis and the Cutter Incident

A national US vaccination programme with the newly licensed IPV had begun on 12 April 1955, with approximately four million doses of the vaccine – manufactured by five different pharmaceutical companies – having been administered to first- and second-grade children across the Union in less than four weeks (Paul, 1971; Blume and Geesink, 2000). But the nascent vaccination programme was called to a sudden halt in early May 1955. Between 18 and 27 April, some 400,000 inoculations with batches of vaccine manufactured by Cutter Laboratories of Berkeley, California, had been administered to the general public, of which an estimated 120,000 were drawn from production pools that contained residual live poliovirus. When cases of poliomyelitis began to appear among recipients of the defective vaccine, Leonard A. Scheele, Surgeon General, requested the manufacturer to recall all outstanding lots of vaccine on Wednesday 27 April. Ten days later, on Saturday 7 May, Scheele recommended a complete suspension of the vaccination programme pending a full assessment of the safety of the vaccines (Langmuir, *et al.*, 1956; Nathanson and Langmuir, 1963a, b).

The Cutter incident was associated with 158 notified cases of paralytic poliomyelitis, with the histograms in **Figure 4.19** showing a time-ordered sequence of the appearance of paralysis in each of three exposure categories. The first cases of paralytic disease were recorded in vaccine recipients on 22–23 April (Figure 4.19A), with cases subsequently appearing in family (30 April; Figure 4.19B) and community (12 May; Figure 4.19C) contacts. The majority of cases of paralysis occurred within a month of the recall of defective vaccine (27 April). Geographically, **Figure 4.20** shows that cases were centred on the states of California (57 paralytic cases) and Idaho (49 paralytic cases) and reflected the unwitting distribution of

defective vaccine by the National Foundation for Infantile Paralysis to school clinics in these states. Defective lots of Cutter vaccine were also used in school clinics in Nevada, Arizona, New Mexico and Hawaii, while the remaining scattered cases were associated with vaccine that had been distributed through commercial channels (Langmuir, *et al.*, 1956).

Cutter Laboratories was not the only manufacturer to experience difficulties in the production of IPV. Coincidental with the Cutter outbreak, a small number of poliomyelitis cases were reported among children in Pennsylvania and Maryland who had received vaccine manufactured by Wyeth Inc. of Philadelphia. But the interruptions caused by the defective Cutter and Wyeth vaccines were relatively brief and, by June, the national vaccination campaign with IPV had resumed (Langmuir, *et al.*, 1956).

False Alarms and Declining Herd Immunity

Occasionally, unfounded or unproven health concerns have shaken public confidence in vaccines. In the 1970s, for example, widely publicised concerns over the safety of pertussis vaccines (including an alleged association with permanent neurological damage that was never demonstrated conclusively; see Baker, 2003) resulted in a dramatic reduction in vaccine uptake in some countries of Europe, North America and elsewhere, with a consequent resurgence of the disease. The MMR controversy in the United Kingdom and oral poliovirus vaccine (OPV) in Nigeria provide more recent examples of the phenomenon and its potential epidemiological consequences.

Developed Countries: The MMR Controversy in the United Kingdom

Although combined measles, mumps and rubella (MMR) vaccine had been licensed in the United States as early as 1971 (Table 4.2), the adoption of the combined vaccine as part of the routine childhood immunisation schedule in the United Kingdom awaited the late 1980s. Following successful trials in three health districts (two in England, one in Scotland), national introduction of combined

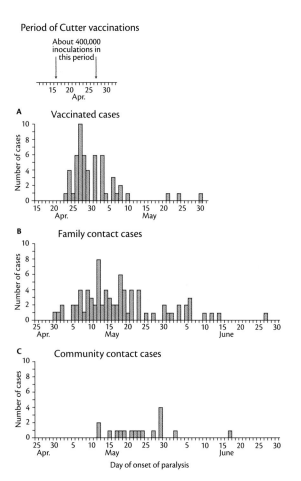

Figure 4.19 Time series of paralytic poliomyelitis associated with the Cutter incident, April–June 1955. Histograms plot, by day of onset of paralysis, the number of recorded cases of poliomyelitis associated with the administration of vaccine manufactured by Cutter Laboratories, California. (A) Cases among vaccine recipients. (B) Cases among family contacts of vaccine recipients. (C) Cases among community contacts of vaccine recipients and their family contacts. *Source*: Smallman-Raynor, *et al.* (2006, Figure 10.2, p. 439), originally redrawn from Langmuir, *et al.* (1956, Figure 1, p. 80).

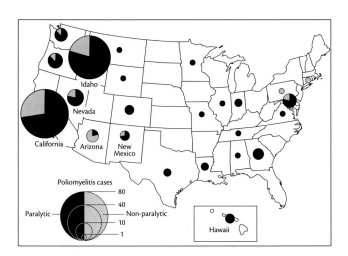

Figure 4.20 Geographical distribution of cases of poliomyelitis associated with the Cutter incident, April–June 1955. Circle areas are drawn proportional to the total number of cases of poliomyelitis recorded in a given state. The proportion of cases in which paralysis was observed is indicated by the shaded sectors. *Source*: Smallman-Raynor, *et al.* (2006, Figure 10.3, p. 440), drawn from data in Langmuir, *et al.* (1956, Table 1, p. 77).

MMR vaccine took place in October 1988 with a target to achieve 90 percent immunisation coverage of children by their second birthday. At the time of the introduction of the MMR vaccine, the measles and rubella components were already in general use in Britain in their monovalent forms, while the mumps vaccine had been licensed for some years. When it was introduced, the triple MMR vaccine had a substantial effect on the three target diseases, notably measles for which available evidence indicated the sustained interruption of indigenous virus transmission by the late 1990s (Ramsay, *et al.*, 2003).

In a controversial paper published in *The Lancet* in 1998, Andrew Wakefield and colleagues described a series of children with developmental disorders that had been referred to the Royal Free Hospital, London, and which pointed to an apparent association between the MMR vaccine and autism. Although subsequent studies in the United States and the United Kingdom failed to identify a link between the MMR vaccine and autism, and Wakefield's original paper was fully retracted by *The Lancet* in 2010, fears over the safety

of the MMR vaccine resulted in reduced vaccine uptake to levels well below those required for herd immunity for the target diseases. From a high of 92 percent in the mid-1990s, MMR vaccine coverage among two-year-olds in England and Wales fell to just 80 percent in 2003–4, 15 percent below the WHO-recommended level for herd immunity (Asaria and MacMahon, 2006). Amid increased calls for a change in national immunisation policy that permitted parents to choose between the triple MMR and single vaccines, measles and mumps re-emerged in epidemic form in the early twenty-first century (**Figure 4.21**).

Measles

Levels of susceptibility to measles grew rapidly. Starting from a position in which indigenous measles virus transmission had been effectively eliminated, 1.9 million school children and 0.3 million preschool children were estimated to be incompletely vaccinated against measles in England by 2004–5. Of these, approximately 1.3 million children aged 2–17 years were deemed susceptible to the disease. Fourteen of the 99 districts and strategic health authorities of England, including 11 London districts, had levels of susceptibility that were sufficiently high to support sustained measles virus transmission, while mathematical modelling pointed to the potential for a measles epidemic of up to 100,000 cases (Hong Choi, *et al.*, 2008). Informed by these estimates, the Health Protection Agency (HPA) announced in June 2008 that the number of susceptible children was sufficient to support the continuous transmission of measles virus and that the disease was once again endemic in the United Kingdom (Health Protection Agency, 2008).

Geographically, the decline in MMR vaccine uptake was especially pronounced in London (**Figure 4.22**), where levels of susceptibility among school children were deemed sufficiently high to support a London-wide epidemic in 2004–5 (**Figure 4.23**). In response, the MMR Capital Catch-up Campaign was launched with the aim of delivering one dose of MMR vaccine to children of

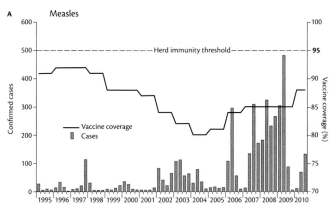

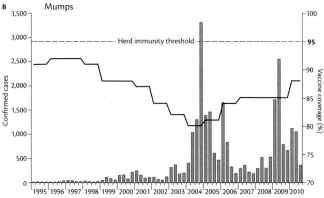

Figure 4.21 Measles and mumps in England and Wales, January 1995–September 2010. Bar charts plot the quarterly count of laboratory-confirmed cases. The quarterly counts for 2010 are based on provisional data. The proportion of the population that had received measles, mumps and rubella (MMR) vaccine at two years of age is plotted as the line traces. (A) Measles. (B) Mumps. The WHO-recommended level of 95 percent vaccine coverage for disease elimination (herd immunity threshold) is indicated. In February 2005, at the height of the 2004–5 mumps epidemic, the HPA temporarily halted the laboratory testing of notified cases in the 1981–86 birth cohort. Testing was resumed in January 2006. The case totals for 2005 in graph (B) therefore exclude a large number of cases that would otherwise have been confirmed by laboratory testing. *Source*: redrawn from Smallman-Raynor and Cliff (2012, Figure 11.5, p. 181), based on data from the Health Protection Agency (HPA).

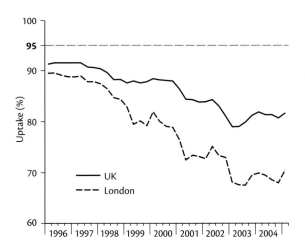

Figure 4.22 Uptake of MMR vaccine, London and the United Kingdom, 1996–2005. Uptake is shown for children at two years of age. The WHO-recommended level of vaccine coverage for measles elimination (95 percent) is represented by the grey horizontal pecked line. While MMR uptake in the United Kingdom (solid line trace) fell steadily from 1997, the decline was most pronounced in London (broken line trace). *Source*: redrawn from Smallman-Raynor and Cliff (2012, Figure 11.6, p. 182), originally from the Health Protection Agency (2006, Figure 4, p. 15).

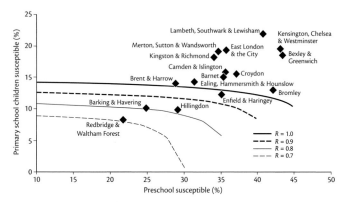

Figure 4.23 Estimated potential for measles virus transmission in districts of London, 2004. The potential for measles virus transmission (assessed according to levels of susceptibility in the population) is summarised by the effective reproduction number, *R*. For the majority of London districts *R* > 1.0, sufficient to generate a London-wide epidemic of measles. *Source*: redrawn from Smallman-Raynor and Cliff (2012, Figure 11.9, p. 183), originally from the Health Protection Agency (2006, Figure 8, p. 20).

primary school age with an incomplete vaccination history. Despite these efforts, measles has continued to spread in parts of the capital. A range of socio-economic factors are believed to have contributed to the low vaccine uptake, including high population mobility and family size, while anecdotal evidence suggests that some parents made an active decision not to have their children immunised.

Mumps

The resurgence of mumps in the early twenty-first century (Figure 4.21B) was a predictable consequence of gaps in eligibility for MMR vaccine that resulted in a cohort of mumps-susceptible children who progressed through secondary school and beyond in the early 2000s. Many were born prior to the implementation of a two-dose MMR programme and they had consequently received only one or no doses of MMR vaccine, thereby creating a pool of susceptibility when they entered university and college settings (Savage, *et al.*, 2005, 2006). The resulting mumps epidemic of 2004–5 spread nationwide and was associated with some 70,000 notified cases (**Figures 4.24A** and **B**). Frequent occurrence of severe complications was a prominent feature of the epidemic. A subsequent epidemic of mumps was observed in 2008–9 and was again associated with several outbreaks in universities and colleges (Figure 4.24C). The lag between the 2004–5 and 2008–9 epidemics may be accounted for by the fact that, since the 2004–5 epidemic, three new cohorts of students had entered the higher education sector, thereby re-establishing a susceptible pool in the confined setting of lecture rooms and halls of residence (Anonymous, 2009).

Developing Countries: Local Cultures and Polio Vaccine Uptake in Nigeria

As described in Section 5.3, the historic resolution that committed the WHO to the global eradication of poliomyelitis was adopted by the Forty-First World Health Assembly in May 1988. This goal was endorsed by the Committee of the WHO Regional Office for Africa in 1989. Eradication activities in Africa were rapidly expanded in 1996 and 1997 so that, by early 1998, most countries of the region had conducted full-scale national immunisation days (NIDs); many countries had established acute flaccid paralysis (AFP) surveillance

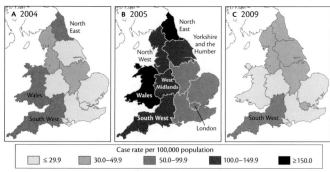

Figure 4.24 Mumps in England and Wales. Maps plot the notified case rate per 100,000 population by Strategic Health Authority for the epidemic years 2004, 2005 and 2009. *Source*: redrawn from Smallman-Raynor and Cliff (2012, Figure 11.10, p. 183), based on data from the Health Protection Agency (HPA).

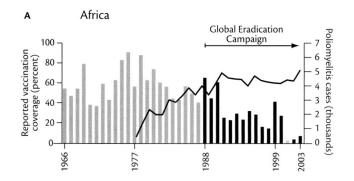

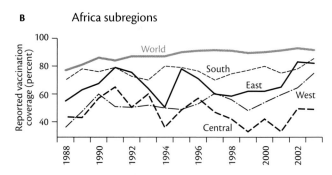

Figure 4.25 Poliomyelitis cases and poliovirus vaccination in the WHO Africa Region, 1966–2003. (A) Annual count of reported cases in the Africa Region (bar chart) and median reported level of national coverage of infants with three doses of poliovirus vaccine (line trace), 1966–2003. (B) Median reported level of national coverage of infants with three doses of poliovirus vaccine in the member states of the WHO Africa subregions, 1988–2003. *Source*: redrawn from Smallman-Raynor, *et al.* (2006, Figures 12.5A and 12.9, pp. 581, 592), originally based on data from WHO Vaccines, Immunization and Biologicals (2005).

systems, while a functional regional laboratory network had also been created (World Health Organization, 1998a).

Some impression of progress towards the interruption of wild poliovirus transmission in the African Region can be gained from **Figure 4.25A**. As the heavy line trace shows, the median reported level of coverage of infants with three doses of poliovirus vaccine increased from 48 percent (1988) to 79 percent (2003), with a corresponding reduction in the number of notified cases of poliomyelitis (bar chart). But marked subregional variations in levels of

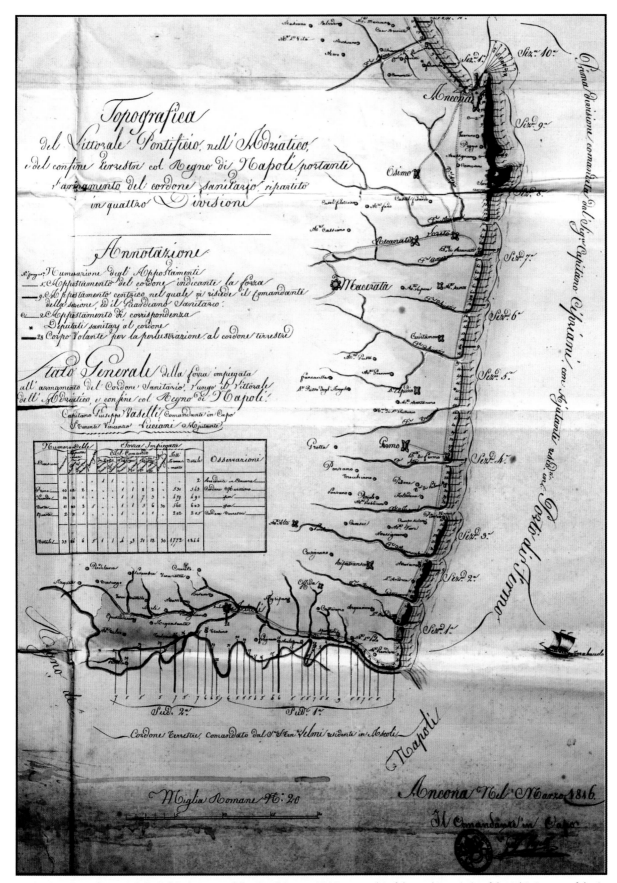

Figure 1.11. Sanitary guard posts of the Adriatic coast of the Papal States. Divisions 1 and 4 of the *cordon sanitaire* of the Adriatic coast of the Santa Sede, 1816. See text for a description of the map elements. *Source*: Appendix 1.1 (15).

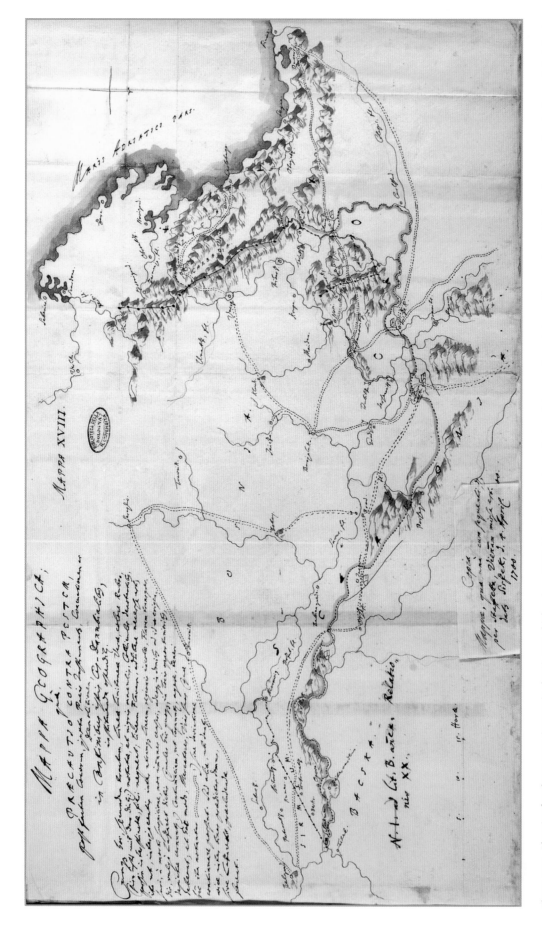

Figure 1.14. Planning for plague containment in the Cis-Danubial regions, 1700. Marsili's map envisages clearing of the area of population and houses, along with the maintenance of trade along strictly defined routes. Lazar houses are marked at road intersections, along with *cordon sanitaire* lines (black lines and dots). *Source:* Appendix 1.1 (23).

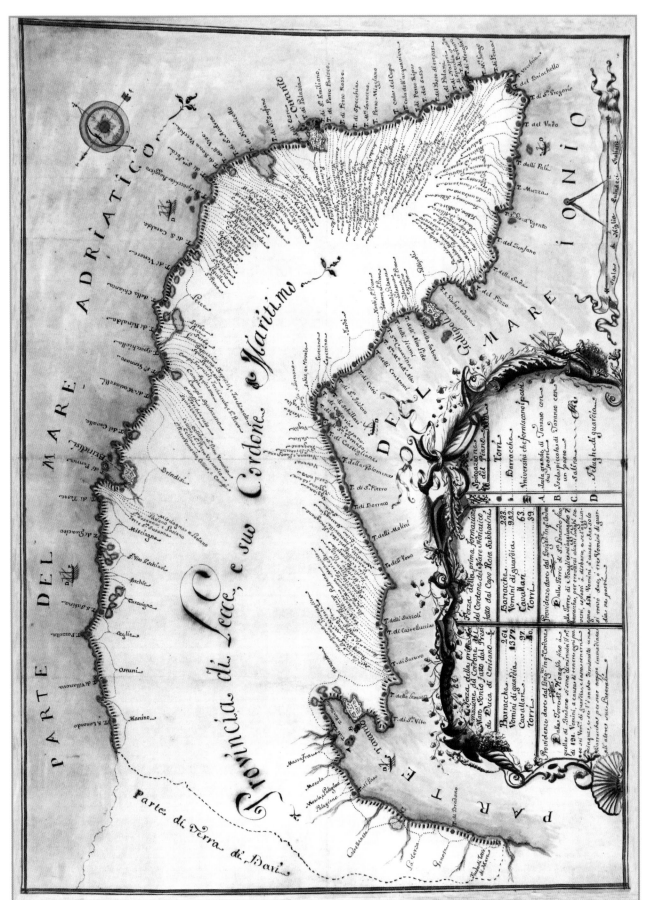

Figure 1.22. Province of Lecce, 1743, *cordon sanitaire*. Distribution of towers and guard huts comprising the *cordon sanitaire*. The entablature gives manning details. *Source:* Appendix 1.1 (18).

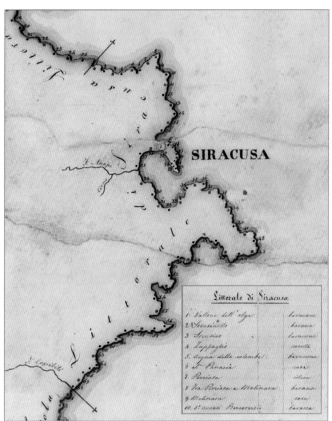

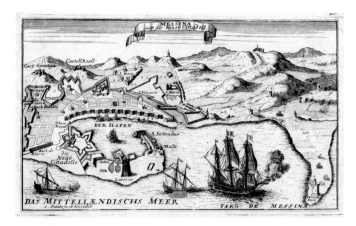

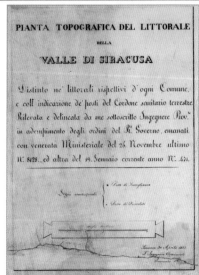

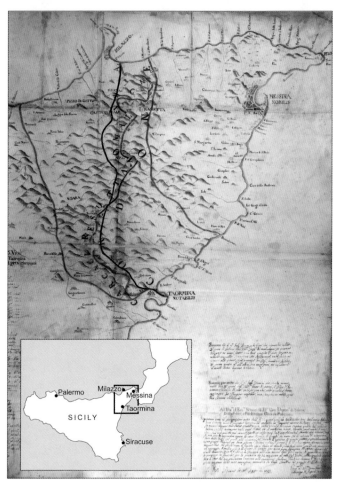

Figure 1.23. Sicily, 1837: defensive isolation. Extracts from a map of southeast Sicily showing (key) *indicazione de' posti del Cordone sanitario terrestre*. The map shows the sanitary observation posts (numbered red and blue dots) for the area around Siracusa (Syracuse). These formed part of a centuries-old circum-island ring of posts designed originally to protect the island from incursions of pirates and the plague. The inset list is part of the full list which gives the mode of construction of each post. *Source*: Appendix 1.1 (21).

Figure 1.24. Plague of Messina, 1743: plague containment. The harbour and fortress of Messina, Sicily, *c.* 1704, and the location of three internal north–south *cordon sanitaire* lines used to isolate Messina from the rest of Sicily during the Plague of Messina. *Source*: (Messina) etching by Gabriel Bodenher, *Messina mitt der Neuen Cittadell*, 1704. (Map) Appendix 1.1 (20).

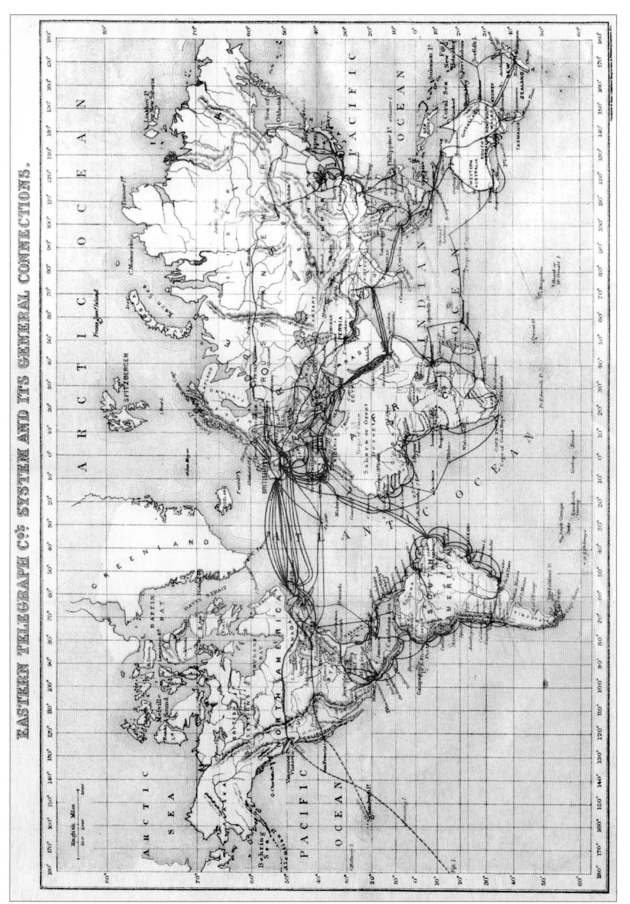

Figure 3.7. Global reach of telegraphic communications at the turn of the twentieth century. Map of submarine telegraph cable routes of the Eastern Telegraph Co., 1901. Formed in 1872 as an amalgamation of several existing cable companies, the Eastern Telegraph Co. was to become the largest cable company in the world, operating 160,000 nautical miles of cable at its maximum.

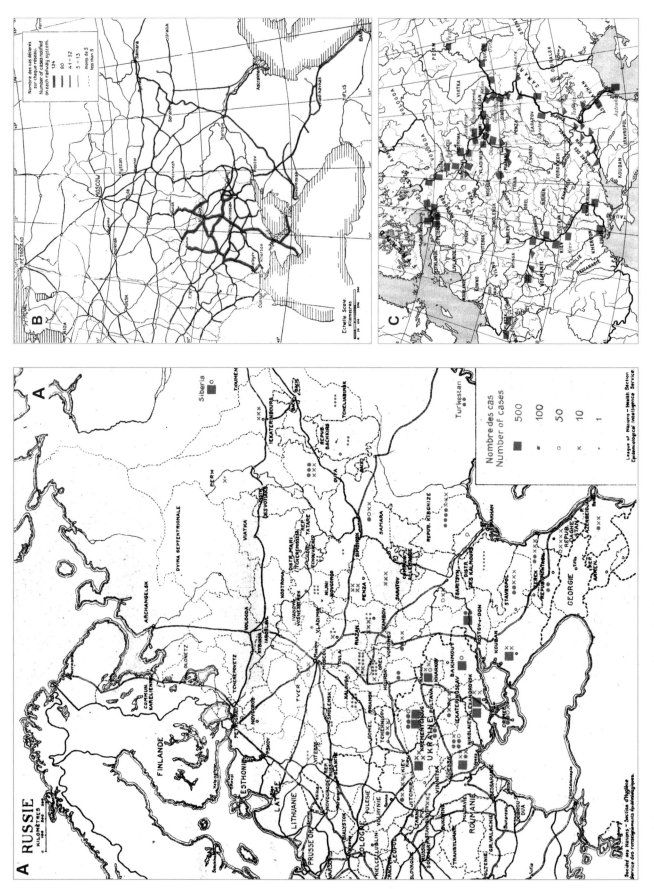

Figure 3.34. Cholera in Russia, January–June 1922. (A) Number of recorded cholera cases in the governments of European Russia, excluding the railways, January–June 1922. (B) Number of cases on the railways, May 1922. Many railway stations contained isolation units. (C) Location of sanitary stations (red squares and triangles) on the principal rivers. *Sources:* (A) League of Nations Health Section (1922a, unnumbered map, between pp. 2–3). (B) League of Nations Health Section (1922b, p. 1; 1922c, unnumbered map, between pp. 7–8). (C) Office International d'Hygiène Publique (1909, Plate VII between pp. 274–5).

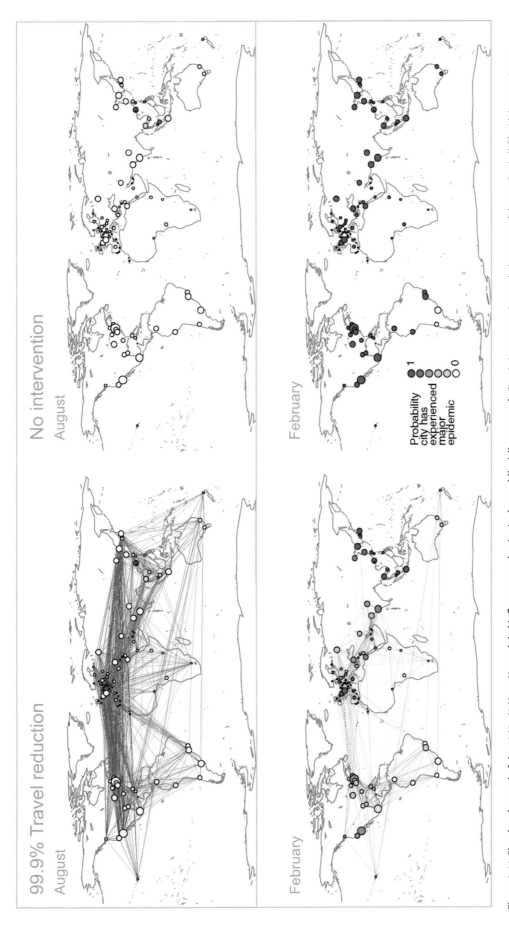

Figure 3.44. Simulated spread of the 1968–69 Hong Kong global influenza pandemic via the world's airline network. Simulations are used to track the course of the pandemic (*left*) with intervention to suspend 99.9 percent of air travel from affected cities and, for comparison (*right*) with no intervention, at two dates – August 1968 and February 1969 – two and eight months respectively after the first cases on 1 June 1968. Blue lines represent surviving flights. Circle areas are proportional to city population size, and shading indicates the probability of each city experiencing a major epidemic (> 1 case per 10,000 people per day). *Source:* Cooper, *et al.* (2006, Figure 4, p. 850).

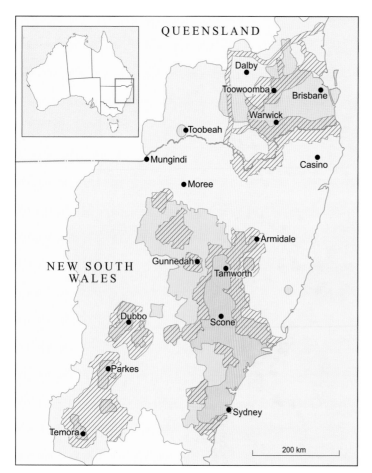

Figure 4.7. Ring vaccination to control the spread of equine influenza in New South Wales and Queensland, Australia, in 2007. The locations of infected premises are identified by the light and dark pink shading; beige-shaded zones, adjacent to the infected zones, had no reported cases. Vaccination buffer zones are represented by the diagonal shading. *Source*: redrawn from Perkins, *et al.* (2011, Figure 1, p. 128).

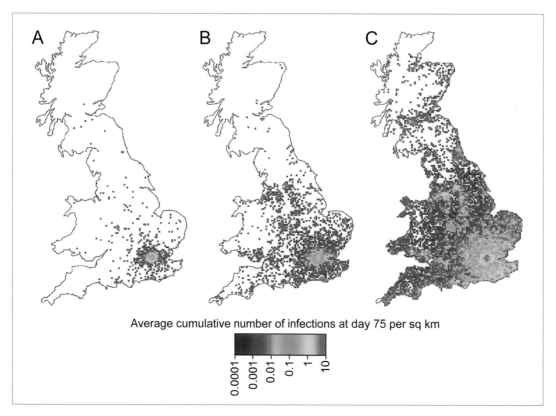

Average cumulative number of infections at day 75 per sq km

Figure 5.25. Smallpox and bioterrorism. The maps show the predicted spread of smallpox following a deliberate release in the vicinity of central London. They give the average number of cumulative infections per square kilometre during the first 75 days of the outbreak under (A) low, (B) medium, and (C) high transmission scenarios. Simulations suggest that case isolation and contact tracing with vaccination would cause rapid cessation of virus transmission under most scenarios. The costs of mass vaccination should only be contemplated at the highest end of the transmission scenarios. *Source*: redrawn from Smallman-Raynor and Cliff (2012, Figure 11.1, p. 178), originally from Riley and Ferguson (2006, Figure 3, p. 12640).

vaccination coverage persisted throughout the period, with relatively high coverage in the subregions of east and south Africa and relatively low coverage in central and west Africa (Figure 4.25B). These variations, in turn, resulted in geographical differences in the timing of poliomyelitis retreat in the African Region. From a baseline position of region-wide endemicity in 1988, endemic activity had ceased in many countries of south Africa by 1994 and east Africa by 1997. By 2002, the disease had been driven out of central Africa while, by 2003, only two countries of the Africa Region (Niger and Nigeria) continued to report the endemic transmission of wild poliovirus.

Nigeria and the decline in poliovirus vaccine uptake

The Global Polio Eradication Initiative was confronted with a number of unprecedented challenges in 2003. Foremost among these was the decision of several Nigerian states – including the northern states of Kaduna, Kano, Niger and Zamfara – temporarily to suspend all supplementary immunisation activities because of rumours over the safety of OPV. While the safety of the vaccine was confirmed to the satisfaction of most parties in March 2004, and the majority of Nigerian states endorsed the resumption of

participation in immunisation activities, the suspensions were associated with a marked increase in the level and geographical extent of poliovirus activity. Between 2002 and 2003, the annual count of confirmed cases of wild poliovirus in Nigeria increased from 202 to 355, while the number of infected states swelled from 15 to 23 (World Health Organization, 2004a, d).

While outbreaks of poliovirus type 3 were recorded in Nigeria in 2003 (World Health Organization, 2004a), it was the upsurge in poliovirus type 1 that was to pose the gravest threat to the Global Polio Eradication Initiative. The maps in **Figure 4.26** relate to the primary surviving genotype of wild poliovirus type 1 in Africa (West Africa-B, or WEAF-B, genotype) and plot the geographical distribution of isolations by year, 2001–3. From an initial focus in northern and central Nigeria and southern Niger in 2001–2, the vectors in Figure 4.26C show that, during 2003, the virus spread beyond the borders of the reservoir states into eight adjacent countries – each of which had been free of indigenous wild poliovirus for at least two years. Notwithstanding the vigorous implementation of vaccination in all eight countries, the net result of the continuing spread of poliovirus was the re-establishment of wild virus transmission in four countries (Burkina Faso, Central African Republic,

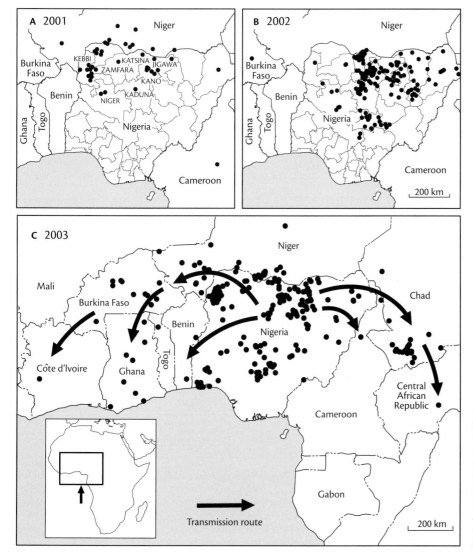

Figure 4.26 Geographical spread of wild poliovirus type 1, West Africa-B (WEAF-B) genotype, Africa, 2001–3. Maps plot the distribution of isolates in (A) 2001, (B) 2002 and (C) 2003. The vectors in map (C) indicate the likely routes of transmission of poliovirus from the Nigerian reservoir in 2003. *Source*: redrawn from Smallman-Raynor, *et al.* (2006, Figure 12.10, p. 595), adapted from maps in *Global Polio Eradication Initiative Virologic Analysis of Serotype 1 (PV1), West Africa-B (WEAF-B) Genotype Monthly Reports (June 2003 and April/May 2004)*, courtesy of Paul Chenoweth, CDC.

Chad and Côte d'Ivoire). In recognition of the gravity of the situation, health ministers of the African Union resolved that 22 west and central African countries should launch emergency synchronised immunisation activities – at an additional cost of US$100 million – in 2004–5 (World Health Organization, 2004b, c).

The spread of wild poliovirus type 1 from Nigeria to other states of west and central Africa marked the first phase of an international spread process that, in 2004–5, extended beyond the strictly defined limits of the Africa Region to include the WHO Eastern Mediterranean (Sudan and Yemen) and South-East Asia (Indonesia) Regions (**Figure 4.27**). The ramifications of the loss in public confidence in OPV in northern Nigeria in 2003, combined with the country's weak public health system infrastructure and programmatic limitations, continue to be felt by the Global Polio Eradication Initiative. Between 2003 and 2011, wild polioviruses of Nigerian origin had been imported into 25 countries, with repeated importations into many countries of west and central Africa (World Health Organization, 2011c).

Spatially Heterogeneous Vaccination Uptake

As noted in Section 4.5, religious groups exempt from immunisation laws form a small but significant risk group for outbreaks of infectious diseases in otherwise highly vaccinated populations. Special epidemiological interest attaches to US Mennonite (Amish) communities. The Amish migrated to the United States in 1709 to escape religious persecution, with the first settlements founded in Pennsylvania. By the late 1970s, Amish communities were located in more than 20 states of the Union, with the total population numbering some 75,000. As Cliff, *et al.* (1993, p. 239) observe, several characteristics of the Amish predispose them to epidemics of common infectious diseases, of which the rejection of immunisation by some sect members is pertinent to the events to be described. When coupled with the high level of national and international socialisation of the Amish and related sects, spatially separated pockets of susceptibility can sustain disease transmission chains over large

(occasionally inter-continental) distances and for extended periods of time. Such was the case for the last recorded outbreak of wild poliovirus in the United States in 1979 (Section 4.5) and, as illustrated here, the analogous events associated with a measles outbreak in 1987–88 (Cliff, *et al.*, 1993, pp. 239–40).

The Amish measles outbreak of 1987–88 had its origin in Lawrence County, Pennsylvania – a county in which no cases of measles had been reported from 1970 until the onset of the outbreak on 5 December 1987 (**Figure 4.28**). The first two cases connected to the outbreak were students from Neshannock school district in Lawrence and their source of exposure to measles virus is unknown. The subsequent sequence of spread among the Pennsylvania Amish is reconstructed in Figure 4.28A. On 21 March 1988, the first cases were reported among Amish students in Mercer County. One virus generation later, measles had reached Indiana and Mifflin Counties. On 4 April, a group of Amish from Lebanon County visited an Amish family in Mifflin County and had contact with a measles patient. Of the visiting group, eight contracted measles from the patient. The disease then spread rapidly through other Amish families in Lebanon so that, by 30 June, 130 cases among 25 Amish families in the county had occurred in some five virus generations. The crude attack rate was 39 percent, and

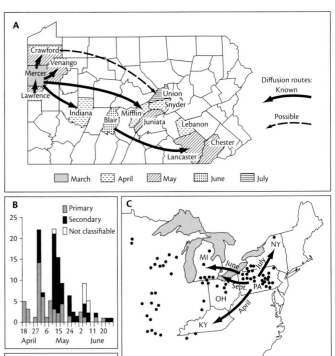

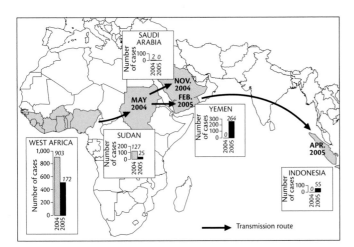

Figure 4.27 The international transmission of West African-related genotypes of wild poliovirus type 1 to Sudan and beyond, 2004–5. Vectors plot the corridors of virus transmission from an imputed origin in west Africa. Bar charts show the number of cases of wild poliovirus detected in infected localities in 2004 and 2005 (1 January–21 June). *Source*: redrawn from Smallman-Raynor, *et al.* (2006, Figure 12.19, p. 616), originally based on information in World Health Organization (2005b, c, d).

Figure 4.28 Pennsylvania measles outbreak, 1987–88: spread in the Amish community. (A) Dates of rash onset of the first Amish case in each county, 1988; vectors identify diffusion routes. (B) Date of rash onset among Amish patients in Lebanon County by exposure status, 1988. (C) Spread to Amish communities in other states, 1988. *Source*: redrawn from Cliff, *et al.* (1993, Figure 9.15, p. 240), based on data from Sutter, *et al.* (1991, Figure 1 and text, p. 13).

74 percent among those susceptible to measles. Amish families in other Pennsylvanian counties also became involved so that, by 30 July 1988, cases were reported among the Amish from 13 counties.

To control the outbreak, special measles vaccination clinics were held in locations convenient to the Amish (schools and homes). In Lebanon County, two clinics were held in May 1988, but attendance was poor and only 14 Amish were vaccinated. Measles spread from the Pennsylvania Amish to other Amish communities in Kentucky (April), Michigan (June), New York (July) and Ohio (September); see Figure 4.28C. All were linked epidemiologically to the Pennsylvania outbreak (Sutter, *et al.*, 1991).

The outbreak illustrates several important themes: the role of schools as diffusion poles, leading to geographically contagious spread; the susceptibility to high attack rates of isolated but linked communities once infection occurs; and the impact of vaccination levels upon the spread of measles. From the viewpoint of measles elimination in the United States, described in Section 4.5, it demonstrates the potential reservoir for virus survival provided by difficult-to-reach, unvaccinated groups. These may be religious sects as discussed here, mobile communities such as gypsies and itinerant populations (Smallman-Raynor, *et al.*, 2006, p. 496) and inner city ethnic groups (for example, the Latinos in Los Angeles studied by Ewert, *et al.*, 1991).

4.7 Conclusion

The range of diseases that can be prevented by routine immunisation has expanded in the post-war decades. In addition to vaccines against the common infectious killers of childhood, vaccines to prevent diseases in later life, including hepatitis B (liver cancer) and human papilloma virus (cervical cancer) vaccines, have been added to the routine infant immunisation schedules of a number of countries. Vaccines for malaria are under development, as are improved vaccines against tuberculosis, while vaccination against HIV may one day be possible. As for the future, Greenwood, *et al.* (2011, pp. 2733–4) observe that:

> If the full, global potential of vaccination is to be achieved, advances must be made in three main areas. Firstly, the fundamental science that leads to new ways of designing vaccines and of delivering them more effectively needs increased support. Secondly, transition of new discoveries in the laboratory into practical vaccines needs to be accelerated. Thirdly, mechanisms need to be developed which make existing vaccines, and the increasing number of new vaccines on the horizon, available to those who need them most, ensuring that every child is reached and that vaccination provides protection for life and not just for childhood.

The development of new vaccines in the early twenty-first century is an expensive process, costing an estimated US$500–1,000 million from first concept to licensed product. There may be as many as 20 vaccines in routine use globally by 2030, costing an estimated US$20 billion a year to apply, compared with the current cost of US$1–2 billion and contributions from recipient countries as well as donors are likely to be required to meet the financial burden (Greenwood, *et al.*, 2011).

To weigh against the high economic costs of vaccine development and delivery, immunisation programmes have resulted in some remarkable public health achievements. In addition to averting many tens of millions of cases of morbidity and premature mortality from common infections worldwide, these achievements have included the global eradication of smallpox, the substantial global retreat of poliomyelitis and, in some countries, the sustained interruption of indigenous measles virus transmission. As described in Section 4.5, the US measles elimination drive of the 1990s has demonstrated that indigenous measles transmission can be interrupted in a large and diverse country with a routine two-dose vaccination strategy, thereby providing support for the feasibility of global measles eradication (Orenstein, *et al.*, 2004). It is to the global eradication of diseases that we now turn.

Appendix 4.1: Vaccine Developments

In this Appendix, we survey the development of vaccines which, today, form a central part of the routine childhood immunisation schedules of many countries against common infectious diseases. Our review draws, in part, on Parish (1968) and Plotkin, *et al.* (2008).

Diphtheria, Tetanus and Pertussis

Diphtheria. The possibility of protecting against diphtheria by inoculation of modified toxin to stimulate the production of antitoxin has been known since the late nineteenth century. In 1890, Emil von Behring and S. Kitasato demonstrated that guinea pigs, when immunised with heat-treated diphtheria toxin, produced antitoxin that prevented the harmful effects of *C. diphtheriae*. In 1907, von Behring established that a suitably balanced preparation of diphtheria toxin and antitoxin could produce safe and lasting immunity to diphtheria in humans while, by the early 1920s, Gaston Ramon at the Pasteur Institute, Paris, had developed a method of diphtheria toxoid production for medical use. The efficacy of large-scale diphtheria immunisation was clearly demonstrated in towns and cities of Canada and the USA in the 1920s and 1930s.

Tetanus. In 1890, von Behring and Kitasato – suspecting tetanus to be the result of a toxin released by the tetanus bacterium – published evidence that would form the basis of tetanus serotherapy. Tetanus antitoxin was found to be a valuable prophylactic for human tetanus and was in use for the treatment of wounds at the start of the twentieth century. Building on the knowledge acquired from studies of diphtheria, Ramon and Zoeller were the first to immunise a human being with a vaccine containing tetanus toxoid. British, French and US troops were vaccinated against tetanus with outstanding success in the Second World War, while the early post-war years marked the introduction of tetanus immunisation to the civil population of many countries.

Pertussis. In 1906, Belgian scientists Jules Bordet and Octave Gengou isolated the bacterium *Bordetella pertussis*, the causative agent of pertussis (whooping cough), which they had first observed in 1900. Bordet and Gengou prepared a pertussis vaccine from killed whole-cell *B. pertussis* preparations in 1912. In 1925, the Danish physician, Thorvald Madsen, tested his pertussis vaccine in children in the Faroe Islands. The vaccine seemed to provide protection against disease. However, another Madsen study, published in 1933, reported that two children died from what may have been reactions to the vaccine. Active work on pertussis vaccines was undertaken in the United States in the period 1926–48, notably by Louis Sauer and Pearl Kendrick, although controversy surrounded their claims of success. In Britain, Medical Research Council (MRC) investigations of the value of pertussis vaccines had begun in 1942 and, by the end of 1952, some two-thirds of local health authorities in England and Wales had received Ministry of Health approval for the establishment of prophylactic schemes.

Combined vaccines. Combined diphtheria–tetanus (DT) and diphtheria–tetanus–pertussis (DTP) vaccines were first licensed in the United States in the late 1940s (Table 4.2). The triple vaccine was adopted in most European countries in the following decade while, in 1974, it was recommended for use by the World Health Organization's Expanded Programme on Immunization (WHO-EPI). During the 1990s, a combined diphtheria–tetanus–pertussis vaccine that used an acellular pertussis vaccine (DTaP), associated with fewer side effects, replaced DTP as the vaccine of choice in the routine childhood immunisation schedules of a number of countries.

Poliomyelitis

Reviews of the history and development of poliovirus vaccines are provided by Parish (1968), Paul (1971), Melnick (1978, 1997) and Salk and Salk (1984). The feasibility of a poliovirus vaccine was first demonstrated in 1934 by Maurice Brodie and John Kolmer. Their independent studies revealed that the immunisation of monkeys with formalin-inactivated (Brodie) and attenuated live (Kolmer) poliovirus produced a potent immune response to the virus. Although further investigations indicated that the resulting vaccines could stimulate antibody production in human beings, both were quickly withdrawn when paralytic disease began to appear in trial vaccinees. The major breakthrough came in 1955 when the success of trials of Jonas Salk's inactivated poliovirus vaccine (IPV) were announced in the United States. Following the temporary suspension of IPV as a consequence of the Cutter incident (Section 4.6), mass immunisation with the inactivated vaccine recommenced in the United States and continued until the early 1960s when Albert B. Sabin's live attenuated oral poliovirus vaccine (OPV) was licensed and adopted as the vaccine of choice (Table 4.2). OPV was subsequently adopted by the WHO-EPI and, since 1988, has formed a central plank of the WHO's Global Polio Eradication Initiative.

Measles, Mumps and Rubella

Measles. The use of human convalescent serum to confer passive immunity against measles was first demonstrated by the Italian, Francesco Cenci, in 1901. In the United States, McKhann and Chu (1933), recommended the use of placental extract (human immune globulin) in place of serum as a reliable source of antibodies against measles. By 1944, Cohen and colleagues at Harvard had developed a human immune serum globulin, the gamma globulin fraction of the appropriate convalescent serum, taken from venous blood placentae. Gamma globulin replaced other products in the passive protection of measles until, in 1954, John Enders and Thomas Peebles at Harvard grew the measles virus in tissue culture. The first measles vaccine was tested in 1958 by a colleague of Peebles, Sam Katz, on children in a school near Boston; the development of symptoms of measles in the test cohort indicated that further attenuation of the live virus was required. The efficacy of a further attenuated vaccine (using the Edmonston-B strain of measles virus) was demonstrated by Enders and colleagues in 1961 and a vaccine using the Edmonston-B measles virus strain was licensed in the United States in 1963. In 1968, a more attenuated measles vaccine (Attenuvax), developed by Maurice Hilleman (Figure 4.2) and which did not require an injection of gamma globulin antibodies to reduce reactions, was licensed for use in the United States (Table 4.2).

Mumps. During the Second World War, Enders worked on a project concerned with active and passive immunisation against mumps in man and, by the 1950s, attenuated live and killed mumps vaccines had been developed and were being implemented with success in some countries. The major breakthrough, however, came in March 1963 when Maurice Hilleman isolated mumps virus from his daughter during her illness. Hilleman attenuated the virus by passing it through chicken eggs and chick cells several times. In 1965, Hilleman and colleagues began to test their experimental mumps vaccine on children in the Philadelphia area. The US Food and Drug Administration licensed Hilleman's mumps vaccine (MumpsVax) in March 1967 (Table 4.2).

Rubella. In 1969, Hilleman modified a rubella vaccine virus that had been obtained from from Paul Parkman and Harry Meyer, scientists at the Division of Biologics Standards. The vaccine entered commercial use in the United States in 1969 (Table 4.2). A decade later, in 1979, the original rubella vaccine was replaced in the United States by Stanley A. Plotkin's newly licensed RA27/3 vaccine, which had been used in Europe for years and which provided superior protection to that of the initial strain.

Combined vaccines. Initial tests on a triple measles–mumps–rubella (MMR) vaccine, undertaken in the United States in 1968, demonstrated that adverse reactions were no greater than seen in single vaccines. Merck's combined MMR vaccine was licensed in the USA in 1971 (Table 4.2), with research indicating that the combined vaccine, properly administered, induced immunity to measles in 96 percent of vaccinated children; to mumps in 95 percent; and to rubella in 94 percent. Combined measles–mumps, measles–rubella and mumps–rubella vaccines were also developed for use in specific target groups at this time (Hilleman, 1992).

Tuberculosis

In 1904, Albert Calmette and Jean-Marie Camille Guérin began to attenuate *Mycobacterium bovis* to the point that it proved non-fatal to guinea pigs. Almost two decades later, in 1921, Calmette and Guérin began the first human tests of their attenuated vaccine preparation that was designated BCG (Bacillus Calmette-Guérin) and, in 1928, the Health Committee of the League of Nations adopted BCG as the tuberculosis vaccine of choice for preventative inoculation. The vaccine was widely used in France, central Europe and the Balkans after its introduction, although it was little employed in the United States until after 1940. The generalised international use of BCG vaccination began after the Second World War when it was administered as part of the International Tuberculosis Campaign of 1948–51, first in Europe and then in other parts of the world.

Other Diseases

Haemophilus influenzae *type b (Hib) disease*. The bacterium *Haemophilus influenzae* was first isolated in 1892 by the German physician Richard Pfeiffer, believing that he had identified the causative agent of influenza. The link between *H. influenzae* and meningitis was established in the United States by Margaret Pittman in 1931; Pittman found that strains of the bacterium that caused meningitis were characterised by a specific polysaccharide. These strains were referred to as *H. influenzae* type b (Hib). Half a century later, in 1985, the first polysaccharide Hib vaccines were licensed in the United States (Table 4.2). The polysaccharide vaccines were subsequently replaced in the US and elsewhere by conjugate Hib vaccines, including polyvalent preparations that also offer protection to diphtheria, tetanus and pertussis and to other diseases.

Hepatitis B. The identification of the hepatitis B virus (HBV) surface protein ('Australia antigen') by Baruch Blumberg in 1965 provided an important stimulus for the development of a hepatitis B vaccine. Maurice Hilleman transformed the Australia antigen into an effective vaccine (Hepatavax B) that was licensed in the United States in 1981. Heptavax was demonstrably effective in preventing hepatitis B although, because of concerns over HIV infection, it was superseded by a recombinant vaccine (Recombivax HB) that did not use human serum in 1986 (Table 4.2).

Meningococcal disease. Polysaccharide vaccines to protect against meningococcal disease were first licensed in the United States in the 1970s (Table 4.2). In the United Kingdom, clinical trials demonstrated that meningococcal C conjugate (MCC) vaccines were immunogenic and safe in all age groups and the first MCC vaccine was licensed in the UK in 1999. In subsequent years, quadrivalent conjugate vaccines to protect against serotypes A, C, Y and W-135 have been developed and introduced into the routine childhood immunisation schedule of some countries.

Pneumococcal disease. Although a killed whole-cell pneumococcal vaccine had been trialled by Almroth Wright in South African gold miners in the early twentieth century, the results of the trials were inconclusive and the vaccine was abandoned. The idea of a vaccine was taken up again by Robert Austrian in the 1960s. Having identified many different serotypes of the pneumococcus, Austrian reported in 1976 that a pneumococcal vaccine had been developed that had proved safe and effective in South African trials. Austrian's polysaccharide vaccine, protective against 14 types of pneumococcal bacteria, was licensed in the United States in 1977. The polysaccharide vaccine, however, did not consistently induce immunity in young children (aged < 2 years) and, in subsequent years, safe and effective conjugate vaccines have been developed and released onto the market.

Rotavirus gastroenteritis. The first vaccine for rotavirus (RotaShield) was licensed and recommended for routine childhood immunisation in the USA in 1998. Following the withdrawal of RotaShield in 1999 on account of its association with potentially fatal intestinal complications, a new vaccine (RotaTeq) was developed and recommended for inclusion in the routine infant immunisation schedule of the United States in 2006.

CHAPTER 5

Eradication

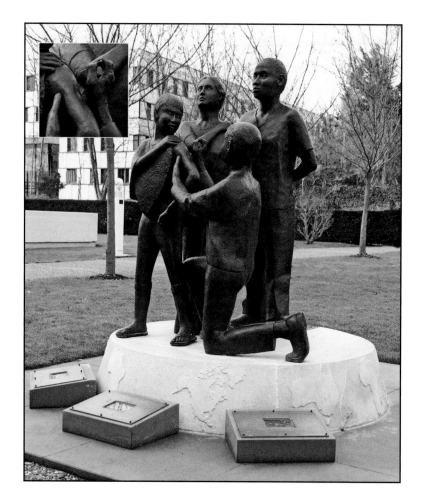

Figure 5.1 The global eradication of smallpox. Statue erected outside the entrance to the main World Health Organization (WHO) building in Geneva, Switzerland. The bronze and stone statue was unveiled on 17 May 2010 by Dr Margaret Chan, Director-General of the WHO, to commemorate the thirtieth anniversary of the WHO's declaration of the global eradication of smallpox. The statue depicts four persons, one of whom is a girl who is about to be vaccinated by a health worker with a bifurcated needle (*inset*). The bifurcated needle was designed to hold freeze dried smallpox vaccine between two prongs, with the vaccine administered by a technique (multiple puncture vaccination) that involved up to 15 insertions delivered in rapid succession in a circle of about 5 mm in diameter. The base of the statue shows the continents, while the plaques surrounding the statue (written in the six official languages of the WHO) state that the eradication of smallpox was made possible through the collaboration of nations.

5.1 **Introduction**

Future nations will know by history only that the loathsome smallpox has existed and by you has been extirpated.

Thomas Jefferson, A Tribute of Gratitude (letter)
to Edward Jenner (14 May 1806, cited in Stanwell-Smith, 1996, p. 509)

As I look back, I realise that smallpox eradication was achieved, but was just barely achieved. Had the biological and epidemiological characteristics of the disease, or the world political situation, been even slightly more negative, the effort might have failed.

Frank Fenner (1986, p. 38)

The idea of eradicating a disease has a long and chequered history (**Table 5.1**). While the vision of a smallpox-free world was articulated in President Thomas Jefferson's well-known letter of gratitude to Edward Jenner in 1806, the first deliberate effort to eliminate a communicable disease at the national level awaited the early twentieth century and the establishment of the Rockefeller Foundation's Sanitary Commission for the Eradication of Hookworm Disease in the United States. Several years later, in 1915, the Rockefeller Foundation established the Yellow Fever Commission with the view to eradicating yellow fever globally. This was the first of six campaigns for the global eradication of human pathogens to be launched over the last 100 years (**Table 5.2**), of which only one (smallpox) has so far achieved the eradication goal (**Figure 5.1**). Elsewhere, in the animal kingdom, the successful eradication of rinderpest (a viral disease of cattle and other ruminants) was declared by the Food and Agriculture Organization (FAO) in October 2010 (Centers for Disease Control and Prevention, 1993b; Roeder, 2011).

Table 5.1 Milestones in the eradication of human diseases, 1800–2010

Period	Disease	Milestones/events
1800–99	Smallpox	1806: President Thomas Jefferson refers to the 'extirpation' of smallpox in his letter to Edward Jenner
	Tuberculosis	1888: Charles V. Chapin urges eradication of TB
	Rabies	1896: Rabies eliminated from England
1900–49	Yellow fever	1901: Yellow fever eliminated from Havana, Cuba
	Hookworm disease	1907: Rockefeller Foundation establishes Sanitary Commission for the Eradication of Hookworm Disease in the USA
	Yellow fever	1915: Rockefeller Foundation establishes Yellow Fever Commission to eradicate the disease
	Tuberculosis	1917: Decision to eliminate bovine TB from USA
	Hookworm disease	1922: Rockefeller Foundation's hookworm campaign begins to phase out owing to limited success
	Yellow fever	1923: Yellow fever reappears in Brazil after an absence of almost one year
	Yellow fever	1928–29: Additional outbreaks of yellow fever in Brazil
	Yellow fever	1934: Proposal to eliminate Aedes aegypti from Brazil
	Tuberculosis	1937: W.H. Frost reports that human tuberculosis is being eliminated from the USA and other countries
	Malaria	1941: Anopheles gambiae eliminated from Brazil
	Yellow fever	1943: Bolivia is first country to proclaim the elimination of Aedes aegypti
	Malaria	1945: Anopheles gambiae eliminated form Egypt
	Yellow fever	1947: PAHO adopts proposal for elimination of Aedes aegypti from Americas
1950–99	Smallpox	1950: Pan American Sanitary Conference approves goal of smallpox elimination in the Americas
	Yaws	1950: Pan American Sanitary Conference approves goal of yaws elimination in the Americas
	Malaria	1951: Malaria eliminated in Sardinia
	Yaws	1954: WHO declares goal to eradicate yaws
	Malaria	1955: Eighth World Health Assembly adopts goal of global malaria eradication
	Smallpox	1958: Eleventh World Health Assembly adopts goal of global smallpox eradication
	Smallpox	1966: Nineteenth World Health Assembly adopts goal of intensified smallpox eradication by 1976
	Malaria	1969: WHO changes malaria eradication policy to one of malaria control
	Smallpox	1970: Smallpox eliminated from the Americas
	Malaria	1975: Europe declared free of malaria
	Smallpox	1977: Smallpox eradicated worldwide
	Measles	1978: USA announces goal to eliminate measles by 1982
	Smallpox	1980: WHO declares the global eradication of smallpox
	Dracunculiasis	1980: India begins national dracunculiasis elimination programme
	Poliomyelitis	1985: PAHO sets goal of poliomyelitis elimination in the Americas by 1990

Table 5.1 (*Continued*)

Period	Disease	Milestones/events
	Measles	1985: Europe sets goal of measles elimination by 2000
	Dracunculiasis	1986: Thirty-ninth World Health Assembly declares goal of dracunculiasis elimination
	Poliomyelitis	1988: Forty-first World Health Assembly declares goal of global poliomyelitis eradication by 2000
	Dracunculiasis	1988: WHO Africa Region sets goal of drancunculiasis elimination from Africa by 1995
	Dracunculiasis	1991: Forty-fourth World Health Assembly declares goal of global dracunculiasis eradication by 1995
	Poliomyelitis	1991: Last case of indigenous wild virus poliomyelitis in the WHO Americas Region
	Onchocerciasis	1991: PAHO resolves to eliminate onchocerciasis morbidity from the WHO Americas Region by 2007
	Poliomyelitis	1994: WHO Americas Region certified poliomyelitis-free
	Measles	1994: PAHO sets target for measles elimination from the WHO America Region by 2000
	Poliomyelitis	1997: Last case of indigenous wild virus poliomyelitis in the WHO Western Pacific Region
	Measles	1997: WHO Eastern Mediterranean Region sets target for measles elimination by 2010
	Poliomyelitis	1998: Last case of indigenous wild virus poliomyelitis in the WHO Europe Region
2000–10	Poliomyelitis	2000: WHO Western Pacific Region certified poliomyelitis-free
	Poliomyelitis	2002: WHO Europe Region certified poliomyelitis-free
	Measles	2002: Indigenous measles virus transmission interrupted in WHO Americas Region
	Measles	2003: WHO Western Pacific Region sets target for measles elimination by 2012
	Measles	2005: WHO Europe Region sets target for measles elimination by 2010
	Measles	2008: WHO Africa Region sets a pre-elimination goal for measles

Source: based on Centers for Disease Control and Prevention (1993b, Table 2, pp. 6–7).

Table 5.2 Eradication initiatives for human disease agents

Disease	Category of agent(s)	Years of eradication effort	Outcome
Yellow fever	Virus	1915–77	Unsuccessful
Yaws	Bacterium	1954–67	Unsuccessful
Malaria	Protozoa	1955–69	Unsuccessful
Smallpox	Virus	1967–79	Successful
Poliomyelitis	Virus	1988–present	Ongoing[1]
Dracunculiasis	Helminth	1991–present	Ongoing[1]

Notes: [1] As of January 2012.

Source: based in part on Aylward, *et al.* (2000, Table 1, p. 1516).

Inevitably, the popularity of eradication as a human disease control strategy has waxed and waned with the successes, setbacks and failures of previous and ongoing campaigns. Many lessons have been learnt from the past (Aylward, *et al.*, 2000) and disease eradication is again at the forefront of global health policy (World Health Organization, 2010b). In the remainder of this introductory section, we define eradication, outline the principal indicators of disease eradicability, and summarise the spatial strategies that may be employed to achieve eradication. In subsequent sections, we chart the successful eradication of smallpox (Section 5.2), the long-running effort to eradicate poliomyelitis (Section 5.3) and the obstacles encountered in other ongoing (dracunculiasis) and failed (yellow fever, yaws and malaria) eradication programmes (Section 5.4). We then look to the prospect of measles eradication (Section 5.5),

the issues posed by bioterrorism (Section 5.6) and the outlook for the ultimate extinction of eradicated disease agents (Section 5.7). The chapter is concluded in Section 5.8.

Defining Eradication

As applied to an infectious disease agent, the term *eradication* has been defined in the literature in a variety of ways and, at times, has been confused with the related term, *elimination*. To achieve uniformity in the definition and application of terms, the Dahlem Workshop on the Eradication of Infectious Diseases, held in March 1997, defined eradication as the

> permanent reduction to zero of the worldwide incidence of infection caused by a specific disease agent as a result of deliberate efforts (Dowdle, 1998, p. 23).

Within this definition, the term eradication is reserved for the complete and permanent worldwide cessation of the natural transmission of a disease agent. Eradication thus represents a distinct stage in disease intervention and is distinguished from the related concepts of *control*, *elimination* and *extinction* as defined in **Table 5.3**.

Indicators of Eradicability

Following Dowdle (1998) and Aylward, *et al.* (2000), the potential of a disease agent for eradication can be assessed on the basis of three principal indicators: (1) biological and technical feasibility; (2) costs and benefits; and (3) societal and political considerations. We consider each indicator in turn.

(1) Biological and technical feasibility

The feasibility of eradicating a disease agent is dependent on a range of biological and technical considerations. These include: (i) the availability of an effective means of interrupting the transmission of the disease agent (e.g. a safe and effective vaccine); (ii) the availability of diagnostic tools of sufficient sensitivity and specificity to detect levels of infection that may result in transmission of the disease agent; and (iii) the absence of a non-human vertebrate reservoir and the inability of the disease agent to amplify in the environment.

(2) Costs and benefits

The decision to eradicate a disease agent is contingent on the costs and benefits of the eradication programme, over and above the costs and benefits arising from alternative intervention scenarios. Costs and benefits can be defined in terms of direct effects (i.e. cessation of morbidity and mortality) and consequent effects (i.e. impact on healthcare systems). As eradication programmes are closely related to other health programmes, emphasis should be placed on the costs and benefits to overall health services.

(3) Societal and political considerations

The success or otherwise of eradication programmes is crucially dependent on societal, political and associated financial commitment to their success. The target disease must be recognised as being of public health importance; eradication must be recognised as a worthy goal by society; and political commitment to eradication is required at the highest level throughout the duration of the eradication programme.

Spatial Strategies for Eradication

Viewed in geographical terms, eradication is the last stage in the progressive spatial contraction of a disease and its causative agent. Drawing on the spatial concepts of disease control in Section 1.4, Cliff and Haggett (1989) discuss a stage-by-stage schema of possible contraction strategies, stressing the ways in which geographical considerations impinge upon control by vaccination. These different spatial control strategies are illustrated in **Figure 5.2**. In the first stage, *local elimination*, the emphasis is on breaking, in some particular location, the infection chain by vaccination. The theoretical basis of disease elimination through vaccination is discussed in Section 4.3, and is illustrated by the mass vaccination programmes for poliomyelitis and measles elimination in the United States in Section 4.5.

Once an area is free from the indigenous transmission of a disease agent, then there is need for the establishment of spatial barriers to disease transmission in the form of *defensive isolation* and *offensive containment*. These barrier concepts are described in Section 1.4

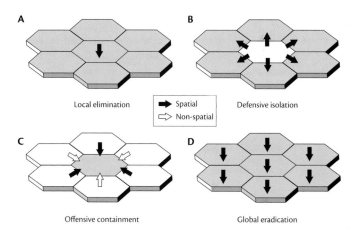

Figure 5.2 Schematic diagram of four spatial and aspatial control strategies to prevent epidemic spread. Infected areas are shaded; disease-free areas are unshaded. The strategies of defensive isolation (B) and offensive containment (C) have already been encountered in Figure 1.20 and are reproduced here as part of the broader suite of spatial control strategies. *Source*: redrawn from Cliff and Haggett (1989, Figure 2, p. 318).

Table 5.3 Definitions of stages of control of infectious agents and their implications for control programmes

| | Stages of control | | | |
	Control	Elimination	Eradication	Extinction
Definition[1]	"The reduction of disease incidence, prevalence, morbidity and mortality to a locally acceptable level as a result of deliberate efforts."	*Disease*: "Reduction to zero of the incidence of a specified disease in a defined geographical area as a result of deliberate efforts". *Infection*: "Reduction to zero of the incidence of infection caused by a specific agent in a defined geographical area as a result of deliberate efforts".	"Permanent reduction to zero of the worldwide incidence of infection caused by a specific disease agent as a result of deliberate efforts."	"The specific infectious agent no longer exists in nature or in the laboratory."
Implication	Continued intervention measures are required to maintain reduction.	Continued intervention measures are required to prevent re-establishment of infection and disease.	Intervention measures no longer needed: all interventions can be halted after certification of eradication.	

[1] Definitions formulated at the Dahlem Workshop on the Eradication of Infectious Diseases (March 1997), cited in Dowdle (1998, p.23).

but, in essence, both seek to limit the spatial spread of a disease agent into disease-free areas.

The final stage of *global eradication* would arise in principle from a combination of the previous three methods: infected areas would be progressively reduced in size, and the coalescence of such disease-free areas would lead, eventually, to the elimination of the disease on a worldwide basis. For vaccine-preventable diseases, eradication therefore rests on a globally coordinated vaccination programme to reduce the sizes of geographically distributed at-risk populations to levels at which the chains of infection cannot be maintained. In terms of the Bartlett model (Section 1.4), this means systematically reducing the wave order of different communities from I to II, and from II to III, eventually bringing the Type III waves into phase so that disease fade-out in all the remaining disease-active areas coincides.

5.2 Smallpox Eradication

At the time of writing, smallpox is the only human disease to have been eradicated globally. As described by Fenner, *et al.* (1988), the practical reality of devising, coordinating and financing a field programme involving more than 30 national governments, as well as some of the world's most complex cultures and demanding environments, proved to be of heroic proportions. Until the mid-1960s, control of smallpox was based primarily upon mass vaccination to break the chain of transmission between infected and susceptible individuals by eliminating susceptible hosts. Although this approach had driven the disease from the developed world, the less developed world remained a reservoir area. Thus between 1962 and 1966, some 500 million people in India were vaccinated, but the

disease continued to spread. Between 5–10 percent of the population always escaped the vaccination drives, concentrated especially in the vulnerable under-15 age group. Nevertheless, the susceptibility of the virus to concerted action had been demonstrated and led to critical decisions at the Nineteenth World Health Assembly in 1966.

The Eradication Campaign

The Nineteenth World Health Assembly committed the World Health Organization (WHO) to a 10-year global smallpox eradication programme which was launched in 1967. As we noted in Section 2.7, the eradication campaign started with mass vaccination, but the importance of surveillance and selective control was soon recognised. Contacts of smallpox cases were traced and vaccinated, as well as the other individuals in those locations where the cases occurred. The success of these strategies may be judged from **Figure 5.3**. By 1970, retreat was under way in parts of Africa. By 1973, smallpox had been eliminated in the Americas while, by 1976, the disease had been pushed out of Southeast Asia and only a part of East Africa remained to be cleared. The world's last naturally occurring case of smallpox was finally tracked down to the Somalian town of Merka in late October 1977 (**Figure 5.4**). After a two-year period during which no further cases (other than laboratory accidents) were recorded, WHO formally announced at the end of 1979 that the global eradication of smallpox was complete (**Figure 5.5**).

Smallpox as a Model for Eradication

It is important to consider how far smallpox is a useful control model for the eradication of other communicable diseases. For

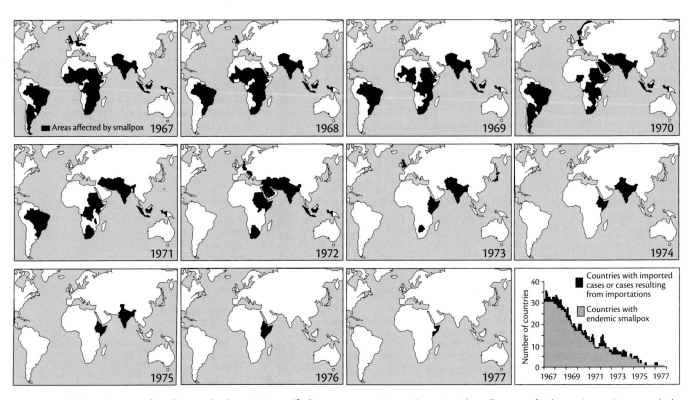

Figure 5.3 Global eradication of smallpox under the WHO Intensified Programme, 1967–77. Countries with smallpox cases for the year in question are marked in black. *Source*: Cliff, *et al.* (1998, Figure 7.25, pp. 374–5), redrawn from Fenner, *et al.* (1988, Figure 10.4 and Plates 10.42–10.51, pp. 516–37 *passim*).

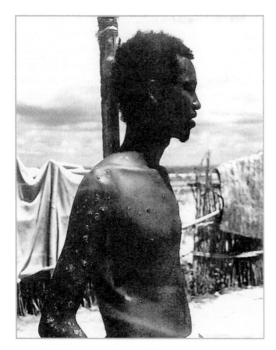

Figure 5.4 The last 'natural' case of smallpox. Ali Maow Maalin, the last case of naturally occurring smallpox in the world, developed a rash on 26 October 1977, in the town of Merka, Somalia. *Source*: Fenner, *et al.* (1988, Plate 22.10, p. 1066).

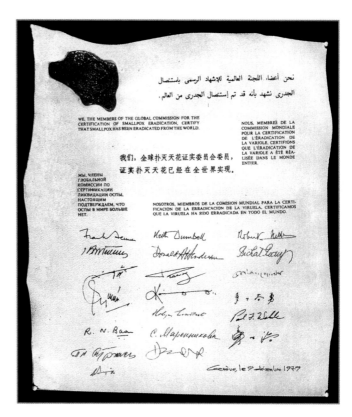

Figure 5.5 Global smallpox eradication document. The official parchment certifying the global eradication of smallpox, dated 9 December 1979. This is arguably the most important document in the history of twentieth-century medicine. *Source*: Fenner, *et al.* (1988, Frontispiece).

whatever the huge difficulties in practice, in principle, smallpox was well suited to global eradication. Fenner (1986) has summarised the biological and socio-political characteristics of smallpox that facilitated global eradication (**Table 5.4**). First and foremost among the biological features, smallpox was such a severe disease that it was clearly worth the effort required for eradication. Second, variola virus was a specific human virus; there is no animal reservoir. Third, sub-clinical infections were virtually unknown, and those that did occur excreted very little virus and were of no epidemiological importance. Fourth, spread usually resulted from direct face-to-face contact with patients with a rash; patients were not infectious during the incubation period or the pre-eruptive phase. If cases were isolated as soon as the rash was apparent, in a setting in which they had contact only with vaccinated or immune persons, the chain of transmission could be broken. Fifth, neither a prolonged carrier state nor recurrence of clinical illness with associated infectivity ever occurred in smallpox; hence the disappearance of acute infections meant that the chance of transmission had been eliminated. Sixth, there was only one serotype of variola virus – over centuries of time and all over the world – and, seventh, since the time of Jenner, there has been an effective live-virus vaccine against smallpox. Additionally, in the 1950s, a freeze-dried vaccine was developed that was stable even under the most adverse conditions (Fenner, 1986).

In addition to the biological features of smallpox, several socio-political factors were also crucial to the success of the eradication campaign. Point 10 in Table 5.4 argues that smallpox imposed a heavy financial burden on the industrialised countries, as well as on those where smallpox was endemic. Quite apart from the disease and death from smallpox itself, the cost of vaccination, plus that of maintaining quarantine barriers, is calculated to have been about

Table 5.4 Biological and socio-political features which favoured the global eradication of smallpox

Biological features
1. A severe disease, with high mortality and serious after-effects
2. No animal reservoir of variola virus
3. Very few sub-clinical cases
4. Cases became infectious at time of onset of rash
5. Recurrence of infectivity never occurred
6. Only one serotype existed
7. An effective, stable vaccine was available
Socio-political features
8. Earlier country-wide elimination showed that global eradication was an attainable goal
9. There were few social or religious barriers to the recognition of cases
10. The costs of quarantine and vaccination for travellers provided a strong financial incentive for wealthy countries to contribute
11. The Intensified Smallpox Eradication Unit of the WHO had inspiring leaders and enlisted devoted health workers

Source: Cliff, *et al.* (1993, Table 16.2, p. 422), originally from Fenner (1986, Table 1, p. 37).

US$1,000 million per annum in the last years of the virus's existence in the wild (Fenner, 1986).

5.3 The Global Polio Eradication Initiative

Although significant differences in the characteristics of smallpox and poliomyelitis render the eradication of poliomyelitis a potentially more difficult task than was the case for smallpox (**Table 5.5**), the feasibility of global poliomyelitis eradication on biological grounds is established in principle (**Table 5.6**). On this basis, the Forty-first World Health Assembly (May 1988) adopted the historic Resolution WHA41.28 that committed the WHO to the global eradication of poliomyelitis by the year 2000 (article 1). The eradication effort was to be pursued in a manner which strengthened the development of the Expanded Programme on Immunization (EPI) and the health infrastructure of member states more generally (article 2). Member states in which at least 70 percent of target populations had already received poliovirus vaccine were invited to formulate plans for the elimination of indigenous wild poliovirus (article 3), while member states with vaccine coverage of less than 70 percent were encouraged to surpass that level as soon as possible (article 4). Member states in which absence of the disease had already been confirmed were requested to sustain their efforts and to share their technical expertise and resources (article 5), while all

Table 5.5 Biological and socio-political characteristics that favoured the global eradication of smallpox: comparisons with poliomyelitis and measles

Features	Smallpox	Poliomyelitis	Measles
Biological			
1. Reservoir host in wildlife	No	No	No
2. Persistent infection occurs	No	No	No
3. Number of serotypes	1	3	1
4. Antigenic stability	Yes	Yes	Yes
5. Vaccine effective	Yes	Yes	Yes
Cold chain necessary	No	Yes	No
Number of doses	1	4	1
6. Infectivity during prodromal	No	Yes	Yes
7. Sub-clinical cases occur	No	Yes	No
8. Early containment of outbreak possible	Yes	No	No
Socio-political			
9. Country-wide elimination achieved	Yes	Yes	Yes
10. Incentive for industrialised countries to assist	Strong	Weak	Weak
11. Records of vaccination required	No	Yes	Yes
12. Improved sanitation required	No	Yes	No

Source: Cliff, *et al.* (1993, Table 16.3, p. 423), originally from Fenner (1986, Table 2, p. 39).

Table 5.6 Biological principles for the global eradication of poliomyelitis

Biological principle	Notes
Poliovirus causes acute, non-persistent infection	The lack of a long-term or persistent carrier state is a key characteristic of poliomyelitis which underpins the feasibility of global eradication. In rare instances, however, persons with primary immunodeficiency disorders have been shown to excrete vaccine virus for six months or more. The long-term excretors have significant implications for when and how OPV use should cease in the wake of the certification of poliomyelitis eradication.
Poliovirus is transmitted only by infectious humans or their waste	Poliovirus is transmitted by droplet spread from the pharynx or by the faecal contamination of hands, eating utensils, food or water. Epidemiological evidence suggests that at least 80 percent of infections with poliovirus are person-to-person (faecal–oral or oral–oral) and that vectors play only a very limited, if any, role in epidemic propagation.
Survival of poliovirus in the environment is finite	While poliovirus may contaminate soil, sewage and surface water, the presence of virus in the environment is the direct result of the recent presence of virus in the human population. Environmental survival is finite; even under favourable conditions, the virus is inactivated in months.
Humans are the only reservoir of poliovirus	Although poliovirus has been identified in shellfish, the virus does not replicate in these organisms and only remains as long as the surrounding waters are polluted. No evidence of infection with poliovirus has been found in domestic and peridomestic animals, while non-human primates are unlikely reservoirs in nature.
Vaccination interrupts poliovirus transmission	Oral poliovirus vaccine (OPV) produces both intestinal and serological immunity to poliovirus, thereby serving to halt the transmission of wild virus in highly vaccinated populations.

Source: based on Dowdle and Birmingham (1997).

member states were urged to intensify surveillance for poliomyelitis and to provide rehabilitation services for as many children as possible who were crippled by the disease (article 6) (World Health Organization, 1988).

Progress Towards Eradication (1988–2010)

The Global Polio Eradication Initiative is founded upon approaches and processes that were developed by the Pan American Health Organization (PAHO) for the elimination of poliomyelitis in the Americas. As summarised in **Table 5.7**, there are four main strands to the global programme: high routine immunisation coverage; national immunisation days (NIDs); acute flaccid paralysis surveillance; and intensive 'mopping-up' immunisation campaigns. Oral poliovirus vaccine (OPV) is the vaccine of choice for both routine and mass immunisation.

The Global Picture

Although the original WHO target date for poliomyelitis eradication (2000) was missed, and there have been further disappointments along the way, substantial progress towards the ultimate goal of poliomyelitis eradication has been made over the years. As **Figure 5.6** shows, the global count of reported poliomyelitis cases tumbled with the continued rise in vaccination coverage, from 34,597 cases (1988) to 1,413 cases (2010). The associated sequence of poliomyelitis retreat over these years is mapped by country according to a three-category classification of disease status (endemic, non-endemic and certified poliomyelitis-free) in **Figure 5.7**. During the

Table 5.7 Strategies for the global eradication of poliomyelitis

Eradication strategy	Notes
High routine infant immunisation coverage with OPV	The aim is to immunise, through routine vaccination services, ≥ 90 percent of infants with four doses of OPV by one year of age. In order to prevent the re-establishment of wild poliovirus through importation, high levels of routine immunisation should also be maintained in poliomyelitis-free regions.
National immunisation days (NIDs)	Supplementary immunisation activities in the form of NIDs provide an effective vehicle for the rapid and massive dissemination of vaccine strains of poliovirus. The aim of NIDs is to interrupt the circulation of wild poliovirus by immunising all members of the target group (generally children aged < 5 years), regardless of prior immunisation status. National immunisation days are conducted in two rounds, separated by 4–6 weeks, with each round being completed as quickly as possible (usually 1–3 days) and with logistic and biological considerations favouring the delivery of rounds in the cool/dry season. Annual NIDs, conducted over 3–5 consecutive years, are generally required to eradicate wild poliovirus in areas where routine immunisation is low. 'Synchronised' NIDs, with immunisation days coordinated between countries, provide an effective platform for international interventions.
Acute flaccid paralysis (AFP) surveillance	The syndromic surveillance strategy, requiring the immediate reporting and rapid laboratory-based investigation of all cases of AFP in children aged < 15 years serves in the detection of typical and atypical cases of poliomyelitis due to both wild and vaccine-derived strains of poliovirus. In addition, AFP surveillance provides a basis for assessment of the quality of disease surveillance for certification purposes. Molecular epidemiologic methods have enhanced the precision and reliability of laboratory-based poliomyelitis surveillance, allowing wild viruses to be classified into genetic families from which inferences on the geographical source of isolates can be drawn.
'Mopping-up' immunisation campaigns	'Mopping-up' immunisation campaigns are used to interrupt the final chains of poliovirus transmission in the last remaining reservoirs, or suspected reservoirs, of wild poliovirus. These localised campaigns involve the delivery of two doses of OPV to all children aged < 5 years in the target area, with the doses separated by one month. To ensure maximum coverage of the target population, vaccine administration is undertaken on a house-to-house basis.

Source: based on Hull, *et al.* (1997).

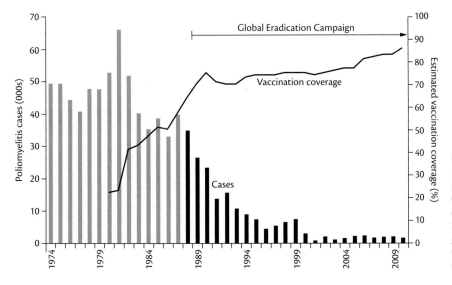

Figure 5.6 Global series of poliomyelitis cases, 1974–2010. The bar chart plots the annual count of poliomyelitis cases as reported to the World Health Organization (WHO). Black bars identify the period covered by the Global Polio Eradication Initiative (1988–2010). Line traces plot WHO/UNICEF estimates of the global coverage of infants with a third dose of poliovirus vaccine (Pol3). *Source*: data from the World Health Organization (www.who.int).

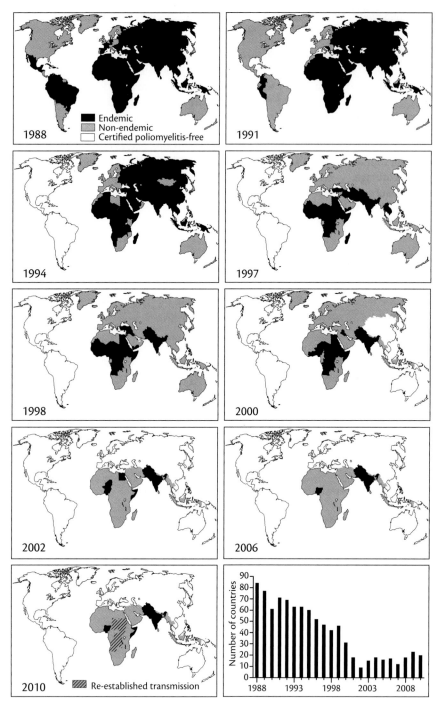

Figure 5.7 Progress towards the global eradication of poliomyelitis, 1988–2010. Countries are classified as endemic (black shading), non-endemic (grey shading) and certified poliomyelitis-free (unshaded). In recognition of the persistent spread (> 12 months) of imported wild polioviruses in some formerly non-endemic countries of the WHO Africa and Eastern Mediterranean Regions, the additional category of re-established transmission is indicated on the map for 2010. Note that re-established transmission was suspected (but not confirmed) for Sudan. The bar chart shows the number of countries that reported cases of poliomyelitis to WHO each year. *Source*: data from the World Health Organization (www.who.int).

course of the 23-year observation interval, the number of poliomyelitis-endemic countries was whittled down from 125 (1988) to four (2010). Wild poliovirus transmission was interrupted in the Americas in 1991 (**Figure 5.8**), the Western Pacific in 1997 and Europe in 1998, with certification of the poliomyelitis-free status of these regions in 1994, 2000 and 2002 respectively (see Figure 4.4). Elsewhere, the scaling up of eradication activities from the mid-to-late 1990s resulted in a marked contraction of the disease in Africa, the Eastern Mediterranean and South-East Asia so that, by 2010, endemic activity had been pushed back to a handful of strongholds in West Africa (Nigeria) and South Asia (Afghanistan, India and

Pakistan) (Figure 5.7). By this time, the global transmission of wild poliovirus type 2 had been interrupted, and all reported cases of wild virus infection were associated with poliovirus types 1 and 3.

Obstacles to Eradication

International Importations and Re-Established Transmission

Throughout the eradication campaign, poliomyelitis-free countries have been under threat from the importation of poliovirus from the remaining endemic regions. The threat has been especially pronounced in those poliomyelitis-free developing countries that, following the cessation of supplementary immunisation activities,

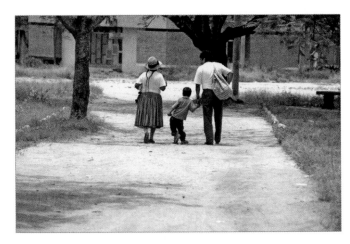

Figure 5.8 The elimination of poliomyelitis in the Americas. This evocative photograph, taken in 1995, shows Luis Fermín Tenorio of Junín, Peru, the last recorded case of wild virus poliomyelitis in the WHO Region of the Americas. *Source*: WHO/PAHO (photograph by A. Waak).

East Asian states, the resurgence of poliovirus activity in connection with the West African state of Nigeria has proved particularly problematic in recent years. As described in Section 4.6, the temporary suspension of immunisation activities in several states of Nigeria in 2003–4 contributed to the spread of wild polioviruses to other countries of the WHO Africa Region and beyond. By 2010, re-established poliovirus transmission (defined as > 12 months of persistent transmission of imported wild polioviruses) was observed in Angola, Chad, Democratic Republic of Congo and, possibly, Sudan (Figure 5.7). To these countries can be added others that recorded outbreaks associated with imported polioviruses in 2010 and 2011, including countries of the WHO Western Pacific (China) and Europe (Kazakhstan, Russian Federation, Tajikistan and Turkmenistan) Regions that had been certified free of wild virus poliomyelitis in earlier years (**Table 5.8**).

Conflict and Security

Wars, particularly in Central America, South Asia and sub-Saharan Africa, have consistently posed one of the single greatest obstacles to the effective implementation of the Global Poliomyelitis Eradication Initiative. In some countries, the war-related disruption of immunisation services has triggered major outbreaks of poliomyelitis and other vaccine-preventable diseases. In the Russian Federation, for example, an outbreak of poliomyelitis in Chechnya during the mid-1990s was consequent upon three years of severe disruption to the health services. Likewise, in Iraq, an outbreak of poliomyelitis in 1999

have experienced a declining level of immunity to the disease. Sample importations of wild poliovirus into poliomyelitis-free countries are illustrated for the period 1999–2003 in **Figure 5.9**. While the map highlights the particular role of India as the source of wild poliovirus in a number of European, Middle Eastern and

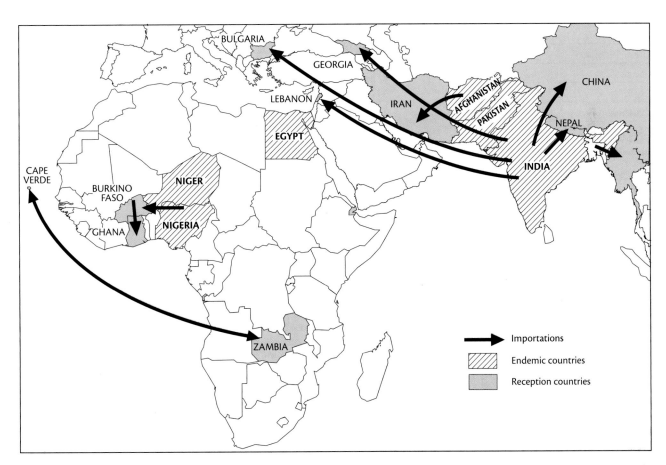

Figure 5.9 Sample importations of wild poliovirus into poliomyelitis-free areas, 1999–2003. Countries in which wild poliovirus was endemic at the end of the observation period are identified by the diagonal shading category. Countries in which importations of wild poliovirus were recorded are identified by the grey shading category. *Source*: redrawn from Smallman-Raynor, *et al.* (2006, Figure 12.17, p. 607), originally from World Health Organization (2003, Figure 9, p. 14).

Table 5.8 Wild poliovirus cases reported to WHO in 2010 and 2011

Country	2010	2011[1]
Endemic		
Afghanistan	25	59
India	42	1
Nigeria	21	45
Pakistan	144	167
Re-established transmission		
Angola	33	5
Chad	26	125
DR Congo	100	87
Outbreak countries		
Central African Republic	0	2
China	0	18
Guinea	0	3
Kenya	0	1
Côte d'Ivoire	0	36
Niger	2	2
Mali	4	7
Congo	441	1
Gabon	0	1
Uganda	4	0
Russian Federation	14	0
Liberia	2	0
Nepal	6	0
Kazakhstan	1	0
Tajikistan	460	0
Turkmenistan	3	0
Senegal	18	0
Mauritania	5	0
Sierra Leone	1	0
Total	1,352	560

Notes: data reported to WHO as of 5 December 2011.
Source: Global Polio Eradication Initiative (www.polioeradication.org).

was associated with continuing unrest in the north of the country (Bush, 2000; Tangermann, *et al.*, 2000). Among those countries in which wild polioviruses continued to be endemic in 2010–11, limited access to conflict-affected areas of Afghanistan (South Region) and Pakistan (Afghan border area) poses a substantial and ongoing threat to the success of the Global Polio Eradication Initiative (Centers for Disease Control and Prevention, 2011d).

Ceasefires and 'periods of tranquillity' have occasionally been negotiated between hostile factions to allow the implementation of disease control and eradication initiatives in conflict-affected areas. Indeed, such health-inspired breaks in fighting have been viewed not only as a means of permitting the delivery of disease intervention measures but also as an informal channel of communication

and peace brokering (Bush, 2000). Examples of states in which ceasefires, periods of tranquillity and various unofficial truces have been negotiated for the purposes of poliomyelitis immunisation include Afghanistan, Angola, Cambodia, El Salvador, Iraq, Myanmar, Sri Lanka and Sudan (World Health Organization, 1997; Tangermann, *et al.*, 2000; Centers for Disease Control and Prevention, 2011d).

Circulating Vaccine-Derived Polioviruses (cVDPVs)

One long-standing public health concern over the use of OPV – the potential for attenuated Sabin strains of poliovirus to revert to the neurovirulence of wild poliovirus and to persist, circulate and cause poliomyelitis outbreaks – was thrown into sharp focus at the turn of the millennium. Between July 2000 and September 2001, 21 cases of paralytic poliomyelitis were identified in the Caribbean island of Hispaniola. The causative agent of the outbreak, which affected both the Dominican Republic (13 cases) and Haiti (8 cases), was found to be a type 1 circulating vaccine-derived poliovirus (cVDPV) – a variant of an attenuated (Sabin) type 1 strain that demonstrated evidence of prolonged replication. With heightened global surveillance for vaccine-derived polioviruses, further outbreaks of cVDPVs have been documented in, among other countries, Afghanistan, Ethiopia, India, Madagascar and the Philippines (Kew, *et al.*, 2004; Centers for Disease Control and Prevention, 2011b).

Global Eradication and the *Strategic Plan 2010–12*

To capitalise on the achievements of the previous 20 years, the Global Polio Eradication Initiative's (2010) *Global Polio Eradication Strategic Plan 2010–12* lays out the milestones to the end of 2012 for the global interruption of wild poliovirus transmission. These milestones include: (1) the interruption of wild poliovirus transmission following importation in countries with outbreaks in 2009 by mid-2010; (2) the interruption of wild poliovirus transmission in countries with re-established transmission (Angola, Chad, Democratic Republic of the Congo and, possibly, Sudan) by the end of 2010; (3) the interruption of wild poliovirus transmission in at least two of the remaining four endemic countries (Afghanistan, India, Nigeria and Pakistan) by the end of 2011; and (4) the interruption of wild poliovirus transmission in all countries by the end of 2012. An interim assessment of progress towards these milestones, provided by the Global Polio Eradication Initiative's Independent Monitoring Board in March–April 2011, concluded that Milestone (1) was 'on track', Milestone (2) had been 'missed', while Milestones (3) and (4) were 'at risk' (World Health Organization, 2011b). At a subsequent meeting, in September 2011, the Board concluded from the evidence that

The GPEI [Global Polio Eradication Initiative] is not on track to interrupt polio transmission by the end of 2012, as had been planned. Indeed … there is substantial risk that stopping transmission will take much longer than the period that remains between now and the end of 2012 (World Health Organization, 2011d, pp. 557–8).

Looking Forwards: Post-Wild Virus Eradication

Assuming that the global interruption of wild poliovirus transmission will be achieved at some future date (**Figure 5.10**), the *Strategic Plan 2010–12* outlines the activities that will be required to certify the achievement and to minimise risks that may arise from two main sources:

(1) vaccine-derived polioviruses, resulting in (i) vaccine-associated paralytic poliomyelitis (VAPP) either in single cases or

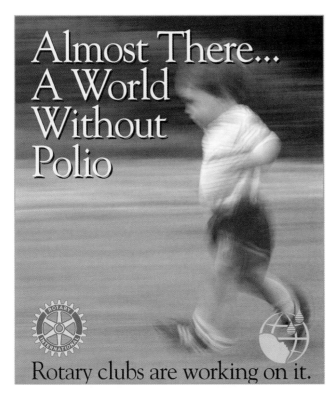

Figure 5.10 Rotary International and the Global Polio Eradication Initiative. Rotary International is one of the four spearheading partners of the Global Polio Eradication Initiative, the others being WHO, US Centers for Disease Control and Prevention and UNICEF. Rotary International established the PolioPlus programme in 1985 and, since that time, the organisation has contributed over US$700 million to the eradication initiative. The poster looks forward to a world without polio. *Source*: Rotary International (www.rotary.org).

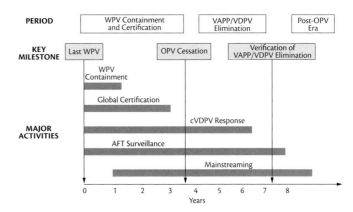

Figure 5.11 Timeline of activities for minimising long-term poliovirus risks following the global interruption of wild poliovirus transmission. AFP = acute flaccid paralysis; OPV = oral poliovirus vaccine; (c) VAPP = (circulating) vaccine-associated paralytic poliomyelitis; VDPV = vaccine-derived poliovirus; WPV = wild poliovirus. *Source*: redrawn from Global Polio Eradication Initiative (2010, p. 58).

outbreaks, (ii) outbreaks due to circulating vaccine-derived polioviruses (cVDPVs) and (iii) long-term excretion of VDPVs by individuals with primary immunodeficiency disorders (iVDPVs);

(2) *wild polioviruses*, resulting from (i) unintentional release from a contained facility (laboratory or vaccine manufacturing site) or (ii) intentional release due to an act of bioterrorism or biological warfare.

Risk minimisation in the post-wild virus transmission era is planned to involve the three stages depicted in **Figure 5.11**, namely:

Stage 1: *Wild Poliovirus Containment and Certification*. This stage involves the destruction or safe storage of infectious or potentially infectious materials, along with the certification of the interruption of global transmission and the containment of wild poliovirus stocks.

Stage 2: *VAPP/VDPV Elimination Phase*. This stage will begin the eventual cessation of the routine use of trivalent OPV in order to eliminate VAPP and the risks of virus re-emergence associated with cVDPVs. AFP surveillance and poliovirus outbreak response capacity will have to be maintained during this phase.

Stage 3: *Post-OPV Era*. This stage is the final stage of the Global Polio Eradication Initiative and will begin with the verification that VDPVs are no longer in circulation.

Ultimately, the *Strategic Plan 2010–12* envisages the transition of existing human resources, physical infrastructure and institutional arrangements away from the Global Polio Eradication Initiative to other priority areas in disease surveillance and control. While the preparatory work for this 'mainstreaming' process can be traced to the 1990s, efforts have been accelerated since 2004 and will continue into the eradication era.

The Long-Term Benefits of Eradication

Economic Benefits

Given the massive investment of time and resources in the Global Polio Eradication Initiative, a fundamental question arises as to the long-term financial benefits that will accrue once the disease has been finally extinguished (cf. Section 6.5). Based on the projected eradication of poliomyelitis by 2005, a cost–benefit analysis by Bart, *et al.* (1996) placed the 'break-even' point – the point at which the financial benefits of eradication exceed the costs – in 2007, with a cumulative global saving of US$13.6 billion by 2040. In a more recent analysis, undertaken for the interval 1970–2050 and with an assumed cessation of poliovirus vaccination after eradication in 2010, Khan and Ehreth (2003) estimate the cumulative global costs of vaccination at US$73 billion and the associated savings in medical care costs at US$129 billion – a net saving of over US$55 billion. Incremental net benefits of a similar order of magnitude (US$40–50 billion) for the period 1988–2035, based on the assumed interruption of wild poliovirus transmission in 2012, have been projected by Duintjer Tebbens, *et al.* (2011).

Human Benefits

Apart from the direct economic benefits of the Global Polio Eradication Initiative, the final elimination of poliomyelitis will relieve the world of a major cause of human suffering and death. Some impression of the magnitude of the long-term human benefits can be gained from **Table 5.9**. Again assuming an eradication date

Table 5.9 Estimated number of poliomyelitis cases and deaths averted, and disability-adjusted life years (DALYs) saved, by routine poliomyelitis immunisation and eradication, 1970–2050

WHO region	Poliomyelitis cases averted (millions)	Poliomyelitis deaths averted (thousands)	DALYs saved (thousands)
Africa	6.89	131	4,426
Americas	9.33	193	10,262
Eastern Mediterranean	4.33	90	3,896
Europe	4.21	88	7,066
South-East Asia	9.05	188	6,762
Western Pacific	7.92	165	7,201
World	41.73	855	39,613

Source: information from Khan and Ehreth (2003, Table 2, p. 704).

of 2010, the table suggests that poliomyelitis control and eradication efforts will avert some 42 million poliomyelitis cases and 855,000 poliomyelitis deaths in the eight decades to 2050. Recognising the crippling nature of poliomyelitis, the avoided morbidity and mortality translates into a long-term saving of 39.6 million disability-adjusted life years (DALYs) (Khan and Ehreth, 2003).

5.4 Other Global Eradication Campaigns

This section examines the several other eradication initiatives that, at various times over the last century, have been launched against human infectious diseases (Table 5.2). We begin with the ongoing campaign to eradicate one of the WHO's 'neglected tropical diseases', dracunculiasis. We then consider the failed efforts to eradicate yellow fever, yaws and malaria.

Campaigns Underway: Dracunculiasis

Dracunculiasis (Guinea worm disease) is a tropical infection of subcutaneous and deeper tissues by the large nematode *Dracunculus medinensis*. Humans are the only known reservoir of *D. medinensis*, with transmission occurring through the ingestion of water from infested wells and ponds. Improving standards of water supply in the first half of the twentieth century reduced the distribution of dracunculiasis. Deliberate campaigns eliminated it from the southern area of the Soviet Union in the 1930s and from Iran in the 1970s. The United Nations-sponsored International Drinking Water Supply and Sanitation Decade of the 1980s called further attention to the disease, and a number of endemic countries (for example, India) began national elimination campaigns. Framed by these developments, the Thirty-ninth World Health Assembly (1986) adopted a resolution calling for the elimination of the disease on a country-by-country basis. This resolution was reinforced when the Forty-fourth World Health Assembly (1991) committed the WHO to the global eradication of dracunculiasis by 1995.

Eradication Feasibility and Strategies

As described by Hopkins and Ruiz-Tiben (1991), a series of biological and socio-political factors make the eradication of dracunculiasis feasible. These include: (1) the easy and unambiguous recognition of the condition; (2) the restriction of the intermediate host (copepods) to water bodies; (3) the availability of simple and cost-effective interventions; (4) the limited geographical distribution and seasonal nature of disease transmission; (5) the absence of an animal reservoir for *D. medinensis*; and (6) the availability of political commitment to the eradication initiative. The principal strategies for eradication are based around the education of at-risk populations, close surveillance and case containment in known endemic villages and the implementation or specific interventions to ensure access to safe water, including the use of filters and the control of copepod populations through the use of temephos insecticide (**Figure 5.12**).

Progress of the Eradication Campaign

Progress towards the global eradication of dracunculiasis is summarised for the period 1991–2010 in **Figures 5.13** and **5.14**. At onset of the eradication initiative in 1991, almost 548,000 cases of the disease were reported from a band of 20 endemic countries that extended from West Africa to the Indian subcontinent (Figure 5.13A). Although the number of reported cases fell rapidly in subsequent years (Figure 5.14), the original eradication target date (1995) was missed and the disease still remained endemic in 13 countries of sub-Saharan Africa at the turn of the millennium (Figure 5.13B). Commitment to the

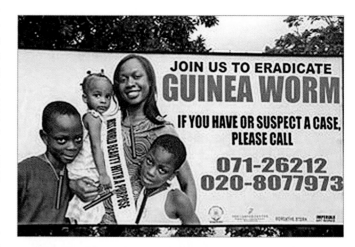

Figure 5.12 Dracunculiasis (Guinea worm disease). A hoarding to promote public awareness of the dracunculiasis eradication campaign in the WHO Africa Region. Note the request for information on actual and suspected cases of the disease, with a view to enhancing surveillance and case containment activities. *Source*: World Health Organization (www.who.int).

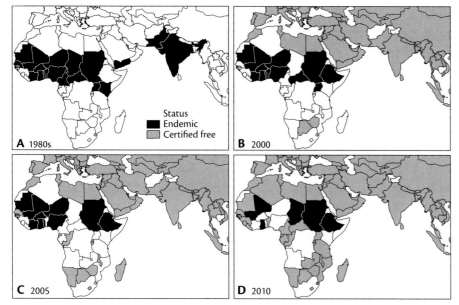

Figure 5.13 Progress towards the global eradication of dracunculiasis, 1991–2010. The situation is shown for the period immediately preceding the onset of the eradication campaign (A) and at the start of 2000 (B), 2005 (C) and 2010 (D). Shading categories identify countries as endemic (black) or certified dracunculiasis-free (grey); other countries (unshaded) were at the precertification stage or were not known to have dracunculiasis but had yet to be certified. *Source*: World Health Organization (www.who.int).

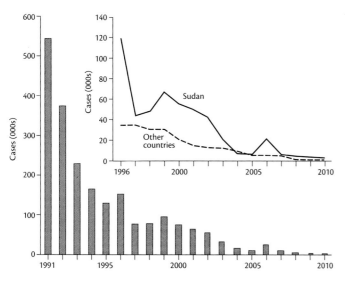

Figure 5.14 Dracunculiasis, 1991–2010. (*Bar chart*) Annual count of reported cases of dracunculiasis worldwide. (*Inset*) Annual count of reported cases of dracunculiasis, Sudan and the rest of the world, 1996–2010. *Source*: data from the World Health Organization (www.who.int).

eradication campaign was maintained throughout the first decade of the twenty-first century such that, by 2010, 180 countries worldwide had been certified free of the disease; indigenous transmission was limited to just five African states (Chad, Ethiopia, Ghana, Mali and Sudan; see Figure 5.13D), with Sudan accounting for the majority of reported cases (Figure 5.14). As of mid-2011, endemic activity had been pushed back to Ethiopia, Mali and the newly-created South Sudan, with insecurity (sporadic violence and civil unrest) in the latter two countries being viewed as the greatest threat to the success of the campaign (Hopkins, *et al.*, 2011).

Failed Campaigns

Of the eradication initiatives in Table 5.2 that have so far been concluded, three (yellow fever, yaws and malaria) ended in failure. The critical factors that contributed to these unsuccessful outcomes are summarised in **Table 5.10** and include: (i) lack of biological and technical feasibility (yellow fever, yaws and malaria); (ii) lack of detailed economic analyses to justify or support the eradication effort (yellow fever and yaws); and (iii) lack of broad-based societal and political support (yellow fever, yaws and malaria) (Aylward, *et al.*, 2000). In the remainder of this section, we review the failed Global Malaria Eradication Programme of 1955–69. Our account draws on Cliff, Smallman-Raynor, Haggett, *et al.* (2009, pp. 243–9).

The Global Malaria Eradication Programme (1955–69)

The development of the insecticide DDT (dichloro–diphenyl–trichloroethane) revolutionised the post-war control of malaria mosquitoes. With the combined virtues of low cost, ready availability and high and long-lasting potency for insects, early reports of the residual application of DDT in parts of southern Europe and the Americas demonstrated the potential for the insecticide to interrupt malaria transmission in endemic areas. Thus prompted, the Eighth World Health Assembly (1955) resolved that the WHO should spearhead a programme for the global eradication of malaria. The resolution was informed by mounting evidence that anopheline mosquitoes were developing resistance to DDT in parts of the world where malaria control programmes had already been implemented, and a desire to achieve worldwide eradication before insecticide resistance became general or widespread (Wright, *et al.*, 1972).

Phases and progress of the campaign

For a given malarious country or region, the eradication campaign was implemented in four phases: (a) *preparatory phase*, characterised primarily by geographical reconnaissance and staff training; (b) *attack phase*, with total coverage spraying of insecticides (DDT and, later, other insecticides); (c) *consolidation phase*, during which total coverage spraying ceased and surveillance was carried out; and (d) *maintenance phase* from the time malaria was eliminated. In addition, anti-larval measures such as marsh draining were used to restrict mosquito breeding grounds, while improved therapeutic and prophylactic drugs were also administered.

Table 5.10 Factors contributing to the failure of disease eradication campaigns

Factor	Yellow fever (1915–77)	Yaws (1954–67)	Malaria (1955–69)
Biological and technical feasibility	Not feasible: animal (non-human primate) reservoir of yellow fever virus.	Not feasible: prevalence and importance of inapparent latent infections was underestimated.	Not feasible: widespread development of vector resistance to insecticides.
Costs and benefits	Economic analyses to justify the campaign were not undertaken until the 1970s.	Economic analyses to justify the campaign were lacking in specific detail.	—[1]
Societal and political considerations	Broad-based political support for eradication was difficult to secure.	Broad-based political support for eradication was difficult to secure.	Political support was secured through the World Health Assembly, although many Member States were not fully aware of their commitments.

Notes: [1]Economic analyses played an important role in justifying the malaria eradication campaign.
Source: based on information in Aylward, et al. (2000, pp. 1515–16).

By 1959, elimination programmes had been launched in 60 of the 148 countries and territories that were classified as malarious, with a further 24 undertaking necessary preparatory work for the launch of elimination initiatives (**Figure 5.15**). Some indication of the subsequent progress of the eradication campaign can be gained from **Figure 5.16**. Between 1959 and 1970, the total population of areas classified in the maintenance phase (malaria eliminated) of the programme grew from ~280 million to ~710 million while, in any given year, a further 500–700 million were resident in areas classified within the consolidation and attack phases (Wright, et al.,

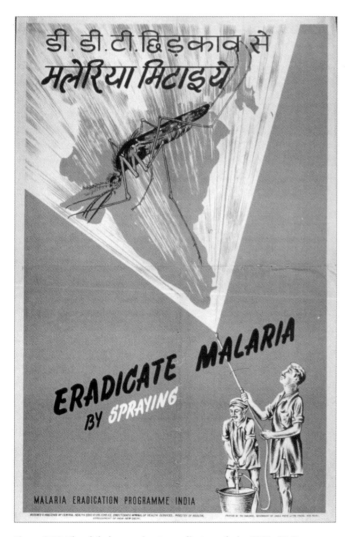

Figure 5.15 The global campaign to eradicate malaria, 1955–69. Poster prepared by the Malaria Eradication Programme, India, c. 1960. The image, which depicts a man spraying insecticide on a larger-than-life mosquito, captures the main strategy of the Global Malaria Eradication Programme in the 1950s and 1960s: the use of DDT and other insecticides to rid the world of malaria mosquitoes. Source: courtesy of the US National Library of Medicine, History of Medicine Division. Copyright owner not known.

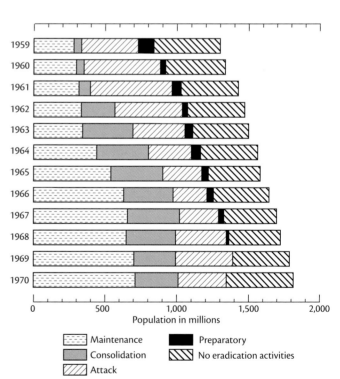

Figure 5.16 Annual distribution of population in areas originally classified as malarious, by phase of the WHO Global Malaria Eradication Programme, 1959–1970. The category 'no eradication activities' includes countries with anti-malaria activities that were not classified as eradication operations. Source: redrawn from Cliff, Smallman-Raynor, Haggett, et al. (2009, Figure 4.33, p. 246), originally from Wright, et al. (1972, Figure 1, p. 77).

1972). Although issues of the feasibility of eradication resulted in the exclusion of most countries of sub-Saharan Africa from the global campaign, large tracts of subtropical Asia and Latin America were all but free of infection by 1965 (Learmonth, 1988; Trigg and Kondrachine, 1998).

The termination of the eradication programme

By the late 1960s, a number of technical and other obstacles to the global eradication of malaria had become apparent. These obstacles included the emergence of substantial vector resistance to DDT and other chlorinated hydrocarbons (**Figure 5.17**), the development of drug-resistant strains of the malaria parasite, logistic difficulties relating to both manpower and the accessibility of areas for insecticide spraying, along with a broad array of other technical, administrative, financial and political issues. In 1969, the Twenty-second World Health Assembly re-examined the eradication strategy, with the conclusion that the aims of the programme should be switched from eradication to control. The effective ending of the malaria eradication initiative resulted in a considerable reduction in financial support for anti-malaria programmes, with the problems compounded by the rise in price of insecticides and anti-malaria drugs with the world economic crisis of the early 1970s (Bruce-Chwatt, 1987; Trigg and Kondrachine, 1998). The epidemic rebound that followed on these developments is illustrated for one country (India) in **Figure 5.18**.

Recent Global Initiatives: The Roll Back Malaria Partnership

Action against malaria has been ramped up in recent years. In 1998, the Roll Back Malaria Partnership (RBM) was launched by the WHO, UNICEF, UNDP and the World Bank with the purpose of coordinating the global response to malaria. The Partnership launched the Global Malaria Action Plan (GMAP) in 2008 as "a blueprint for the control, elimination and eventual eradication of malaria", with the specific objective of reducing the number of *preventable* deaths from malaria worldwide to "near zero by 2015" and with the overall vision of a 'world free from the burden of malaria' (World Health Organization, 2011e, p. 3) (**Figure 5.19**). Malaria control also forms a key target of the UN Millennium Development Goal 6 – to halt and to begin to reverse the incidence of malaria and other major diseases by 2015 (Target 6.C). As we describe in the following section, malaria is not deemed to be eradicable with current technology, although there are aspects of its occurrence that are susceptible to elimination.

5.5 Prospects for Future Eradication

International Task Force for Disease Eradication (ITFDE)

The ITFDE was established in 1988 by a grant from the Charles A. Dana Foundation to the Carter Center at Emory University,

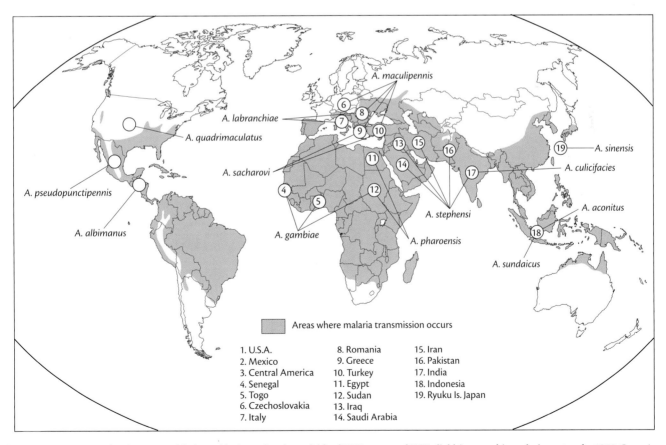

Figure 5.17 Documented resistance to chlorinated hydrocarbon insecticides (DDT group and HCH-dieldrin group) in malaria vectors by 1970. Countries in which vector resistance had been detected (circles) are shown against the global distribution of malaria transmission at the onset of the eradication initiative (shading). Resistant *Anopheles* species in a given country are named. *Source*: redrawn from Cliff, Smallman-Raynor, Haggett, *et al.* (2009, Figure 4.35, p. 250), based on information in Wright, *et al.* (1972).

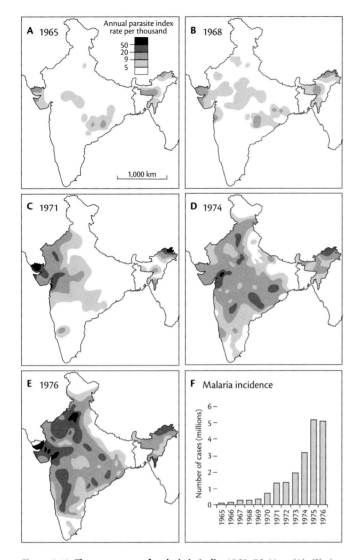

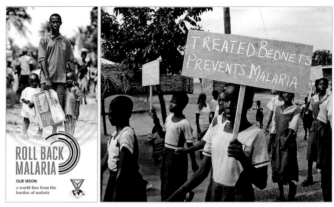

Figure 5.19 The Roll Back Malaria Partnership. (*Left*) The Roll Back Malaria Partnership was formed in 1998 as the global framework for implementing coordinated action against malaria. This promotional poster shows a man holding a long-lasting insecticidal net (LLIN), treated with insecticide and designed to be draped over a bed to protect the user against malaria mosquitoes. (*Right*) Treated bed nets form a key element in efforts to control malaria transmission in endemic areas. *Source*: World Health Organization (www.who.int).

Figure 5.18 The resurgence of malaria in India, 1965–76. Maps (A)–(E) plot the annual parasite index (number of malaria cases per 1,000 population per year) by malaria control area for sample years. The annual incidence of malaria in India is plotted in graph (F). From residual foci of disease activity in central, northeastern and western parts of India in 1965, the map sequence displays a spatial resurgence of malaria activity that, in the words of Chapin and Wasserstrom (1983, p. 273), constituted a "major ecological disaster". Widespread tolerance to organochlorines in some important malaria vectors has been identified as one of the factors that contributed to the resurgence (Chapin and Wasserstrom, 1983; Learmonth, 1988; Sharma, 1996). *Source*: redrawn from Cliff, Smallman-Raynor, Haggett, *et al.* (2009, Figure 4.34, p. 248), based on Learmonth (1988, Table 10.1 and Figure 10.9, pp. 210, 212–13).

Atlanta, with the remit of evaluating diseases as potential candidates for future eradication. Following the cessation of funding in the 1990s, the group was reconstituted with the support of the Bill and Melinda Gates Foundation in 2000. By April 2008, the ITFDE had conducted detailed assessments of 34 infectious diseases. Endorsing existing WHO target diseases for global eradication, the ITFDE concluded that seven diseases (dracunculiasis, lymphatic filariasis, measles, mumps, poliomyelitis, rubella and taeniasis/cysticercosis) were eradicable or potentially eradicable with current technology, while aspects of a further eight diseases could be eliminated (**Table 5.11**). The remaining 19 diseases were variously

deemed by the ITFDE not to be eradicable under the present circumstances (e.g. diphtheria, tuberculosis and yellow fever) or not to be eradicable (e.g. African trypansomiasis and Buruli ulcer) (**Table 5.12**).

Regional Elimination Campaigns: Measles

In addition to those infectious diseases listed in Table 5.2 that are subject to ongoing global eradication campaigns, concerted action against a number of other diseases (including lymphatic filariasis, malaria, measles, onchocerciasis and yaws) has resulted in their retreat from large areas of the globe. Of these diseases, special attention has focused in recent years on measles as a potential candidate for global eradication.

The Regional Elimination of Measles

Prior to the widespread availability of measles vaccine in the world's poorer countries, an estimated 2.6 million people died of the disease each year. This situation changed as the WHO's Expanded Programme on Immunization (EPI) was rolled out from the 1970s and 1980s (Section 4.4). Between 1980 and 2010, the annual number of notified measles cases worldwide fell from 4.21 million to 0.33 million – a decline that was accompanied by a similarly sharp reduction in the WHO's estimates of global measles deaths. Five of the WHO Regions have used these developments as a springboard for regional elimination initiatives. In 1994, the WHO Americas Region established the target of eliminating measles from the Western Hemisphere by 2000. Similar elimination initiatives have subsequently been established in the WHO Regions of Europe (elimination target date: 2010), Eastern Mediterranean (2010), Western Pacific (2012) and Africa (2020), with only South-East Asia having yet to establish a target date for elimination.

Progress towards the WHO regional elimination goals is illustrated in **Figures 5.20** and **5.21**. The elimination of measles in the Americas was achieved in 2002, albeit with subsequent small outbreaks associated with measles virus importations. Major setbacks to measles elimination have been encountered elsewhere, however, including numerous and prolonged outbreaks of measles in Africa

Table 5.11 International Task Force for Disease Eradication: candidate diseases for eradication or elimination (status: April 2008)

Disease	Annual toll worldwide	Chief obstacles to eradication	Conclusion
Eradicable and potentially eradicable diseases			
Dracunculiasis	<10,000 infected; few deaths	Sporadic insecurity	Eradicable
Lymphatic filariasis	120 million cases	Weakness of primary healthcare systems in Africa; increased national/international commitment needed	Potentially eradicable
Measles	780,000 deaths	Lack of suitably effective vaccine for young infants; cost; public misconception of seriousness	Potentially eradicable
Mumps	Unknown	Lack of data on impact in developing countries; difficult diagnosis	Potentially eradicable
Poliomyelitis	2,000 cases of paralytic disease; 200 deaths	Insecurity; low vaccine coverage; increased national commitment needed	Eradicable
Rubella	Unknown	Lack of data on impact in developing countries; difficult diagnosis	Potentially eradicable
Taeniasis/cysticercosis	50 million cases; 50,000 deaths	Demonstration of elimination on national scale	Potentially eradicable
Diseases/conditions of which some aspects could be eliminated			
American trypanosomiasis	10–12 million infections	Difficult diagnosis, treatment; animal reservoirs	Not eradicable; can stop vector-borne transmission to humans in some areas
Hepatitis B	250,000 deaths	Carrier state; infections *in utero* not preventable; need routine infant vaccination	Not now eradicable, but could eliminate transmission over several decades
Malaria	> 300 million cases; > 1 million deaths	National and international commitment; weak primary healthcare systems; drug and insecticide resistance; non-specific diagnoses	Not now eradicacable; elimination possible in Hispaniola
Neonatal tetanus	560,000 deaths	Inexhaustible environmental reservoir	Not now eradicable, but could prevent transmission
Onchocerciasis	37–40 million cases; 340,000 cases of blindness	Lack of macrofilaricide and test for living adult worms	Could eliminate associated blindness in Africa, and probably transmission in the Americas
Rabies	52,000 deaths	No effective way to deliver vaccine to wild animals that carry the disease	Could eliminate urban rabies
Trachoma	150 million cases; 6 million cases of blindness	Link to poverty; inadequate rapid assessment methodology and diagnostic test for ocular infection	Could eliminate associated blindness
Yaws and other endemic treponematoses	Unknown	Lack of political will; inadequate funding; weaknesses in primary healthcare systems	Could eliminate transmission nationwide, as illustrated by India

Source: information from Centers for Disease Control and Prevention (1993b, Table 3, pp. 8–9) and the International Task Force for Disease Eradication (www.cartercenter.org).

and Europe and the continued high burden of the disease in some parts of South-East Asia. These developments have been attributed to sub-optimal coverage with measles-containing vaccine (see, for example, Section 4.6) and to the deleterious impact of funding gaps on vaccination campaigns (Bellini and Rota, 2011).

Integrated approaches: measles and rubella elimination in the Americas

In the drive to eliminate measles from the Americas, the Pan American Health Organization (PAHO) recommended that measles vaccines should also contain rubella antigen. In September 2003, having successfully interrupted the indigenous transmission of measles virus, PAHO adopted a target for the regional elimination of rubella by 2010. The rubella elimination strategy has used a combined measles-rubella vaccine, with the dual function of increasing population immunity to rubella virus whilst maintaining high levels of immunity to measles virus. The last endemic case of rubella in the Americas was detected in 2009 (Andrus, *et al.*, 2011) (**Figure 5.22**).

Accelerated Measles Control and Eradication

The Measles Initiative was established in 2001 as a collaborative effort of the WHO, UNICEF, the American Red Cross, the United States Centers for Disease Control and Prevention (CDC) and the United Nations Foundation to support governments and communities in the implementation of measles vaccination campaigns and surveillance (**Figure 5.23**). With an effective global partnership in place, the Sixty-third World Health Assembly resolved in May 2010

Table 5.12 International Task Force for Disease Eradication: diseases deemed not to be eradicable (status: April 2008)

Disease	Annual toll worldwide	Chief obstacles to eradication
Diseases that are not eradicable under the present circumstances		
Ascariasis	1 billion infections; 20,000 deaths	Eggs viable in soil for years; laborious diagnosis; widespread
Cholera	Unknown	Environmental reservoirs; strain differences
Diphtheria	Unknown	Difficult diagnosis; multiple-dose vaccine
Hookworm disease	740 million cases; 10,000 deaths	Increased national and international commitment; monitoring impact of interventions
Leprosy	225,000 cases	Need for improved diagnostic tests and chemotherapy; social stigma; potential animal reservoir
Meningococcal meningitis	614,000 cases; 180,000 deaths	Lack of serogroup A conjugate vaccine; cost
Pertussis	40 million cases; 400,000 deaths	High infectiousness; early infections; multiple-dose vaccine
Rotaviral enteritis	80 million cases; 870,000 deaths	Inadequate vaccine
Schistosomiasis	200 million infections	Reservoir hosts; increased snail-breeding sites; need simple diagnostic test for intestinal disease
Tuberculosis	8–10 million new cases; 2–3 million deaths	Need for improved diagnostic tests, chemotherapy and vaccine; wider application of current therapy
Visceral leishmaniasis	500,000 cases	Inadequate surveillance, drug supply and knowledge of vector breeding sites; weak primary healthcare systems
Yellow fever	> 10,000 deaths	Sylvatic reservoir; heat-labile vaccine
Diseases that are not eradicable		
African trypanosomiasis	300,000–600,000 infections	Reservoir hosts; difficult treatment and diagnosis
Amoebiasis	500 million cases; 40,000–110,000 deaths	Asymptomatic infections; difficult diagnosis, treatment
Bartonellosis	Unknown	Asymptomatic infections; difficult diagnosis, treatment
Buruli ulcer	Unknown	Inadequate surveillance, early detection and treatment; need field diagnostic test and orally administered treatment
Clonochiasis	Unknown (20 million cases in China)	Animal reservoir; asymptomatic infections; carrier state
Enterobiasis	Unknown	Widespread; mild disease
Varicella zoster	Unknown (3 million cases in USA)	Latency of virus; inadequate vaccine

Source: information from Centers for Disease Control and Prevention (1993b, Table 3, pp. 8–9) and the International Task Force for Disease Eradication (www.cartercenter.org).

to move towards the eventual eradication of measles. Although no date for the eradication of the disease was set, the Assembly did endorse a series of targets to be realised by 2015 for accelerated measles control. These targets include: > 90 percent coverage with a first dose of measles-containing vaccine at the national level, and > 80 percent coverage at the regional level; reduction of annual measles incidence to < 5 cases per million with this level to be maintained; and, within the framework of Millennium Development Goal 4 (MDG 4 – *to reduce child mortality*), to reduce measles mortality by 95 percent as compared with estimated levels for 2000 (Bellini and Rota, 2011).

Feasibility of global measles eradication

Although measles does not share all the criteria of the smallpox eradication 'model' (Table 5.5), the feasibility of global measles eradication is endorsed by the ITFDE (Table 5.11). Humans are the sole reservoir of the virus; accurate diagnostic tests for measles virus infection exist; and an effective and affordable intervention (vaccine) is available (Bellini and Rota, 2011; Moss and Strebel, 2011). The elimination of measles from the Americas has demonstrated

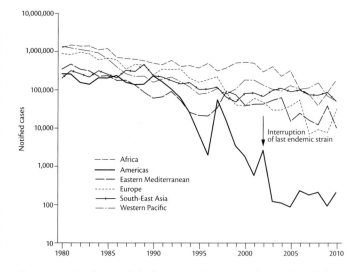

Figure 5.20 Measles trends in the WHO regions. Annual count of notified cases of measles in each WHO region, 1980–2010. See Figure 2.31 for a map of the regions. *Source*: data from the World Health Organization (www.who.int).

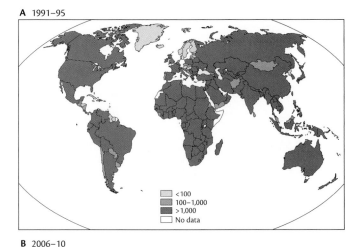

A 1991–95

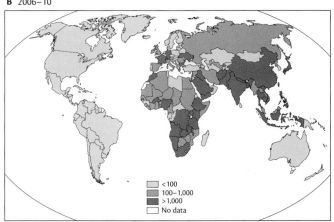

B 2006–10

Figure 5.21 World maps of measles incidence. Maps plot the average annual count of measles cases reported by WHO member states. (A) 1991–95. (B) 2006–10. *Source*: data from the World Health Organization (www.who.int).

the programmatic and operational feasibility of the interruption of measles virus transmission over large geographical areas (Figures 5.20 and 5.21), while economic and health system analyses also validate the feasibility of measles eradication. To these criteria can be added the broad platform of support that has already been established for an eradication initiative (World Health Organization, 2010b; Keegan, *et al.*, 2011). The principal challenges to measles eradication are likely to be logistical, political and financial, with rapid urbanisation and increasing population density, wars and conflicts serving as major obstacles (Keegan, *et al.*, 2011; Moss and Strebel, 2011).

5.6 Hostile Threats: Disease Eradication and Bioterrorism

Once a disease agent has been eradicated, strategies are required to minimise the risk of the reintroduction of the agent into the human population. Recognising that certain international terrorist groups have a declared intent to develop unconventional (Chemical, Biological, Radiological and Nuclear or CBRN) weapon capabilities, the identification of bioterrorism as one of the foremost risks for national and global security has highlighted the threat that attaches to the deliberate release of disease agents (Morens, *et al.*,

2004). Although a large number of viral, bacterial and other disease agents have been posited as possible agents for biological weapons and bioterrorist attacks (World Health Organization, 2004e), a series of factors (including cultivation and effective dispersal, transmission dynamics, environmental stability, infectious dose size and availability of prophylactic and therapeutic measures) suggests that relatively few agents have strategic potential. Among these, smallpox (variola) virus has received particular attention in the literature (Smallman-Raynor and Cliff, 2004).

Smallpox

The Emergency Preparedness and Response (EPR) Program of the US Centers for Disease Control and Prevention (CDC) classifies variola major virus (smallpox) alongside *Bacillus anthracis* (anthrax), *Clostridium botulinum* toxin (botulism), *Yersinia pestis* (plague), *Francisella tularensis* (tularemia) and the viruses associated with certain haemorrhagic fevers (Ebola, Lassa, Machupo and Marburg) as Category A agents for use in biological attacks (Centers for Disease Control and Prevention, 2008). These agents are considered to pose a high-priority risk to national security because they can be easily disseminated or transmitted from person-to-person; they can result in high mortality rates; they have the potential for major public health impacts that might cause public panic and social disruption; and they require special action for public health preparedness.

Particular concern attaches to variola major virus as a Category A biological weapons agent on account of the status of smallpox as an eradicated disease. Routine vaccination against smallpox ceased on the eradication of the disease in the late 1970s, and global immunity has consequently waned in the ensuing years. Under such circumstances, smallpox bioweapons have the potential to spark pandemic transmission of the viral agent, even more so given the lack of familiarity with the disease among recent generations of physicians.

Planning for a Deliberate Smallpox Release: The United Kingdom

In the United Kingdom, guidelines for smallpox response and management in the event of a deliberate smallpox release were published by the Department of Health in 2003. The guidelines detail the establishment of nine Regional Smallpox Diagnosis and Response Groups (RSDRGs) in England, one for each public health region, and one each for Scotland, Northern Ireland and Wales. The groups are headed by a Regional Epidemiologist, with each group having at least five Smallpox Management and Response Teams (SMART) to respond to suspected and probable cases of smallpox. Designated Smallpox Care Centres will provide observation and treatment facilities for suspected and confirmed cases. Designated Smallpox Vaccination Centres will deliver vaccine to target groups while, to assist the implementation of vaccination strategy and other actions, a six-level system of smallpox alert has been established (**Figure 5.24**).

Control under different transmission scenarios

Spatial forecasts of smallpox transmission from initial seedings in the vicinity of central London, generated for three representative scenarios (low, medium and high) of the average number of secondary infections generated by an infected person in a susceptible population, are provided by Riley and Ferguson (2006) (**Figure 5.25**, located in the colour plate section). Their results imply that rapid

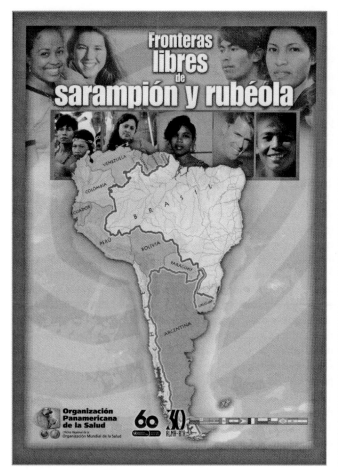

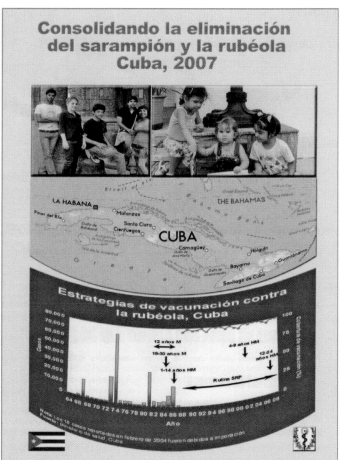

Figure 5.22 The elimination of measles (sarampión) and rubella (rubéola) in the Americas. (*Left*) Pan American Health Organization poster, "Borders free from measles and rubella." (*Right*) Cuban Ministry of Health poster, "Consolidating the elimination of measles and rubella in Cuba, 2007." Cuba had eliminated measles in 1993 and rubella in 1995 through the implementation of routine vaccination and two mass vaccination campaigns in 1985 and 1986 that targeted children, adolescents and adults. In response to a mumps outbreak, a vaccination campaign with measles, mumps and rubella (MMR) vaccine was launched in 2007. Coverage of the target group (males and females aged 12–24 years) was 97 percent and contributed to the maintenance of measles and rubella elimination. The lower graph relates to rubella and shows vaccination coverage (line trace, right-hand axis) and the number of reported cases (bar graph, left-hand axis). *Source*: Castillo-Solórzano, *et al.* (2009, unnumbered plates, pp. 29, 87).

isolation of cases on presentation of rash would be sufficient to bring low- and medium-transmission scenarios under control. Regional or national mass vaccination would only need to be considered for the highest transmission scenarios. A rather different problem would arise if the smallpox release occurred elsewhere in the world and the virus spread to the United Kingdom as a result of multiple independent importations that were dispersed over time. Under such circumstances, mass vaccination may become a more attractive scenario.

Poliomyelitis

Unlike smallpox, poliomyelitis is not generally viewed as representing an immediate bioterrorist threat because of the currently high levels of immunity to poliovirus. This situation will, however, change with OPV cessation in the post-certification era (Sutter, *et al.*, 2004). While the containment of poliovirus stocks, with a view to limiting both the accidental and intentional release of the virus, forms a central component of the Global Polio Eradication Initiative's *Strategic Plan 2010–2012* (Section 5.3), the ability to

synthesise poliovirus from stretches of mail-order DNA on the basis of a genetic blueprint from the Internet (Cello, *et al.*, 2002) has raised fresh concerns over the bioterrorist threat:

> As a result of the World Health Organization's vaccination campaign to eradicate poliovirus, the global population is better protected against poliovirus than ever before. Any threat from bioterrorism will arise only if mass vaccination stops and herd immunity against poliomyelitis is lost. There is no doubt that technical advances will permit the rapid synthesis of the poliovirus genome, given access to sophisticated resources (Cello, *et al.*, 2002, p. 1018).

"The potential for viral synthesis," Cello, *et al.* conclude, "is an important additional factor for consideration in designing the closing stages of the poliovirus eradication campaign" (*ibid.*).

5.7 Towards Extinction

Table 5.3 draws a fundamental distinction between *eradication* and *extinction*, the latter term describing the state in which a disease agent no longer exists in nature or the laboratory. To date, only

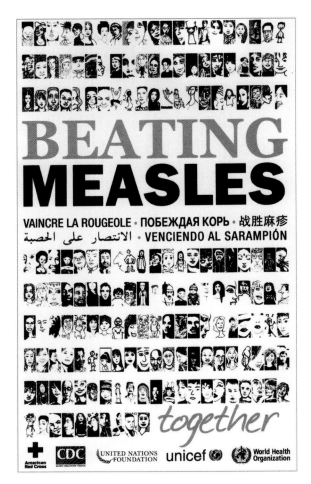

Figure 5.23 Poster for the Measles Initiative. The Measles Initiative was established in 2001 as a collaborative effort of the WHO, UNICEF, the American Red Cross, the United States Centers for Disease Control and Prevention (CDC) and the United Nations Foundation to promote the global control of measles. *Source*: Castillo-Solórzano, *et al.* (2009, unnumbered plate, p. 23).

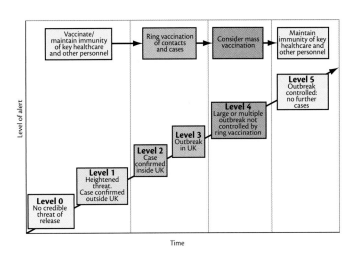

Figure 5.24 Alert levels for a deliberate release of smallpox virus in the United Kingdom. The Department of Health's *Guidelines for Smallpox Response and Management in the Post-Eradication Era* (2003) identify six levels of alert in the event of a deliberate release of smallpox, with each level associated with a specific vaccination strategy and other actions to contain and control the event. Vaccination activities at Levels 0 and 1 centre on the maintenance of immunity in key healthcare workers and other personnel. Levels 2 and 3 are associated with the implementation of ring vaccination strategies in outbreak-affected areas (Section 4.3). If ring vaccination fails to control the outbreak, Level 4 marks the possible implementation of mass vaccination. Finally, Level 5 is associated with the continuing maintenance of immunity in key healthcare workers and other personnel in the post-outbreak period. *Source*: redrawn from Smallman-Raynor and Cliff (2012, Figure 11.21, p. 189), based on Department of Health (2003).

smallpox (variola) virus has reached the status of a disease agent on the brink of extinction.

The Destruction of Known Variola Virus Stocks

WHO-sanctioned stocks of variola virus are currently held in the laboratories of the CDC in Atlanta, USA, and the State Research Centre for Virology and Biotechnology in Koltsovo, Russian Federation. A long-running debate over the ultimate fate of these last known virus stocks has been informed by a range of scientific, political and ethical considerations, with the potentially calamitous consequences of a release – accidental or otherwise – forming one line of argument for their destruction (Butler, 2011; Lane and Poland, 2011). Following a major review of variola virus research by the WHO Advisory Committee on Variola Virus Research (ACVVR) in 2010, the Sixty-fourth World Health Assembly (2011) endorsed the decision of previous Assemblies that existing virus stocks should be destroyed once vital research has been completed. In the light of a further review of variola virus research, a possible date for the destruction of WHO-sanctioned stocks will be considered at the Sixty-seventh World Health Assembly in 2014. While the destruction of these stocks would

mark a step towards virus extinction in the terms of Table 5.3, the possible existence of other (undeclared) laboratory stocks of live variola virus cannot be ruled out. The situation is further complicated by the recognition that variola virus, like poliovirus, can be reconstructed in the laboratory from published gene sequences (Lane and Poland, 2011).

5.8 Conclusion

The concept of disease eradication has had a chequered history, occasionally finding favour and then falling into disrepute as a global health strategy over the last 100 years (Table 5.1). Commenting on the eradication concept in the 1990s, the International Task Force for Disease Eradication (ITFDE) observed that

> The main obstacle to the concept's current acceptance is that if the concept of eradication is invoked against inappropriate or unattainable targets, it can be brought into disrepute. The declared targets of 'elimination' of neonatal tetanus by 1995 and of leprosy by 2000 are potential examples of such dangers. Care should be taken to reserve use of the terms 'eradication' and 'elimination' only for carefully chosen diseases that have a high likelihood of being eradicated (Centers for Disease Control and Prevention, 1993b, p. 23).

As we have seen in this chapter, the success or otherwise of a global eradication campaign is contingent not only on issues of biological and technical feasibility, but also on issues of economic costs and benefits and, crucially, societal and political commitment. Historically, these criteria have determined the failure of some campaigns (yellow fever, yaws and malaria), the success of others (smallpox) and, on the basis of these past experiences, the judicious selection of target diseases for the future. From the list of potentially eradicable diseases identified by the ITFDE, measles was singled out by the 2010 World Health Assembly as a likely successor to poliomyelitis and dracunculiasis for global eradication. But successful eradication campaigns raise fresh dilemmas. Once a disease has been eradicated, difficult decisions need to be made over the ultimate fate of the remaining laboratory stocks of the associated pathogen – a dimension of disease eradication that the global community has been grappling with in respect of smallpox virus for three decades.

CHAPTER 6

Intervention: Modelling, Demographic Impact and the Public Health

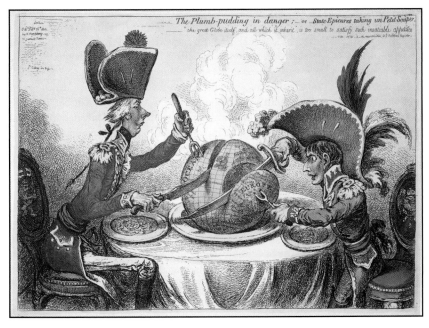

Figure 6.1 The Plumb Pudding in Danger. Pitt and Napoleon exercise their own version of intervention at the global scale in James Gillray's famous political caricature of 1805. In the image, Pitt slices a chunk of ocean, while Napoleon helps himself to Europe – allegories of the respective areas of influence of the two countries. *Source*: Wellcome Library, London.

6.1 Introduction

… It follows that epidemic theory should certainly continue to search for new insights into the mechanisms of the population dynamics of infectious diseases, especially those of high priority in the world today, but that increased attention should be paid to formulating applied models that are sufficiently realistic to contribute directly to broad programmes of intervention and control.

N.T.J. Bailey, *The Mathematical Theory of Infectious Diseases and its Application.* London: Griffin, 1975, p. 27

… The history of malaria contains a great lesson for humanity – that we should be more scientific in our habits of thought, and more practical in our habits of government. The neglect of this lesson has already cost many countries an immense loss in life and in prosperity.

Ronald Ross, *The Prevention of Malaria.* London: John Murray/New York: Dutton, 1910, p. 48

The timely and effective application of the interventions described in previous chapters – quarantine, isolation and vaccination – to control the geographical spread of an outbreak of an infectious disease is not as straightforward as Pitt and Napoleon found it for global domination at the beginning of the eighteenth century (**Figure 6.1**). And so, as we saw in Sections 2.6–2.8, the implementation of control strategies today is commonly guided and adapted in real time by sophisticated, continuous surveillance systems which collect geo- and temporally-coded disease data. The advent of geographical information systems (GIS) and the ready availability of powerful computing hardware and software at all levels of public health delivery systems in both developed and developing economies has added a new dimension – mathematical and statistical modelling – to the development of spatially-targeted interventions. The kinds of models described in, for example, Bailey (1975), Anderson and May (1991), Daley and Gani (1999), Diekmann, *et al.* (2000) and Grassly and Fraser (2008), linked to high-grade surveillance, permit scenarios for disease spread to be explored, along with the efficacy of different intervention strategies. Properly conceptualised and calibrated models can allow the time trends of communicable diseases to be established and enable geographical control questions to be examined. Will this epidemic grow or fade? Will it be like one of the really great pandemics of infectious diseases which from time to time have swept from continent to continent around the inhabited world, like plague in the fourteenth century, cholera in the nineteenth century, influenza in 1918–19 and HIV/AIDS from the late 1970s? Or will it be like severe acute respiratory syndrome (SARS) and be the equally interesting dog which did not bark in the night? How rapidly will it spread? Where will it spread from and to? How may intervention strategies be developed to make the most effective use of resources?

In this chapter, we discuss and illustrate modelling for communicable diseases which may provide some answers to these questions. We begin in Sections 6.2 and 6.3 with the most basic question of all: will this infectious disease outbreak burgeon over time and space, or will it simply fade away? The models are illustrated by application to twentieth-century influenza and poliomyelitis data from a variety of different geographical locations and spatial scales (the United States, France, Iceland, the United Kingdom and Australia). We then move on in Section 6.4 to look at spatial forecasting models which may be deployed to answer the question of "where from

and where to?" for a growing epidemic, drawing upon examples from the epidemiological laboratory of Iceland.

The book is concluded in Sections 6.5 and 6.6. Here we review global aspirations through to 2015 for controlling the spread of communicable diseases, including a cost–benefit analysis of the programme and the likely demographic impacts of control.

6.2 The Basic Reproduction Number, R_0

The *basic reproduction number*, R_0, is one of the key concepts in epidemiology. Critical reviews of the history, development and use of the concept are provided by Dietz (1993), Heesterbeek (2002) and Heffernan, *et al.* (2005). Heesterbeek and Dietz (1996) regard the basic reproduction number as "one of the foremost and most valuable ideas that mathematical thinking has brought to epidemic theory". As described in Heffernan, *et al.*, R_0 was originally developed for the study of demographics (Böckh, 1886; Sharp and Lotka, 1911; Dublin and Lotka, 1925; Kuczynski, 1928). It was independently studied for vector-borne diseases such as malaria (Ross, 1911; MacDonald, 1952) and directly transmitted human infections (Kermack and McKendrick, 1927; Dietz, 1975; Hethcote, 1975). It is now widely used in the study of infectious disease.

We use the concepts and notation of the *SIR* models described in Section 1.4. In a population which is entirely susceptible, R_0 is the number of other individuals infected by a single infected individual during his or her entire infectious period. However, only very rarely will a population be totally susceptible to an infection in the real world. Many human communicable diseases (e.g. measles) confer lifelong immunity upon those attacked. In these circumstances, the *effective reproduction number* estimates the average number of secondary cases per infectious case in a population made up of both susceptible and non-susceptible hosts. It can be thought of as the number of secondary infections produced by a typical infective, and it is the basic reproduction number discounted by the fraction of the host population that is susceptible.

From these definitions, it is clear that when $R_0 < 1$, each infected individual produces, on average, less than one new infected individual, and we therefore predict that the infection will be cleared from the population, or the microparasite will be cleared from the individual. If $R_0 > 1$, the pathogen is able to invade the susceptible population. This threshold behaviour is the most important and useful aspect of the R_0 concept (see Appendix 6.1). In an epidemic, we can determine which control measures, and at what magnitude, would be most effective in reducing R_0 below one, providing important guidance for public health initiatives. The magnitude of R_0 is also used to gauge the risk of an epidemic or pandemic in emerging infectious disease. For example, the estimation of R_0 was of critical importance in understanding the outbreak and potential danger from SARS (Choi and Pak, 2003; Lipsitch, *et al.*, 2003; Lloyd-Smith, *et al.*, 2003; Riley, *et al.*, 2003). It has been likewise used to characterise bovine spongiform encephalitis (BSE) (Woolhouse and Anderson, 1997; Ferguson, *et al.*, 1999; de Koeijer, *et al.*, 2004), foot-and-mouth disease (FMD) (Ferguson, *et al.*, 2001; Matthews, *et al.*, 2003), novel strains of influenza (Mills, *et al.*, 2004; Stegeman, *et al.*, 2004) and West Nile virus (Wonham, *et al.*, 2004). The incidence and spread of dengue (Luz, *et al.*, 2003), malaria (Hagmann, *et al.*, 2003), Ebola (Chowell, *et al.*, 2004) and scrapie (Gravenor, *et al.*, 2004) have also been assessed using R_0 in recent literature. Topical issues such as the risks of indoor airborne infection (Rudnick and Milton, 2003) and bioterrorism (Kaplan, *et al.*, 2002; Longini, *et al.*, 2004) also draw upon this concept.

Herd Immunity

For a communicable disease to be controlled, by whatever means, R_0 in the population must be maintained below unity. Today, this is generally by vaccination. *Herd immunity* occurs when a significant proportion of the population (or the herd) has been vaccinated, and this provides protection for unprotected individuals. See Fine (1993) for a review of the concept. The larger the number of people in a population who are vaccinated, the lower the likelihood that a susceptible (unvaccinated) person will come into contact with the infection. It is more difficult for diseases to spread between individuals if large numbers are already immune, and the chain of infection is broken (cf. Section 1.4).

The *herd immunity threshold, HIT,* is the proportion of a population that needs to be immune in order for an infectious disease to become stable in that community. If this is reached, for example as a result of immunisation, then each case leads to a single new case and the infection will become stable within the population ($R_0 = 1$). If the threshold is bettered, then $R_0 < 1$ and the disease will die out. *HIT* is defined as:

$$HIT = (R_0 - 1)/R_0 = 1 - (1/R_0) \qquad (6.1)$$

This is an important measure used in infectious disease control and in immunisation and eradication programmes.

In the first decade of the new millennium, there have been several global alerts about the health risks posed by newly-emerging and re-emerging diseases (Cliff, Smallman-Raynor, Haggett, *et al.*, 2009, p. 668). Especial concern has been expressed about both SARS and the likelihood of a new global pandemic of influenza with the killing power of the 1918–19 H1N1 pandemic – a concern heightened by the emergence of two novel strains of the influenza virus, highly pathogenic avian influenza (HPAI/A/H5N1) in 2003–5 and swine flu (A/swine/H1N1) in 2009. In the event, all have thankfully had limited impact in terms of human mortality although the World Health Organization raised the alert for H1N1 to the final phase of its six-phase severity scale. As Anderson (*Times Higher*, 9 January 2004) has drily remarked in the context of SARS, "Next time we may not be so lucky", and so we look here at the values for R_0 for the 1918–19 and 2009 influenza outbreaks, not least because both were caused by varieties of H1N1.

Spanish Influenza: Australia, 1918–19

The great influenza pandemic of 1918–19, caused by a new virus strain H1N1, occurred in three waves: spring and early summer 1918 (Wave I); autumn 1918 (Wave II); and winter 1918–19 (Wave III); see **Figure 6.2**. Here, we provide a brief overview of the global dispersal of the three waves. Our account draws on the study of Patterson and Pyle (1991).

Wave I (Spring and Early Summer 1918)

Wave I of the influenza pandemic was attributed at the time to Spain by France and vice versa, and to Eastern Europe by the Americans. But, whatever the truth, the disease acquired its popular name of *Spanish influenza* at this stage. Some of the first records

of influenza activity can be traced to US Army recruits at Camp Funston, Kansas, where an epidemic of influenza first manifested in early March 1918. By the end of July, all continents had been reached. Wave I was comparatively mild.

Wave II (Autumn 1918)

During the summer of 1918, the virus mutated into a more lethal strain and a second, more severe, form of the disease emerged. Pneumonia often developed quickly, with death usually coming two days after the first indications of influenza. The exact geographical origins of Wave II are, like Wave I, unknown although western France is generally viewed as the source. The first reports can be traced to the French Atlantic port of Brest, a landing point for American troops, in late August. From here, ships appear to have carried the disease to coastal locations of North America, Africa, Latin America, South Asia and the Far East by September. New Zealand was infected in October by ships from the United States while Australia remained largely free of the disease until January 1919.

Wave III (Winter 1918–19)

In the aftermath of Wave II, a third influenza wave – of intermediate severity to the preceding waves – appeared in the winter of 1918–19. While relatively little is known of the origin and spread of this tertiary wave, the pandemic appears to have finally run its course by the spring of 1919.

Australia

Australia's involvement in the First World War was on a massive scale in relation to its small size. From a population of some five million, over 300,000 troops served in Europe, and the problems of bringing the survivors home in the autumn and winter of 1918 – at the very height of the influenza pandemic – was on a similarly massive scale. In the early part of October 1918, with the health authorities of Australia cognisant that a virulent form of influenza was within striking distance of the country, instructions were issued for the port quarantining of all vessels with cases of influenza aboard (Cumpston, 1919, p. 7). So began Australia's six-month maritime defence against the great influenza pandemic. The medical officer who successfully led the strategy was J.H.L. Cumpston (**Figure 6.3**), Director of Quarantine and later Australia's first Commonwealth Director-General of Health.

The quarantine record

Records have survived for 228 vessels arriving in Australia between October 1918 and April 1919, of which 79 (35 percent) documented cases of influenza (Smallman-Raynor and Cliff, 2004, Table 11.7, p. 584). **Figure 6.4** plots, by week of arrival in Australia, the distribution of the 79 infected vessels according to the inferred place of virus acquisition: Pacific Rim (chart A); Europe (B); and other locations (C). Vessels on which cases of influenza were documented after arrival in Australia and which, in the absence of quarantine, would have served as potential sources of infection for the population of Australia, are indicated by the black shading. Figure 6.4 suggests a temporal shift in the geographical source of maritime influenza, from the Pacific Rim in October–December 1918 (chart A) to Europe in January–April 1919 (chart B). This temporal shift was associated with the arrival of generally larger, and more heavily crowded, troopships from Europe via Suez in the latter period.

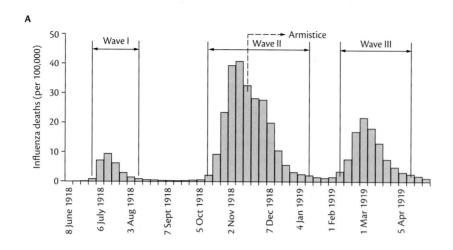

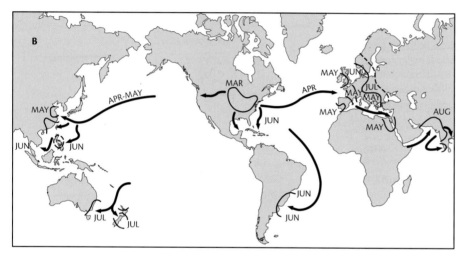

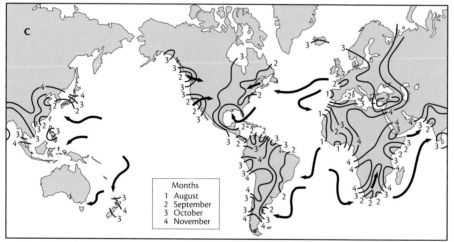

Figure 6.2 Spanish influenza, 1918–19. (A) Weekly influenza death rate per 100,000 population, London and the county boroughs of England and Wales, June 1918–April 1919. The three wave form of the pandemic is clear. The global diffusion of the first two waves is mapped in (B) and (C). (B) Wave I, spring and early summer 1918. (C) Wave II, Autumn 1918. *Sources*: (A) Smallman-Raynor, *et al.* (2002, Figure 1, p. 457), (B) and (C) Smallman-Raynor and Cliff (2004, Figure 11.4, p. 583).

Evidence from infected troopships

The influenza records for four troopships (*Devon*, *Medic*, *Boonah* and *Ceramic*), arriving at Australian ports between November 1918 and March 1919, are shown in **Figure 6.5**; the vessels involved are illustrated in **Figure 6.6**. Some impression of the conditions that prevailed on the ships can be gained from the eyewitness accounts of senior officers. According to one anonymous officer aboard the *Medic*, the scene

… was remarkable. A score or more of stalwart young men lay helpless about the after well-deck, awaiting transport to the improvised and overflowing hospitals in the troop-decks. That they lay there was not due to any neglect or delay on the part of the busy stretcher-bearers, but to the extraordinarily sudden and disabling onset of the disease. One smart, well set-up young soldier came up a companion-ladder close to where I stood, held on for a few seconds to a rail, and then sagged slowly down till he assumed the characteristic flattened sprawl on the deck. There was no pretence or "old-soldiering" about

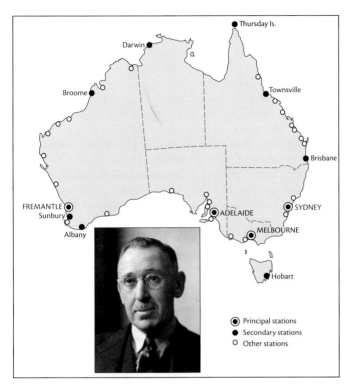

Figure 6.3 Quarantine administration, Commonwealth of Australia, at the end of the First World War. Australia's principal and secondary quarantine stations are marked, along with other ports of entry at which quarantine officers were stationed. The photograph is of J.H.L. Cumpston (1880–1954), Australia's first Commonwealth Director-General of Health, 1921–45. Cumpston oversaw the health of Australia and the troops she put in arms in two world wars. He produced a number of service handbooks on diseases in Australia from 1788 to 1920. The findings were summarised in a book, *Health and Disease in Australia*, completed in 1928. This was not published until 1989, when the work was edited and introduced by Milton Lewis as part of Australia's bicentennial celebrations. *Sources*: (*Map*) drawn from *The Quarantine Annual*, 1930, Office International d'Hygiène Publique, League of Nations; (*photograph*) National Library of Australia.

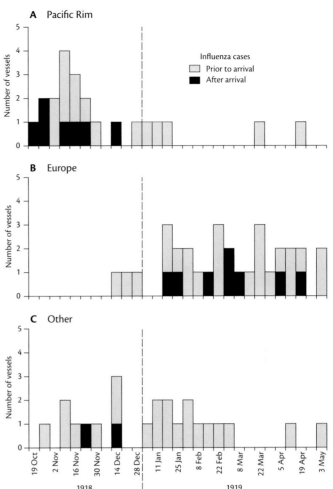

Figure 6.4 Maritime quarantine and 'Spanish influenza', Australia, 1918–19. Graphs plot, by overseas source of infection, the weekly count of vessels infected with influenza and quarantined on arrival at Australian ports, October 1918–May 1919. (A) Pacific Rim. (B) Europe. (C) Other. Vessels on which cases of influenza were recorded after arrival in Australia, and which may therefore be assumed to have maintained an unbroken chain of infection aboard ship, are indicated on each graph by the black shading. *Source*: Smallman-Raynor and Cliff (2004, Figure 11.5, p. 585).

it. The men were literally being knocked down by a profound systematic intoxication of extraordinarily rapid onset (Anonymous, cited in Cumpston, 1919, p. 53).

As Figure 6.5 shows, the influenza curve for the *Medic* followed a broadly similar course to other troopships, with two marked features of the frequency distribution of cases:

◆ a generally log-normal nature. Cases peaked within three to 10 days of start of voyage, with a long positive tail to the distribution;

◆ recurring secondary cycles of cases within general lognormal shape. Statistical analysis using the autocorrelation function (ACF) suggests that there is a periodicity in the time series of about four days, roughly corresponding with the known serial interval of the disease.

The long journey from Europe gave Cumpston time to organise a quarantine system. Boats reporting influenza were isolated in harbour, and troops were not allowed ashore until they were free of the disease. Once soldiers were landed and returned to their homes, they found that interstate travel was also restricted to inhibit transmission – by armed guards in the case of the land border between

Queensland and New South Wales. The effect of these measures was to ensure that peak death rates in Australia were about an eighth of those in the United States, and a quarter of those in South Africa and New Zealand. Such was the success of the influenza control measures, concluded Cumpston, that

during the last three months of 1918, maritime quarantine had the effect of holding at the sea frontiers an intensely virulent and intensely infective form of influenza, which not only caused disastrous epidemics in New Zealand and South Africa, but actually arrived at the maritime frontiers of Australia, and caused alarming epidemics amongst the personnel of vessels detained in quarantine (Cumpston and Lewis, 1989, pp. 318–19).

Although the effectiveness of the quarantine measures of late 1918 has been questioned (McQueen, 1975), epidemiological evidence does point to a delay of several months in the spread of virulent influenza in Australia. So, on the basis of recorded mortality, Cumpston traced the start of the Australian epidemic to

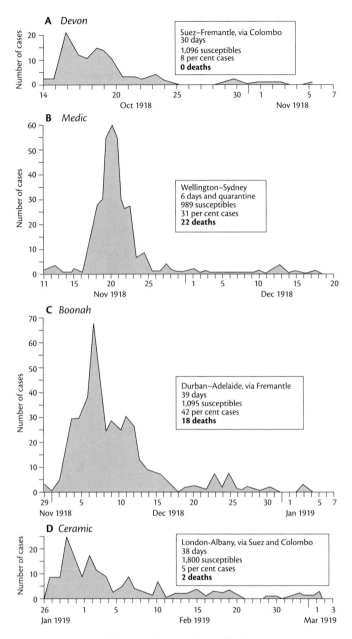

Figure 6.5 The role of ships in dispersing 'Spanish' influenza, 1918–19.
Number of cases of influenza reported daily on four troopships repatriating troops from Europe to Australia in the aftermath of the First World War. (A) *Devon*. (B) *Medic*. (C) *Boonah*. (D) *Ceramic*. *Source*: Cliff, *et al.* (2000, Figure 5.9, p. 194).

early 1919. The first influenza deaths were reported in the state of Victoria (January), to be followed thereafter by New South Wales (February), South Australia (March), Queensland (April), Western Australia (June) and Tasmania (August). In explaining the timing of the epidemic sequence, Cumpston noted that:

> Western Australia and Tasmania are the two States having the least human contact with the two [earliest] infected States, New South Wales and Victoria; they were the two States which most vigorously applied inter-State quarantine restrictions; and they were the States latest infected in the series (Cumpston and Lewis, 1989, p. 119).

Lessons from Epidemics at Sea

A number of writers have commented on the potential epidemiological value of the Australian experience in sea transport and naval vessels in the First World War. Cumpston (1919) argued that a troopship is a self-contained highly insulated and concentrated herd. In Australian transports, this herd remained together on the voyage to or from England for a period of eight weeks, far longer than other transports (for example, US and Canadian troops crossing the Atlantic). The herd was reasonably homogeneous in its susceptible history, and used to suffering a wide range of protective and prophylactic expedients and experiments (for example, shore quarantine, prompt diagnosis and isolation, immunisation and treatment). As Butler (1943, p. 671) has commented:

> Every new case was reported on pain of severe disciplinary action, a skilled staff, professional and clerical, was often available; and provision could easily have been made for the collecting, assembling, and manipulation of a large number of reasonably comparable experiences.

Cumpston's assertion is borne out by Vynnycky, *et al.* (2007). Using the morbidity data from the *Devon*, *Boonah* and *Medic* as confined settings, they compared the estimated basic and effective reproduction numbers for the 1918 pandemic with the numbers calculated for open settings in European and American cities. Several different estimation methods based on the growth rate and the final size of the pandemic were used. They found that the effective reproduction number was in the range 2.1–7.5 for confined settings like the *Devon* and 1.2–3.0 in community-based settings (**Figure 6.7**). Further, assuming that 30 percent and 50 percent of individuals were immune to Spanish influenza after the first and second waves respectively, Vynnycky, *et al.* estimated that, in a totally susceptible population, an infectious case could have led to 2.6–10.6 further cases in confined settings and 2.4–4.3 in community-based settings. These findings confirm the greater dangers of transmission in confined environments and the relatively low transmissibility of the 1918 Spanish influenza virus in open settings which has been found by other studies (for example, Mills, *et al.*, 2004; Chowell, *et al.*, 2006).

Pandemic Influenza A/Swine/H1N1, 2009

The novel strain of influenza, A/swine/H1N1 claimed its first suspected cases in Mexico during March, 2009, and spread to the United States (California) in early April. By 12 May 2009, 5,251 cases of the new influenza had been officially reported to the World Health Organization (WHO) from 30 countries, with most of the identified cases exported from Mexico (Fraser, *et al.*, 2009). Boëlle, *et al.* (2009) estimated the basic reproduction number from the epidemic curve in Mexico using several methods and concluded that the number was less than 2.2–3.1 in Mexico. Fraser, *et al.* (2009) arrived at a value in the range 1.34–2.04 using data for La Gloria, Mexico. These comparatively low rates are in line with or slightly below the rate estimated by Vynnycky, *et al.* for the 1918 pandemic in community settings. This seems to imply that it is sustained person-to-person transmission which is essential for pandemic development of influenza rather than catastrophically high basic reproduction numbers. We look more closely at the development of the swine flu pandemic in the US in Section 6.3. See Anderson (2009) for a discussion of the 2009 pandemic in the United Kingdom.

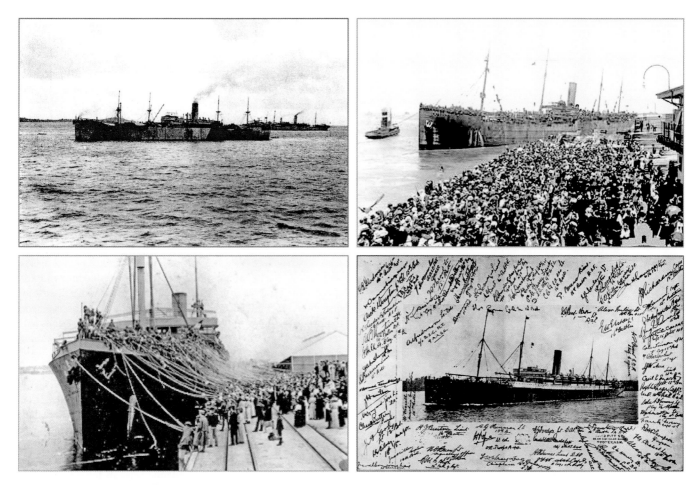

Figure 6.6 Australia and the influenza pandemic of 1918–19. Four troopships which carried 'Spanish' influenza from the European Theatre or South Africa to Australia in the aftermath of the First World War. (*Upper left*) Troopship *Devon* (foreground) in First World War camouflage with troops aboard, 1915. (*Upper right*) Troopship *Medic*. HMAT (His Majesty's Australian Transports) *Medic* (A7) departs Melbourne assisted by a tug, and watched by a crowd of well-wishers on the wharf, 16 December 1916. (*Lower left*) Troopship *Boonah* (HMAT A36) departing from Brisbane during World War One, 1916. Image shows a large crowd gathered to wave farewell to the troops. The ship is decorated with streamers. (*Lower right*) Signed photograph of the troopship HMAT A40 *Ceramic*, the troopship that took the 16th Battalion from Melbourne to Egypt in late December 1914. On this, the *Ceramic*'s first trip as a troopship, the dangers of epidemics of infectious diseases in confined spaces was illustrated. "The first death of a member of the batallion occurred this day [20 January 1915] when Private C.R. … died of pneumonia following measles" (Longmore, 1929, p. 29), and "On January 20, a sick return showed that there were 10 cases of pneumonia, 13 of measles, 7 of influenza, and 15 with other diseases in hospital, a total of 45 or 1.7 per cent. of the troops on board. During this period of the trip all hands were vaccinated and inoculated, to the obvious disgust and temporary discomfort of the troops" (Longmore, 1929, p. 21). *Sources*: (*Upper left*) National Maritime Museum, Greenwich. (*Upper right*) Australian War Memorial website. Photographer Josiah Barnes. (*Lower left*) John Oxley Library, State Library of Queensland, Australia. Photographer unknown. (*Lower right*) Longmore (1929, between pp. 18–19).

6.3 The Spatial Basic Reproduction Number, R_{0A}

Swash–Backwash Models

If we are dealing with the spread of a communicable disease through a system of geographical areas like counties or countries, we need to be aware of Tobler's (1970, p. 236) First Law of Geography – "everything is related to everything else, but near things are more related than distant things", a point reinforced by Gould (1970, pp. 443–44):

Why we should expect [spatial] independence of observations that are of the slightest intellectual interest or importance in geographic research I cannot imagine. All our efforts to understand spatial pattern, structure and process have indicated that it is precisely the lack of independence – the interdependence – of spatial phenomena that

allows us to substitute pattern, and therefore predictability and order, for chaos and apparent lack of interdependence – of things in time and space.

Unfortunately, this leaves us with a problem as far as R_0 is concerned because its formulation is aspatial. The best we can do when dealing with a system of areas is either to evaluate it for the set of areas taken as a whole, or independently for each geographical unit in the set. We thus need a spatial analogue of R_0 which takes account of the First Law and which gives a sense of whether an infectious disease will propagate epidemically through a system of areas or die out.

We have demonstrated elsewhere using measles and poliomyelitis data that the spatial extent of infected units within a geographical area, and the time taken from the start of an epidemic for a communicable disease to reach each unit, may be used to measure

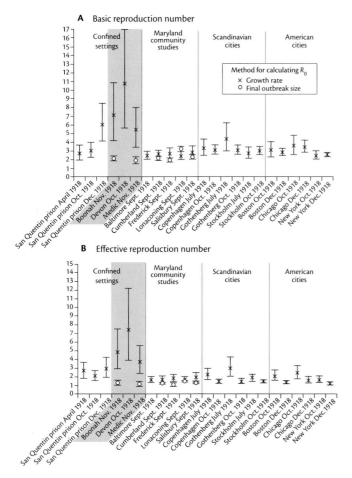

Figure 6.7 Effective and basic reproduction numbers for Spanish influenza, 1918. Morbidity data from cities in Europe and America for community-based and confined settings. Several different methods based on the growth rate and final size of the epidemic have been used to estimate the effective and basic reproduction numbers for the 1918 (Spanish) influenza virus. The effective reproduction number (the average number of secondary infectious cases produced by a typical infectious case in a given population) for the 1918 influenza virus was in the range 1.2–3.0 and 2.1–7.5 for community-based and confined settings, respectively. The basic reproduction number (the average number of secondary infectious cases resulting from a typical infectious case in a totally susceptible population) was in the range 2.4–4.3 and 2.6–10.6 cases in community-based and confined settings, respectively. *Source*: Vynnycky, *et al.* (2007, Figure 2, p. 885).

the spatial velocity of an epidemic wave (Cliff and Haggett, 1981; Trevelyan, *et al.*, 2005; Cliff and Haggett, 2006). In this section, we propose a robust spatial version of R_0, which we denote by R_{0A}, for estimating the spatial velocity of a communicable disease as it passes through a system of areas. It enables us to determine whether a disease will grow spatially or fade out. R_{0A} is robust because it uses only the binary presence/absence of disease reports rather than the actual number of reported cases/mortality.

The Model

Our account is taken from Cliff, Smallman-Raynor, Haggett, *et al.* (2009, pp. 555–58). A single epidemic wave in any large geographical area is a composite of the waves for each of its constituent sub-areas. That is, the composite wave at the larger geographical scale (say, a country) can in principle be broken down into a series of

multiple waves for its constituent sub-areas (say, its regions) at the smaller geographical scale.

Assuming that both the sub-areas and the time periods are discrete, we use the following notation:

A = Area covered by an epidemic wave in terms of the number of sub-areas infected where a_i is a sub-area in the sequence 1, 2, . . . a_i . . . A

T = Duration of an epidemic wave, defined in terms of a number of discrete time periods, t_j, in the sequence 1, 2, . . . t_j . . . T.

Q = Total cases of a disease recorded in a single epidemic wave measured over all sub-areas and all time periods. Thus q_{ij} is the number of cases recorded in the cell formed by the i-th sub-area and the j-th time period of the $A \times T$ data matrix.

To illustrate the method, we assume in **Figure 6.8** a simple epidemic wave where $A = 12$, $T = 10$ and $Q = 122$. Thus in Figure 6.8A we begin with a hypothetical map which is converted into a 12×10 space–time data matrix in which 122 recorded cases of a disease are distributed to simulate an array typical of an epidemic wave. Note that, whereas this overall wave is continuous (no time periods with zero cases), for individual sub-areas the record may be discontinuous with one or more time periods with zero cases.

For any one of the rows in the data matrix in Figure 6.8A, two cells can be identified which mark the 'start cell' and the 'end cell' of a recorded outbreak; if the infection only lasts for one time period, the start and end cell are the same. Figures 6.8B and C analyse these start and end cells. In Figure 6.8B the 12×10 matrix is rearranged so as to position the start cells in an ascending temporal order. This line of cells (dark shading) defines the position of the leading edge (*LE*) marking the start of the epidemic wave in the different sub-areas. To the left and above this line lies a zone of cells (light shading) which have yet to be infected and thus may be regarded as areas to which the epidemic has yet to spread.

Equally, the 12×10 matrix can be organised as in Figure 6.8C, so as to arrange the end cells in ascending temporal order. This line of cells (dark shading) defines the position of the trailing edge or following edge (*FE*), marking the completion of the epidemic waves in each of the different sub-areas. To the right and below this line lies a zone of cells which have ceased to be infected and which thus may be regarded as areas which have recovered from infection.

Both the edges, *LE* and *FE*, can be combined as in Figure 6.8D to identify cells which are in susceptible, S, infected, I, and recovered, R, states. The resulting graph may be regarded as a *phase transition* or *SIR diagram*. It has two roles: first, it defines the boundaries of the two phase shifts from susceptible to infective status ($S \Rightarrow I$) and from infective to recovered status ($I \Rightarrow R$) and second, it integrates the three phases, S, I, and R, as areas within the graph. As discussed in Cliff and Haggett (2006), the phase diagram assumes characteristic configurations depending upon the velocity, duration and ultimate spatial extent of an epidemic wave as it passes through a region.

Three model parameters relating to the phase diagram are especially useful. We refer to these here as V_{LE}, and V_{FE}, the velocities of the leading and following edges of the wave which are functions of the average temporal position of the edges in the phase diagram; and R_{0A}, here defined as the *spatial basic reproduction number*. The relevant equations are summarised in Appendix 6.1.

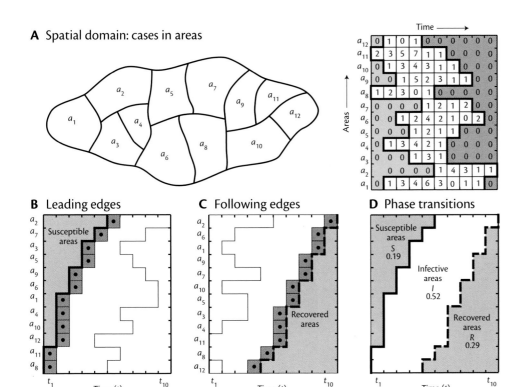

Figure 6.8 Calculating R_{0A}: hypothetical 12-area example. (A) Base map with areas reference coded as $a_1 \dots a_{12}$, and associated space–time data matrix with reported cases for each area given in cells. (B) Matrix rearranged to order leading edges, LE and (C) following or trailing edges, FE. (D) Leading and following edges plotted as a phase-transition diagram with susceptible (S), infected (I) and recovered (R) integrals for areas. *Source*: Cliff, Smallman-Raynor, Haggett, *et al.* (2009, Figure 10.3, p. 556).

Spatial Basic Reproduction Number

In the notation of Figure 1.17, the aspatial basic reproduction number, R_0, is defined as the ratio between the infection rate, β, and the recovery rate, μ. That is, $R_0 = \beta/\mu$ and, as we have noted, it is interpreted as the average number of secondary infections produced when one infected individual is introduced into a wholly susceptible population. In the spatial domain, as shown in Figure 6.8D, the S, I and R integrals define the boundaries of the two phase shifts from susceptible to infective status ($S \Rightarrow I$) and from infective to recovered status ($I \Rightarrow R$). The spatial basic reproduction number, R_{0A}, is the average number of secondary infected areas produced from one infected area in a virgin region. The integral S parallels β in that a small value indicates a very rapid spread. The integral R parallels the reciprocal of μ in that a large value indicates very rapid recovery. As detailed in Appendix 6.1, we can compute R_{0A} as the ratio of $S_A:R_A$. Values of R_{0A} calibrate the velocity of spread (the larger the value, the greater the rate of spread).

Cyclical Re-Emergence: Spotting Influenza Pandemics

To illustrate the use of R_{0A}, we begin by applying it to the task of separating out influenza pandemic seasons from the normal run of influenza years over the course of the twentieth century. Three different spatial scales of data are used: France, a continental country (population 52 million in 1970); Iceland, an isolated island location (population 205,000 in 1970); and Cirencester, a small market town served by a single general practitioner, Edgar Hope-Simpson, for the second half of the century (population 15,000 in 1970). Then we combine the notion of different spatial scales within a single country by examining the potentially pandemic A/swine/H1N1 global outbreak of 2009 in the United States.

France: A Continental Country

As described in Cliff, Smallman-Raynor, Haggett, *et al.* (2009, pp. 558–9), it is possible for the 113-year time window from 1887 to create two matrices giving the time series of monthly influenza mortality for two geographical frameworks: (i) $n = 51$ towns with populations over 30,000 (**Figure 6.9**) × 168 months, 1887–1900 and (ii) $n \approx 90$ *départements* × 1,188 months, 1901–99. These two matrices form the basis for the analysis reported as follows.

Figure 6.10 illustrates the temporal pattern of recorded deaths from influenza in France over the period. Figure 6.10A shows the seasonal distribution of mortality, with its winter peak characteristic of northern hemisphere countries. For this reason, in the analysis which follows, we have used as our temporal unit an *influenza season* running from 1 July through to 30 June of the following year, rather than calendar years which split months of high influenza mortality across year boundaries. Figure 6.10B charts the annual time series. In Europe, as described by Dowdle (1999), pandemics (marked) occurred as follows within this 113-year window:

(i) 1889. First deaths were reported in France in November 1889; the peak month was January 1890. The pandemic occurred in three successive waves in most parts of the world, producing mortality and morbidity greater than had been seen in decades. H2N? was the likely strain.

(ii) 1900. Dowdle (1999) has queried whether this was truly a pandemic. Excess mortality was reported in North America and in England and Wales but not globally. H3N? was the likely strain.

(iii) 1918–19. This occurred in three waves as follows – Wave I: April–July 1918; Wave II: August–November 1918; Wave III: March 1919 (Patterson and Pyle, 1991). It produced mortality

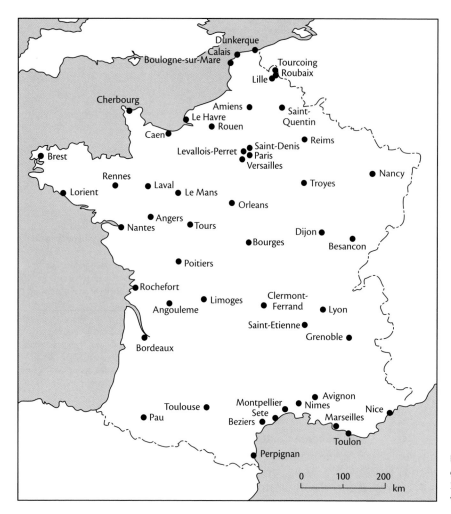

Figure 6.9 Towns of France, 1887. Geographical distribution of 51 towns with populations in excess of 30,000 used to estimate the spatial velocity of influenza waves in France, 1887–1905.

unequalled in recorded history – up to 50 millions or more worldwide. H1N1 was the likely strain.

(iv) 1957. This pandemic occurred in two main waves – Wave I: February–December 1957; Wave II: October 1957–January 1958 (Cliff, *et al.*, 2004). H2N2 was the causative virus.

(v) 1968–69. Wave I: 1968–69 (30 percent of deaths); Wave II: 1969–70 (70 percent of deaths). Wave I primarily affected North America and to a lesser extent Europe. In Wave II the situation was reversed and was associated with significant drift in the N surface antigen (Viboud, *et al.*, 2005). H3N2 was the causative strain.

Figure 6.10B shows that, as in most countries of the world, the 1918–19 pandemic stood alone in France in terms of mortality caused. While the long-term trend in mortality is steadily downwards, nevertheless it is the case that pandemic years generally experienced heightened mortality as compared with adjacent years.

The time series illustrated in Figure 6.10B reinforces the need for robust methods of analysis. Influenza mortality appears to have run at a much higher level between 1887 and 1900, than in the rest of the time series. However, this is an artefact of the recording method; from 1887–1900, influenza mortality in France was estimated from excess pneumonia deaths, whereas in the rest of the series, it was recorded directly.

Figure 6.11A plots the results for the spatial basic reproduction number, R_{0A}, and the two edge parameters, V_{LE}, and V_{FE}, along with the linear regression trend lines. It shows that the long term trend in R_{0A} was slowly downwards over the last century; i.e. the rate of geographical propagation of influenza epidemics gradually diminished, probably reflecting less intense epidemics arising from (i) improved standards of living and healthcare, and (ii) no shift of virus strain since 1969. This century-long declining trend in R_{0A} is reflected in a similar decline in the leading edge (*LE*) velocity parameter, and a rising trend in the following edge (*FE*) parameter implying that epidemics have arrived later and ended sooner in each influenza season; influenza seasons have become of shorter duration.

Within these long term trends, however, the pandemic seasons of 1900, 1918–19, 1957 and 1968–69 showed a locally raised R_{0A}. In the case of 1889, this is not evident, while the rise to a higher level in 1969 persisted for four seasons. In the latter case, this is consistent with the description by Viboud, *et al.* (2005) of the 1968–69 pandemic as a "smouldering pandemic". From the late 1980s, R_{0A} oscillated wildly, suggestive of locally intense epidemics in each influenza season involving only a few *départements* rather than the entire country.

Table 6.1 highlights the difference between pandemic and non-pandemic seasons in France. The 103 seasons for which data were available have been classified into three groups: (a) pandemic-

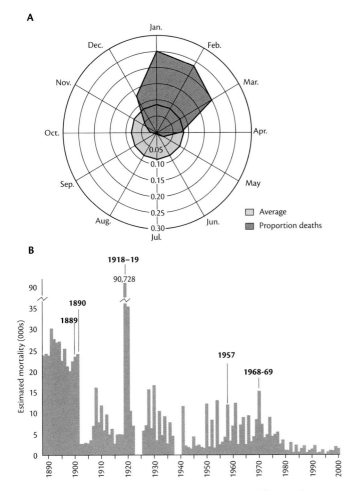

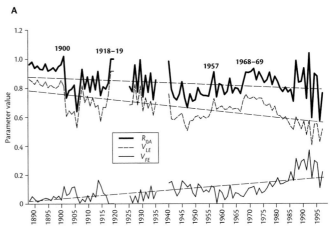

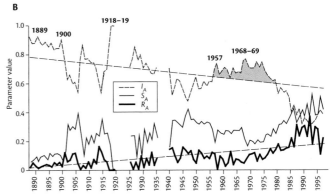

Figure 6.10 Influenza mortality in France, 1887–1999. (A) Radar chart showing the proportion of deaths reported in each month over the period (dark shading). The average monthly proportion is marked by light shading. (B) Time series of annual deaths from influenza reported in French records. For 1901–5, the national series of deaths by cause was recorded for towns whose populations exceeded 5,000 rather than 30,000.

Figure 6.11 Swash model parameters for influenza in France, 1887–1999. (A) Time series plots of calculated values for the spatial basic reproductive number, R_{0A}, and for the edge velocity parameters, V_{LE} and V_{FE}. (B) Time series of the infected (I), susceptible (S) and recovered (R) integrals. Linear regression trend lines are also shown.

affected (11), (b) high-intensity inter-pandemic (54), with death rates greater than the lowest pandemic season, and (c) low-intensity inter-pandemic (38), with death rates lower than the lowest pandemic season. The average velocity of the leading edge ($\bar{t}_{LE}$, equation A1 in Appendix 6.1) for the three groups is (a) = 2.39 months, (b) = 3.59 months and (c) = 4.93 months. The results for V_{LE} in Table 6.1 confirm that pandemic seasons had higher velocities than inter-pandemic years. This higher velocity was maintained even compared with inter-pandemic influenza seasons of similar intensity levels as pandemic seasons. Moreover, pandemic seasons appeared to be of greater spatial intensity (larger R_{0A}) and were slower to clear (lower following edge velocities).

The plots of the susceptible and recovered integrals in Figure 6.11B show rising trends over the twentieth century, and this is consistent with the generally declining trend in the infective integral. As noted in Figure 6.10B, these trends imply declining intensity of influenza epidemics over the century-long study period. Again the pandemic years bucked the trend with raised infective integral values. The main other variations in the long term fall in the infectives integral occurred following the arrival of Asian influenza in 1957,

when the infected integral remained above the trend (shaded in Figure 10.6B) for the next quarter of a century, and then, from the mid-1980s, when the integral remained resolutely below the trend line. The extended period of higher values for the infectives integral post-1957 may be attributed to the combined action of three effects: (i) the long interval since the last major strain shift (40 years since 1918); (ii) the shift from H2N2 to H3N2 in 1968–69; and (iii) the re-emergence in 1976 of Russian influenza (strain of H1N1) which has been co-circulating with the Hong Kong strain ever since. Together these effects meant that a greater proportion of the French population was likely to be susceptible to one or other of the mix of circulating strains than if just a single strain had been present over the period. After a generation, with no new major strains emerging, herd immunity appears to have caught up from the mid-1980s, leading to a general collapse of nationwide epidemics.

Iceland: An Island Location

This subsection is based upon Cliff, Smallman-Raynor, Haggett, *et al.* (2009, pp. 566–72). Since 1895, Iceland has required direct notification of influenza cases by physicians. This concern for data collection stems from the island's early history which was marked by disastrous externally-introduced epidemics, including the 1843 influenza outbreak which, although lasting only two

Table 6.1 French influenza seasons, 1887–1999. Values of swash model parameters for 103 influenza waves classified by intensity of mortality

Type of influenza wave	Mortality (mean/100,000 population per season)	Start $\bar{t}_{LE}$ (mean in months)	Velocity (V_{LE})	End $\bar{t}_{LE}$ (mean in months)	Velocity (V_{FE})	R_{0A} (mean)
Pandemic (a) (n = 11)	27.29	2.39	0.80	11.45	0.05	0.93
Interpandemic:						
High intensity (b) (n = 54)	14.91	3.59	0.70	11.20	0.07	0.84
Low intensity (c) (n = 38)	3.14	4.93	0.59	10.12	0.16	0.80

Notes:

(a) Pandemic seasons of 1889–91, 1900, 1918–19, 1957–58 and 1968–69.

(b) High intensity = Deaths per 100,000 population greater than the least-intense pandemic season.

(c) Low intensity = Deaths per 100,000 population less than the least intense pandemic season.

Data unavailable for seasons 1920–24 and 1936–39.

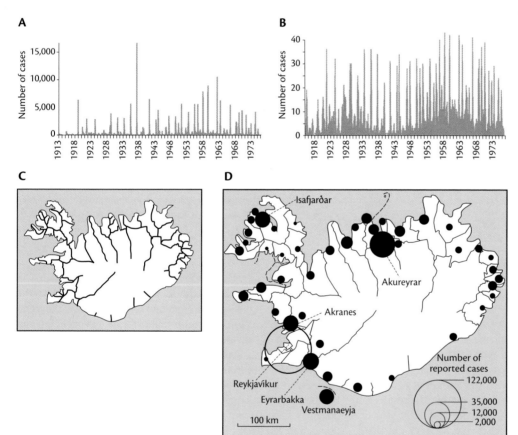

Figure 6.12 Reported influenza morbidity in Iceland. (A) Monthly records for total reported influenza cases from January 1913 to December 1976. (B) Monthly record of the number of Icelandic medical districts reporting one or more cases of influenza, January 1915 to December 1976. (C) Map of boundaries of Icelandic medical districts for the year 1945. (D) Cumulative total of reported monthly influenza cases for each Icelandic medical district in the period January 1915 to December 1976. Circles are drawn proportional to the cumulative number of cases but note the special position of the capital city, Reykjavík. All influenza data based on *Heilbrigðisskýrslur* (*Public Health in Iceland*).

months, doubled the expected death rate for the year (Schleisner, 1851). Annual totals and other summary data have been published in that country's annual public health reports (*Heilbrigðisskýrslur*) since that date with, for influenza, national monthly morbidity time series available from 1913 (**Figure 6.12A**). For the 61-year period spanning the middle of the twentieth century from 1915 (Figure 6.12B), monthly data are broken down to a local level for some 50 medical districts (Figure 6.12C). This allows application of the swash model to estimate the changing spatial and temporal velocity of influenza epidemics over the period.

Over the whole 61 years studied, Iceland's doctors reported 530,276 cases of influenza, half of them from Reykjavík and immediately surrounding areas (Figure 6.12D). Although reported cases are likely to be under-estimates, the broad shape of outbreaks in both space and time is readily discernible. The distribution throughout the year shows clear peaks in March–April with the low periods in August–September, a pattern which, as we have seen for France in Figure 6.10A is typical of many northern latitude countries. However, the sub-Arctic climate of Iceland pushes the peak influenza months slightly later in the influenza season than in France, and so we use for Iceland a slightly different definition of season, running from September 1 through to August 31 of the following year.

The swash–backwash model was applied to Iceland as a whole. The time series of both edges is shown in **Figure 6.13A**. Despite marked year to year variation, the average trend shown by the linear regression line for the leading edge is distinctly upward implying that waves have speeded up over time, i.e. influenza waves moved around the island faster at the end than at the beginning of the study period. By contrast the position of the following edge when influenza incidence ceased in any influenza season has remained essentially unchanged. This implies that the duration of reported influenza incidence grew slowly longer, from around 2.5 months in 1915–16 to nearly 4.0 months in 1975–76 (Figure 10.8B), a finding which differs from that for France.

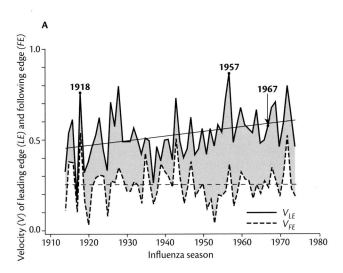

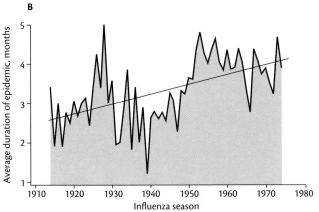

Figure 6.13 Velocity of epidemic waves in Iceland for the influenza seasons 1915–16 to 1975–76. (A) Velocities of the leading edge (*LE*, solid lines) and following edge (*FE*, pecked lines) are shown as the velocity ratios, V_{LE} and V_{FE}, defined in Appendix 6.1 equation (A2). *V* is in the range, $0 \leq V \leq 1$. The larger the value of *V*, the faster the edge. (B) The widening time gap between the two edges illustrated in (A) is confirmed in this graph which plots the average duration of each district's epidemic wave in months. In both (A) and (B) the trend lines were determined by OLS linear regression.

Three of the 61 seasons studied were associated with pandemics of influenza A (the Spanish, Asian and Hong Kong pandemics). **Figure 6.14** uses data on the spatial extent of influenza in each season to plot the position of the pandemic front with reference to the three seasons which immediately preceded or followed it. In the Spanish and Asian pandemics the front stands out clearly but in the third (Figure 10.9C) the Hong Kong front appears, as in France, to have been spread over two seasons.

Although pandemic years had large numbers of influenza cases, they were not the largest recorded over the period. The 1937–38 season had the largest number of cases (21,977) and the highest monthly rate and, as Figure 6.12A shows, monthly case numbers in several inter-pandemic years exceeded those with pandemics. For Iceland in **Table 6.2**, as for France in Table 6.1, we have divided the 61 seasons into three groups: (a) pandemic (3); (b) high-intensity inter-pandemic (24), with case rates greater than the lowest pandemic season; and (c) low-intensity inter-pandemic (34), with case rates lower than the lowest pandemic season. The average velocity of the leading edges (*LE*) for the three groups is (a) = 2.83 months, (b) = 5.53 months and (c) = 6.03 months. Echoing the results for France, this suggests that pandemic seasons have higher velocities than inter-pandemic years, and that this higher velocity is maintained even compared with inter-pandemic influenza seasons of similar intensity levels as pandemic seasons. Table 6.2 also shows that values for R_{0A}, when calculated for the three categories of influenza season, (a), (b) and (c), defined above produced the same differentials as the leading and following edge parameters.

Thus application of the swash–backwash model to Iceland's influenza morbidity records has shown that (i) the onset of waves speeded up over the period 1914 to 1975 and (ii) waves in three viral shift (pandemic) seasons spread significantly faster and were of longer duration than other equally large waves in non-shift (inter-pandemic) seasons. These are identical to the results reported for France. It suggests that both the swash model and the findings are robust across the transfer of geographical scales from a large country (France) to a small country (Iceland), and from a continental to an island setting. To test transferability across geographical scales further, we now apply the model at the smallest of our spatial scales by looking at influenza waves between 1947–48 and 1975–76 in the English market town of Cirencester.

Cirencester: A Small English Town

Cirencester is a small market town lying between Gloucester and Swindon in the English Cotswolds. It had a population of about 12,000 in 1957, rising to 15,000 by 1970 and 18,000 in 2011 (**Figure 6.15B**). Based in the town, R.E. Hope-Simpson ran a general practice covering an area of about 210 km² from a centrally located surgery. In this practice, individual patients were identified and influenza was diagnosed and studied by a single doctor and his partner over a 30-year period following the end of the Second World War. The panel consisted of between three and four thousand patients and Hope-Simpson kept very detailed records of the incidence of several infectious diseases, but especially influenza, for each patient. Working with the help of his wife and later with the support of the UK's Medical Research Council and the Public Health Laboratory Service he set up an Epidemiological Research Unit in Cirencester. By converting cottage rooms at his surgery in Dyer Street, he established a laboratory to permit identification of the viruses isolated from his patients. As a result, this unique practice became

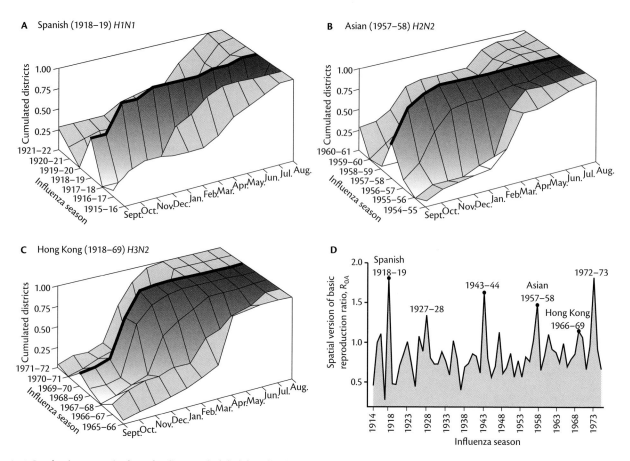

Figure 6.14 Pandemic seasons in the Icelandic records. (A)–(C) Profiles showing the cumulative number (scaled to unity) of medical districts reporting influenza cases by month as a measure of the spatial extent of influenza in Iceland for the three shift seasons of 1918–19, 1957–58 and 1968–69. In each case the profile for the shift season is compared with the profiles of the three preceding and three following non-shift seasons. (D) Value of the spatial version of the basic reproduction number, R_{0A}, for Iceland for the influenza seasons 1915–16 to 1975–76. Peaks are associated with the three viral shift years for influenza A (1918–19, 1957–58 and 1968–69) and for three other non-shift seasons (1927–28, 1943–44, and 1972–73).

Table 6.2 Icelandic influenza seasons, 1915–16 to 1975–76. Swash model parameters for Iceland's 61 influenza waves

Type of influenza wave	Morbidity (mean cases/ season)	Start ($\bar{t}_{LE}$) (mean in months)	Velocity (V_{LE})	End ($\bar{t}_{LE}$) (mean in months)	Velocity (V_{FE})	Duration (mean in months)	R_{0A} (mean index)
Pandemic waves (a) ($n = 3$)	11,027	2.83	0.76	7.03	0.41	3.82	1.48
Interpandemic waves:							
High intensity (b) ($n = 24$)	10,113	5.53	0.54	9.14	0.24	3.56	0.84
Low intensity (c) ($n = 34$)	2,302	6.03	0.50	9.04	0.25	3.10	0.80

(a) Three pandemic seasons of 1918–19, 1957–58 and 1968–69.

(b) High intensity = Cases per 100,000 population greater than the least-intense pandemic wave.

(c) Low intensity = Cases per 100,000 population less than the least intense pandemic wave.

internationally known and it provides an unrivalled window into the behaviour of influenza epidemics at the micro-scale.

Hope-Simpson recorded every case of influenza identified in the practice, along with the causative strain of the virus and the geo-coordinates of the patient. Figure 6.15A maps the geographical framework used by Hope-Simpson for data collection, along with a block diagram (Figure 6.15C) of the cases reported in each influenza season, 1946–74. The earlier appearance of influenza in the town in the pandemic seasons of 1957–58 and 1968–69 is striking. This appearance of an early peak at times of antigenic shift in the causative virus can be related to the larger stock of susceptibles available for immediate infection on such occasions.

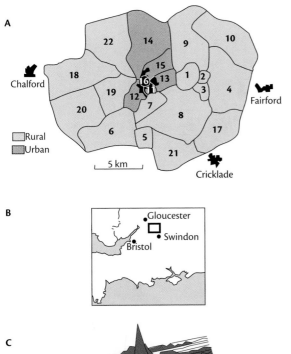

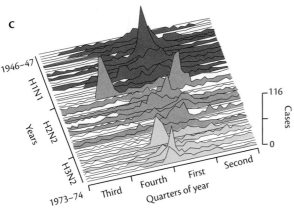

Figure 6.15 **Influenza waves in an English GP practice.** The country practice of a local doctor, Edgar Hope-Simpson, near Cirencester, England. Hope-Simpson made a special study of influenza in the area for some 50 years. (A) Boundaries of the 22 geographical units used by Hope-Simpson for data collection. (B) Location map of Cirencester. (C) Block diagram of cases of clinically-diagnosed influenza A weekly, 1946–74. The earlier appearance of influenza in the pandemic seasons of 1957–58 and 1968–69 is striking, as is the greater number of cases reported. *Source*: data from R.E. Hope-Simpson in Cliff, *et al.* (1986, Figures 3.1, 3.12, pp. 48, 65).

In **Figure 6.16**, the results of applying the swash–backwash model to the Hope-Simpson data from 1963–75 are summarised. They echo those already obtained for France and Iceland, with a sharp upturn in R_{0A} and an increase in the leading edge velocity in the second season of Hong Kong influenza (1969). Thereafter R_{0A} fell slowly to reach pre-1968 levels by 1973.

United States: The Swine Flu Outbreak of 2009

As noted in Section 6.2, the first cases of influenza caused by a novel influenza virus, subsequently typed 2009 swine A/H1N1 influenza, were reported in the state of Veracruz, Mexico, in March 2009, although the evidence suggests that there had been an ongoing epidemic for months before it was officially recognised. The Mexican government closed most of Mexico City's public and private

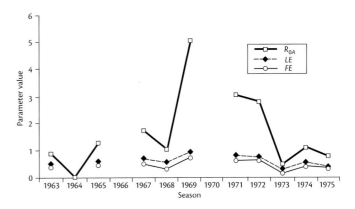

Figure 6.16 **Cirencester, England: the 1968–69 pandemic of influenza in the Hope-Simpson general practice.** Values of the reproductive number, and leading and following edge velocities for the swash–backwash model, 1963–75. As in France and Iceland, influenza moved more rapidly and struck earlier in 1968 than in non-pandemic seasons.

facilities in a futile attempt to contain the spread of the virus. The first cases in the United States were reported from California in April 2009. Rapid global diffusion of the new strain continued from the Mexican epicentre so that, on 11 June 2009, WHO declared the world to be at stage six of its six-phase pandemic alert scale. The crisis continued through into 2010, although the new strain had largely run its course by the turn of the year. The US Public Health Emergency for 2009 H1N1 influenza expired on June 23 2010 and, on 10 August 2010, WHO declared an end to the 2009 H1N1 pandemic globally. The new strain has subsequently behaved like normal seasonal influenza and is likely to be around for many years. In the US, the CDC estimates that between 43 million and 89 million cases (mid-range 61 million) of 2009 H1N1 occurred between April 2009 and April 10 2010; that there were between about 195,000 and 403,000 (mid-range 274,000) H1N1-related hospitalisations; and that there were between 8,870 and 18,300 (mid-range 12,470) 2009 H1N1-related deaths. US cases surged when schools reopened for the autumn term. The global impact of the pandemic is illustrated in **Figure 6.17** and for the United States in **Figures 6.18** and **6.19**.

Figure 6.20 plots the values of the spatial basic reproduction number, R_{0A}, and the leading edge parameter, $\bar{t}_{LE}$, of the swash model for weeks 27–39 (second week of July–first week of October of the five normal influenza seasons, 2004–5 to 2008–9, and for the first swine flu influenza season, 2009–10). Note the substantially higher velocity through the US population for the new swine flu strain as compared with normal seasonal influenza at all three spatial scales as evidenced by the larger values of R_{0A} and smaller values of $\bar{t}_{LE}$ in the 2009–10 season. The time window plotted covers the start of each influenza season and the reopening of schools, colleges and universities in the Fall.

Discussion

In this section, a spatial version of R_{0A} has been developed in the context of what we have called a *swash–backwash model*. This has been applied to records of influenza from France (1887–1999), Iceland (1916–75), Cirencester (1963–75) and the United States in 2009, locations of vastly different geographical scales and settings. But common threads have been found: pandemic influenza at all spatial scales appeared (i) earlier than normal in the influenza

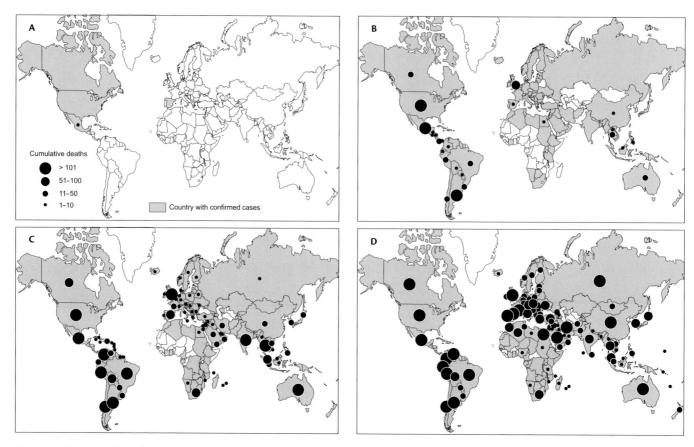

Figure 6.17 Pandemic (A/swine/H1N1) influenza, 2009. Countries, territories and areas with laboratory confirmed cases and cumulative number of deaths reported to the World Health Organization, Geneva, from the start of the pandemic. (A) 27 April 2009. (B) 22 July 2009. (C) 25 October 2009. (D) 21 March 2010. *Source*: WHO Global Health Observatory Map Gallery.

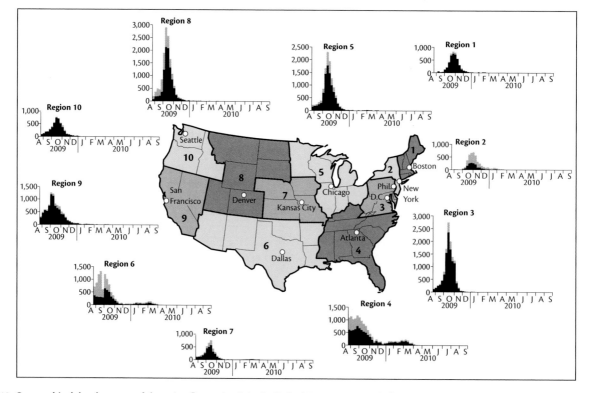

Figure 6.18 Geographical development of the swine flu pandemic in the United States, 2009–10 influenza season. Each histogram shows the number of positive influenza virus isolates by Department of Health and Human Services regions reported by WHO/NREVSS Collaborating Laboratories. The preponderance of swine flu A(H1N1), shown in black, as opposed to normal seasonal strains (grey) is evident in all regions. *Source*: data from US Centers for Diseases Control, Influenza Division.

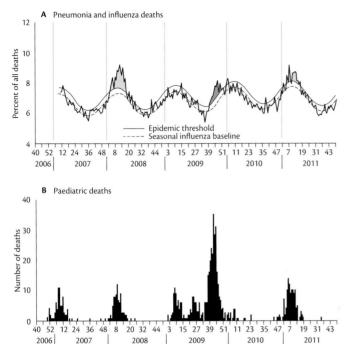

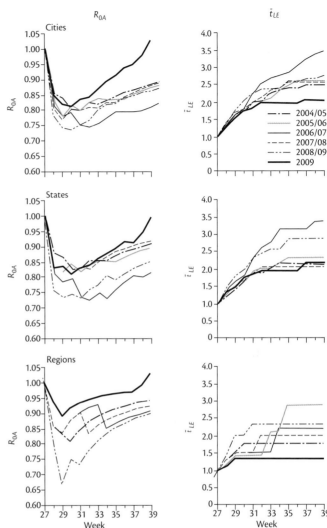

Figure 6.19 Pneumonia and influenza mortality in the United States, 2007–11. (A) The percentage of all deaths due to pneumonia and influenza in 122 US cities is plotted against the US national seasonal influenza baseline and the 95% confidence band above which epidemics (shaded) are declared. While the 2009–10 season in the round does not appear exceptional compared with adjacent seasons, especially 2008, the epidemic of swine flu in the fall of 2009 stands out as the largest autumn influenza event in this time series. (B) Number of influenza-related paediatric deaths. The high infant mortality during the swine flu season as compared with normal seasonal influenza in adjacent seasons is evident. *Source*: data from US Centers for Diseases Control, Influenza Division.

Figure 6.20 Swine flu, United States, 2009–10. Values of the swash model parameters, R_{0A} and $\bar{t}_{LE}$, for the first 39 weeks (July–October) of each of the influenza seasons, 2004–5 to 2008–9, and for the first swine flu season, 2009–10 at three geographical scales. (A) 122 cities comprising the ILINet (influenza-like illnesses) PI (pneumonia–influenza) mortality dataset. (B) Fifty states. (C) Ten United States Department of Health and Human Services regions. *Source*: data from Centers for Disease Control, ILINet website.

season and (ii) spread spatially more rapidly than normal. If our findings are confirmed elsewhere, this will have wider implications for public health measures. It would suggest that any new influenza pandemic in the twenty-first century, whether emerging from highly pathogenic avian influenza, swine influenza, or other sources, will give little lead time if the public health is to be protected. This conclusion underscores the role of surveillance and virus watch systems, issues which we considered in Chapter 2 and for which we now provide a practical example.

Pandemic Detection

As recent WHO reports have stressed, among the critical needs of any epidemic forecasting model if it is to be useful in informing control strategies is the ability to predict an epidemic's likely spatial spread at some point relatively early in its unfolding history. Here we test the capability of the swash model for this purpose. We use the French influenza data. A positive outcome would imply that the swash–backwash model has a potential use as part of a disease early-warning system.

The following experiment was devised:

(i) In month 2 (August) of a given influenza season, the swash model parameters, R_{0A}, V_{LE} and V_{FE}, defined in Appendix 6.1 in equations (A2) and (A7), were calculated and plotted.

(ii) In each successive month through to the end of the influenza season, the data set was updated as new data arrived. The model parameters were recalculated and plotted.

(iii) The experiment was applied to the following groups of influenza seasons, each centred around a pandemic year(s): (a) 1887–92; (b) 1896–1902; (c) 1914–20; (d) 1955–59; (e) 1966–72.

Figure 6.21 plots the results for R_{0A} when the approach was tested for the group (c) seasons, centred on the 1918 pandemic. This pandemic spread over three influenza seasons (Wave I in the spring of 1918 in the 1917–18 season, Wave II in the autumn of 1918 in the 1918–19 season, and Wave III in the spring of 1919, affecting both the 1918–19 and 1919–20 seasons; cf. Figure 6.2). The plots for R_{0A} show that, for the main part of the pandemic (Waves II and

III), R_{0A} ran at a consistently higher level from September than in immediately preceding and succeeding seasons. From the viewpoint of online monitoring, public health officers would have had early warning from the beginning of the 1918–19 season that the impending influenza experience was likely to be unlike anything they had encountered in the war years.

Figure 6.22 summarises the results of the experiment for all the pandemic seasonal groups, (a)–(e). Each chart plots the median values of the model parameters obtained in each seasonal group for (i) the virus shift season(s) and (ii) the non-shift seasons. From October in the influenza seasons studied, this diagram shows that the spatial basic reproductive number, R_{0A}, was consistently greater in virus shift seasons than in other seasons. For the leading edge parameter, V_{LE}, velocity of spread was also greater in shift seasons than in other seasons except for 1889. For the following edge parameter, V_{FE}, no consistent picture emerges from Figure 6.22.

When a new strain of human influenza A appears, the population will have at best limited natural resistance, resulting in a much larger stock of susceptibles for infection than normal. Under these circumstances, pandemic influenza may occur, with the new strain running rapidly through the population. *Ceteris paribus*, characteristic features of virus shift seasons are likely to be (i) high levels of morbidity and mortality compared with 'normal' influenza seasons, manifested in larger values of R_{0A}, and (ii) rapid geographical spread (large values for V_{LE}). The expected behaviour of the following edge parameter, V_{FE}, is not clear. In shift seasons, long spatial occupancy would lead to a low value for V_{FE}, whereas rapid passage through and clearing of an area, which is feasible with a new virus strain, would yield a small value for V_{FE}. Indeed, the ambiguous behaviour of V_{FE} is confirmed by a correlation of 0.07 between R_{0A} and V_{FE} for the French data.

The results presented in this subsection broadly match expectation. **Figure 6.23** shows that, in shift years, epidemics occurred earlier in the season and that they were, for the 1918, 1957 and 1968 shifts, more sharply peaked than in adjacent seasons. Figure 6.22A displays a long-term decline in the reproduction number

for influenza which was linked to declining velocity of spread (the correlation coefficient between R_{0A} and V_{LE} is 0.77). The localised peaks in R_{0A} and in epidemic velocity set against the century-long falling trend all occurred in virus shift seasons and their immediate aftermath.

Swash Model and Other Infectious Diseases
Poliomyelitis in England and Wales, 1919–71

The historical geography of poliomyelitis as a twentieth-century emerging disease is described in Smallman-Raynor, *et al.* (2006). **Figure 6.24** plots the monthly time series of reported cases of poliomyelitis per 100,000 population in England and Wales, 1919–71. The upsurge of epidemic poliomyelitis after the Second World War until the impact of mass vaccination against the disease kicked in from the 1960s is dramatic (see Smallman-Raynor, *et al.*, 2006, pp. 317–51 and pp. 482–6). In this epidemic sequence, that of 1947 was by far the largest and most severe. From an apparent onset in the late spring of 1947, the epidemic spread across the entire country, attacking both urban and rural populations with force. At the height

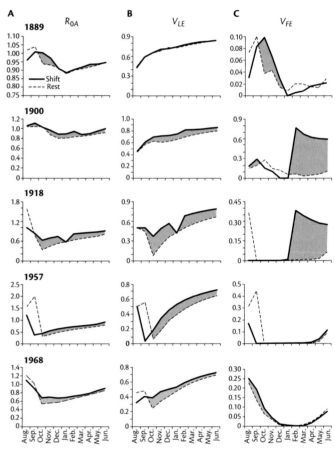

Figure 6.22 Real-time detection of influenza pandemics in France, 1887–1999. Median values of (A) the spatial basic reproduction number, R_{0A}, (B) the leading edge parameter, V_{LE}, and (C) the following edge parameter, V_{FE}, for the swash–backwash model applied to continually updated influenza mortality reports in France for the following groups of influenza seasons: (a) 1887–92; (b) 1896–1902; (c) 1914–20; (d) 1955–59; (e) 1966–72. In each group, influenza seasons were classified as *shift* if they were affected by a new strain of influenza virus and *rest* otherwise. Months in which the parameter values for shift seasons exceeded those for rest are shaded.

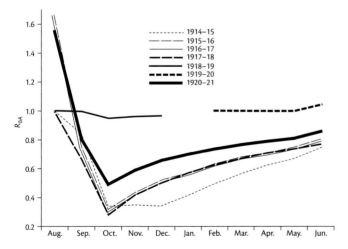

Figure 6.21 Real-time detection of the 1918–20 influenza pandemic in France. Time series plot of the values of the spatial basic reproduction number, R_{0A}, for the swash–backwash model applied to continually updated influenza mortality reports in France for the 1914–20 influenza seasons.

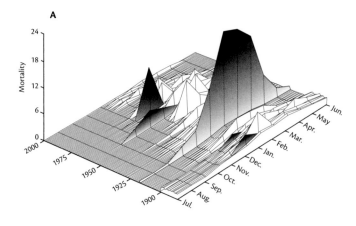

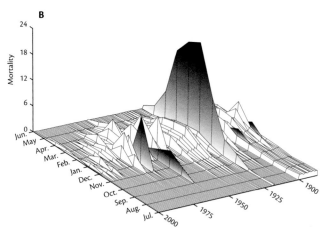

Figure 6.23 Block diagram of influenza seasons in France, 1887–1999. The recorded monthly mortality from influenza in France is plotted by season. Viral shift years have been highlighted. Outbreaks in shift years generally start earlier and commonly had larger mortality than non-shift seasons. The block has been drawn from two different viewpoints to highlight these features.

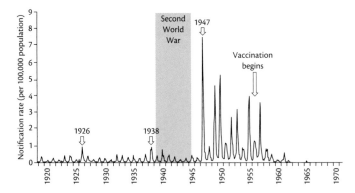

Figure 6.24 Poliomyelitis in England and Wales, 1919–71. Monthly number of notified cases of poliomyelitis per 100,000 population. *Source*: data from the General Register Office.

of the epidemic, in late August and early September, more than 600 cases of poliomyelitis were recorded each week. All told, the epidemic was associated with some 7,655 civilian and 735 military cases – a toll far in excess of the 1,600 or so notifications associated with the previous epidemic high of 1938. As Gale (1948) observes,

it was not simply that the local intensity of the 1947 epidemic was greater than ever before; the geographical reach of the epidemic, too, exceeded all previous experience of the disease.

Origin and course of the epidemic

The events of the summer and autumn of 1947 were not wholly unanticipated by the medical community of England and Wales, although some purveyed complacency. As early as 28 June – a full month before the usual seasonal upturn in poliomyelitis – *The Medical Officer* observed that notifications of poliomyelitis in the week ending 14 June were "higher than usual for the time of year," adding that "an upward trend is expected" (Anonymous, 1947a, p. 260). A few weeks later, and with the count of poliomyelitis notifications still rising, readers of *The Lancet* were alerted to a Ministry of Health memorandum that warned of "an unprecedented prevalence" of poliomyelitis in the months ahead (Anonymous, 1947b, p. 155). The deepening fears of the medical community were underscored by an editorial comment in *The Medical Officer*. "The brisk rise in notification of poliomyelitis in the late spring of the present year," the editorial noted, "gives us much uneasiness … Nobody can foretell what poliomyelitis is going to do, but an epidemic on an extensive scale appears to be due in this country" (Anonymous, 1947c, p. 23). "Unfortunately," the editorial added, "we can do nothing about it, for there is no proof that any measures to control the disease have any value."

Figure 6.25 confirms the pandemic-like qualities of the 1947 outbreak as compared with the previous three poliomyelitis upswings and the one which followed in 1948. It attacked the geographical mesh of boroughs and districts more completely, more rapidly (R_{0A}, LE), and persisted longer (time between LE and FE) than any of the other four outbreaks. **Table 6.3** gives the swash parameters defined in Appendix 6.1 for the five polio seasons between 1944 and 1948. As with influenza, the swash model picks out the extraordinary poliomyelitis epidemic of 1947 from its neighbouring, less intense, polio years.

6.4 Forecasting for Intervention

Any intervention against the spread of a communicable disease is likely to be more effective, to be more likely to succeed, and to make the best use of resources if the intervention can be targeted. Targeted interventions become feasible if we can forecast where to and how rapidly a communicable disease is spreading through a set of locations. In this section we look at possible ways to forecast spread from the point(s) of introduction of a disease (the disease impulse) to other areas (the response). To provide a common geographical framework for the discussion, the country of Iceland is used as an epidemiological laboratory. Our discussion focuses upon approaches to the disease forecasting problem rather than upon mathematical details of model fitting for which appropriate references are provided.

Iceland as an Epidemiological Laboratory

A number of reasons make Iceland particularly valuable as an arena within which to test geographical models of communicable disease spread:

1. Quality of Data

Iceland's public health and epidemiological records are among the highest quality in the world in terms of their completeness,

Table 6.3 Poliomyelitis in England and Wales, 1944–48. Values of the swash model parameters for the poliomyelitis outbreaks in each year at the county borough and district scale

		N of infected units	t_{LE}	t_{FE}	V_{LE}	V_{FE}	S_A	I_A	R_A	R_{0A}
1944	All units	256	13.64	15.30	0.48	0.41	0.49	0.10	0.41	0.87
1945	All units	321	13.94	17.72	0.46	0.32	0.50	0.18	0.32	0.74
1946	All units	283	13.34	16.31	0.49	0.37	0.47	0.15	0.37	0.84
1947	All units	1113	10.29	18.50	0.60	0.29	0.36	0.35	0.29	0.90
1948	All units	532	13.66	18.41	0.47	0.29	0.49	0.22	0.29	0.72

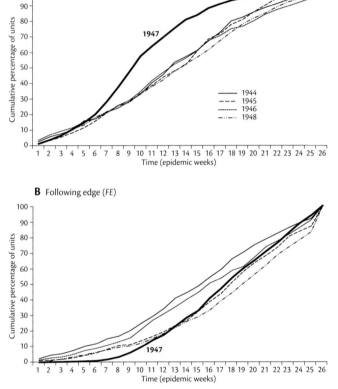

Figure 6.25 Poliomyelitis in England and Wales, 1944–8: leading and following edges of poliomyelitis activity in England and Wales. Graphs plot the cumulative percentage of administrative units (county, metropolitan and municipal boroughs, urban districts and rural districts) that first notified (leading edge, *LE*; graph A) and last notified (following edge, *FE*; graph B) cases of poliomyelitis in the epidemic year of 1947 (heavy line trace) and in the corresponding weeks of the four non-epidemic years of 1944–46 and 1948.

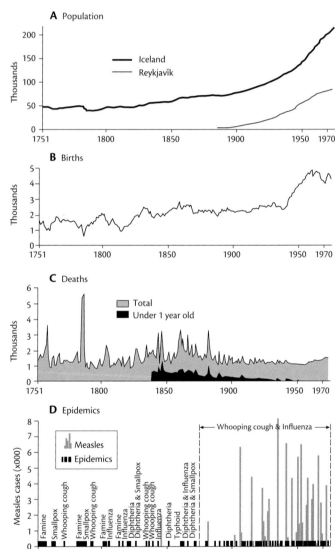

Figure 6.26 Iceland demography and communicable disease history, 1751–1970. Annual population total, births, deaths and major epidemics of communicable diseases. *Source*: Cliff, *et al.* (1981, Figures 3.8 and 3.9, pp. 47–48).

geographical granularity and temporal resolution. For many human communicable diseases, mortality and morbidity counts are available on a monthly basis for around 125 years in some 50 geographical areas; for some diseases the record goes back on a similar basis to the middle of the eighteenth century. **Figure 6.26** summarises the general demographic history of Iceland from that date, along with the occurrence of the major epidemics of communicable diseases until the last quarter of the twentieth century by which

time mass vaccination had all but eliminated them. Population size was stable at around 40–60,000 for the period 1751–1900, when a remarkable growth set in; the population approximately quadrupled between 1900 and 1970 to about 200,000. Up to 1950, this growth was concentrated mainly in the capital, Reykjavík. Since then, Reykjavík and the rest of Iceland have grown in population at about the same rate. The decline in infant mortality since 1850 and the higher birth-rates of the twentieth century (especially since 1940) are the main reasons for Iceland's population growth.

Throughout its history, neither the island as a whole nor any individual settlement approached the critical community size required to maintain endemically the spectrum of human infectious diseases (Section 4.3). As a result, epidemics of infectious diseases in Iceland have been spatially and temporally separated, with inter-epidemic intervals during which either no or only isolated cases occurred. **Figure 6.27** illustrates the point by plotting Iceland's twentieth-century time series for three diseases – measles, rubella and pertussis. Thus for a significant outbreak of one of these diseases to occur on an Icelandic farmstead, the disease agent had to cross several hundred miles of sea, travel from a seaport or airport to the rural community, and eventually to the farm itself. Once the susceptible

population was exhausted, the agent disappeared from the island until the susceptible population grew again by births to a sufficient size to sustain a new outbreak. This temporal and spatial separation of outbreaks facilitates both the development and testing of forecasting models.

2. Population Distribution

Iceland is a large island (about the size of southern England or the state of Indiana) located just south of the Arctic Circle. Its 1990 population was somewhat over 250,000. It is the least-densely settled country in Europe and the harsh environment of the interior plateau has restricted population to the peripheral lowlands (diagonal shading in **Figure 6.28**). This diagram maps the geographical distribution of Iceland's population by medical districts using proportional circles and squares. The percentage change in population that has taken place over the last century is also shown. A pattern familiar across Western Europe – of rural depopulation on a large scale – is evident. The biggest single settlement is the capital, Reykjavík, which has been growing both absolutely and in its share of Iceland's total population. In 1901 its 6,700 inhabitants accounted for less than a tenth of the island's 78,000; by 1990, Reykjavík had grown to 100,000 out of a total of 256,000. The overall impression is of population distributed around the coast much like the beads on a necklace. The degree of isolation of settlements around the coast means that it is often possible to treat such communities as separate epidemiological cells from a modelling point of view, giving a spatial equivalent to the discrete epidemic waves in time evident in Figure 6.27.

3. Physician Reports

Historically, Icelandic legislation required the principal physician of each of the country's c. 50 medical districts to submit an annual report to the Chief Medical Officer of Health in Reykjavík. The reports contain contact tracing information for each epidemic of an infectious disease to have affected the district that year. The reports give, in varying detail, information on the origin of the outbreak

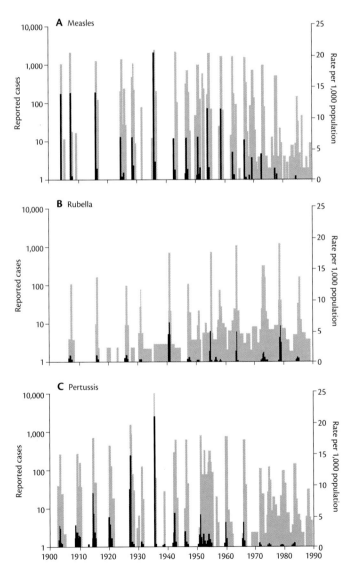

Figure 6.27   Epidemic diseases in Iceland, 1900–90. Monthly time series of reported cases (grey, log scale) and rate per thousand population (black, arithmetic scale) of measles, rubella and pertussis. *Source*: Cliff, *et al.* (2000, Figure 6.3, p. 245).

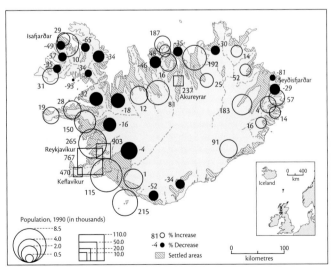

Figure 6.28   Iceland population distribution. Settled areas of Iceland with 1990 medical district populations shown by proportional circles and squares. Medical district boundaries plotted as pecked lines. Percentage population change, 1900–90 indicated numerically. *Source*: Cliff, *et al.* (2000, Figure 6.2, p. 243).

and its local spread. They are much fuller prior to 1945 than thereafter. **Figure 6.29** maps the results of this contact tracing for all epidemics of measles, rubella and pertussis which have affected Iceland since 1900. The last map, D (*All*), pools the results for the three diseases. The principal vectors fan out from the capital, Reykjavíkur (population 95,000 in 1990), to the three main regional towns in Iceland of Akureyrar (population 15,000), Ísafjarðar (population 3,600) and Seyðisfjarðar (population 1,000) – cascade or hierarchical diffusion. Local spread from these centres into their hinterlands (contagious diffusion) is illustrated by the vectors within the diagonally shaded areas on each map, and is most clearly seen on map *All* around Akureyrar.

Lag Maps

The number of steps in the particular pathway followed as an epidemic moves from one geographical area to another will clearly affect its time of arrival. Using lag maps, this subsection shows the impact of Iceland's internal pathways upon spatial timing. Measuring epidemic velocity has attracted theoretical attention because of its importance for possible preventive measures; the spread of slow-moving waves may be simpler to check than that of rapidly moving waves. Basic references are Mollison (1991) and

van den Bosch, *et al.* (1990). If we are dealing with a simple spatial process where the epidemic spreads with a well-defined wave front (as in the case of the studies by Mollison (1977)), then the physical concept of distance travelled over time may be appropriate. However, where the wave front is not a well-defined line, and where the susceptible population through which the epidemic moves is both discontinuous in space and has sharp variations in density, then alternative definitions of velocity must be sought.

Calculation of Lag Maps

For epidemic ℓ, code the first month in which a disease was reported anywhere in Iceland as month 1 and, for medical district i, note the month in which the disease was reported in that medical district as month 2, or 3, or 4, etc. Denote this month as $t_{i\ell}$. The desired quantities are then

$$\bar{t}_i = (1/n)\sum_\ell t_{i\ell}, \ell = 1, 2, \ldots, n, \tag{6.1}$$

where i is subscripted over the 47 medical districts.

Figure 6.30 plots the $\{\bar{t}\}$ for three of the Icelandic diseases separately (measles, rubella and pertussis) and for an average map, where the average has been calculated from the results for

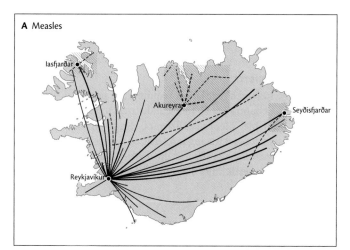

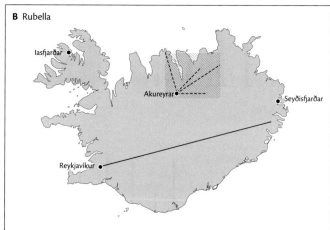

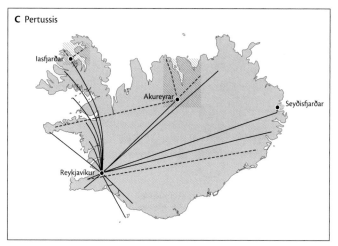

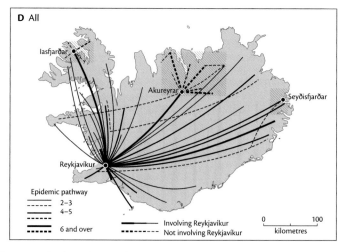

Figure 6.29 Iceland: internal epidemic pathways. Observed transmission routes between Icelandic settlements for measles, rubella and pertussis, 1900–90. Vectors show the number of times the diseases were recorded in *Heilbrigðisskýrslur* (Public Health in Iceland) as passing between linked medical districts. *Source*: Cliff, *et al.* (2000, Figure 6.4, p. 247).

the three separate diseases and influenza; data for 1900–90 have been used. Circle sizes are proportional to the 1990 populations of medical districts. Circles have been coloured black on the map in which they first appear and have been left as open circles thereafter. A similar pattern is seen across the diseases. Reykjavík and the Reykjavík region are reached early; the principal regional capitals of Akureyri, Ísafjörður and Seyðisfjörður are attacked at the second stage; and epidemic decay occurs in the smaller and more remote settlements of the fjord areas of eastern and northwest Iceland. This is consistent with the pathway diagrams in Figure 6.29, and yields a schematic space–time model like **Figure 6.31**.

Models of Disease Spread

With the spatial and temporal structure of epidemic spread in Iceland over the twentieth century in mind, we can now turn to modelling such space–time patterns and we use two approaches:

1. The first is to try to capture the process and build a spatial *SIR* model. Here the particular difficulties are (i) obtaining reliable estimates of the susceptible population and (ii) constructing a model in which the mixing parameter, β, between *I* and *S* in Figure 1.17 can vary over space and time. The homogeneous

mixing assumption of Figure 1.17 is clearly not tenable when both cascade and contagious disease diffusion occurs. Such spatial inhomogeneities in the spread process are usually handled via a *compartment model* in which homogeneous mixing is allowed within the compartments or boxes, but different interaction rates are estimated between the compartments. See, for example, Baroyan, *et al.* (1969, 1971, 1977). The mixing parameters themselves may also change over time as intervention to control spread occurs.

2. The second is to use time series methods in which the main emphasis is upon identifying structural regularities in the data and projecting these forward spatially and temporally. These methods tend to be less data hungry than *SIR* models but do not handle non-stationary processes in time and space very easily. They accordingly run the risk that an unexpected change in the process over time will cause serious errors of forecast.

We now give examples of the results which may be obtained with each approach. The data used are monthly reported measles cases by medical district in Iceland, 1945–74. See Cliff, *et al.* (1981) for details of the data.

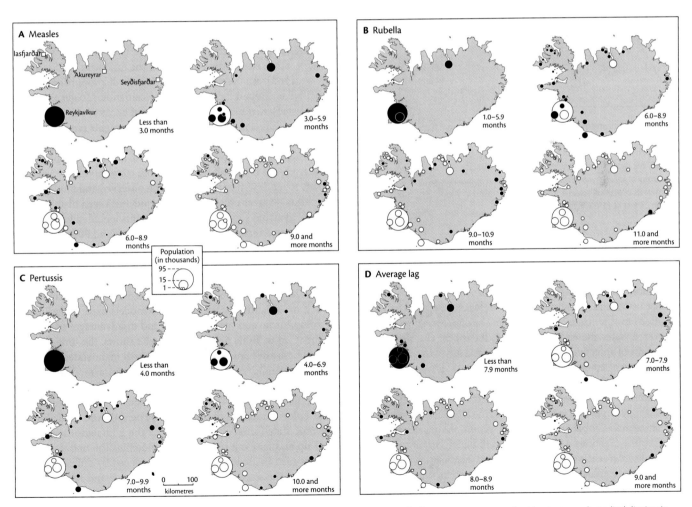

Figure 6.30 Time lag maps for infectious diseases in Iceland, 1900–90. Average time in months from commencement of epidemics to reach medical districts in different parts of Iceland. On each map, medical districts reached for the first time are shown as solid circles. Districts appearing on earlier maps appear as open circles on later maps. Circle sizes are proportional to 1990 medical district populations. (A) Measles. (B) Rubella. (C) Pertussis. (D) Average across all three diseases and influenza. *Source:* Cliff, *et al.* (2000, Figure 6.12, p. 264).

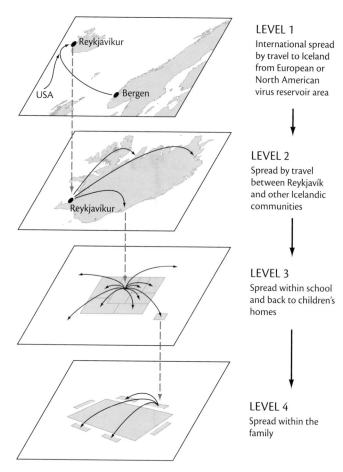

LEVEL 1
International spread by travel to Iceland from European or North American virus reservoir area

LEVEL 2
Spread by travel between Reykjavík and other Icelandic communities

LEVEL 3
Spread within school and back to children's homes

LEVEL 4
Spread within the family

Figure 6.31 Communicable disease diffusion in Iceland. Hypothetical sketch of the spread of an infectious disease agent from an international source down to a farm family in rural Iceland. The arrows indicate possible contacts. At levels 1 and 2, the movements are likely to be young adults; at 3 and 4, children. The synchrony of Iceland with Europe and the United States as international sources which seed infectious diseases in Iceland is discussed in Weinberger, *et al.* (2012). *Source:* Cliff, *et al.* (1981, Figure 3.14, p. 54).

SIR Models

Cliff and Ord (1995, pp. 153–64) have adapted the basic *SIR* model of Section 1.4 to examine epidemic return times for measles outbreaks in Iceland's medical districts between 1945 and 1974. In addition to the transitions between infected, susceptible and recovered states shown in Figure 1.17, the model also allowed for migration of infectives into each medical district to approximate the priming of epidemics between geographical areas as shown in Figure 1.18. Estimation of likely epidemic return times to different geographical areas, especially if they are disease-free, will become increasingly important in the context of the UNICEF/World Health Organization's Global Immunization Vision and Strategy (GIVS) programme (Sections 4.4 and 6.5). It will be important to link the model to intervention strategies. Planned vaccination campaigns, for example, feedback to affect epidemic return times.

Figures 6.32 and **6.33** show the results obtained for the eight medical districts which comprise Iceland's northwest fjords region. The time periods used for model fitting and for *ex-post* forecasting of the time gap in months between the penultimate and ultimate epidemics in the measles time series of each district are marked on

Figure 6.32. The bar graphs in Figure 6.33 show that the observed return times lay within the upper and lower ten percent points of the estimated distribution for return times in all eight districts, but that the correspondence between individual observed and 50th percentile forecast values was poor in two districts (Þingeyrar and Reykhóla).

Observed epidemic return times for measles across Iceland in the post-1945 period have been generally 36–60 months (3–5 years), often a little shorter in the capital, Reykjavík, and sometimes longer in very small settlements. This is expected from Figure 1.18. **Table 6.4** gives the results for the return times model if the analysis is extended from northwest Iceland to the whole country. In the table, settlements have been classified according to their time lag in months behind Reykjavík to be reached by measles outbreaks (cf. Figure 6.30A) after virus arrival in Iceland: group 1 settlements, six months or less; group 2, 6–9 months; group 3, over nine months. The classification reflects the geographical structure for disease propagation shown in Figure 6.29. The entry point into Iceland for most communicable diseases is Reykjavík, from which spread to regional centres – Akureyri (group 1), Ísafjörður (group 2) and Seyðisfjörður (group 3) – occurs, with localised spread from thence into regional hinterlands.

The return times model was fitted to each settlement group separately. Parameter estimates were calculated using all the epidemic intervals except the last in the study period, and these estimates were then used to generate *ex-post* forecasts of the waiting time in months to the last measles epidemic in the time window. Reykjavík was excluded from the analysis because of its disproportionate population size compared with any other settlement (eight times the next biggest town in the mid-1970s), and because this city generally led the diffusion process. The other settlements ranged down in size from c. 15,000 population. As Table 6.4 shows, despite low correlations between the point estimates, the average 50th percentile point from the model shows reasonable correspondence with the average for each settlement group. Both observed and model means reflect the 3–5-year cycle for measles epidemics seen historically in Iceland. In all but eight of the 44 settlements included in the analysis, observed return times fell within the 10th and 90th percentage points of the model estimates.

Spatial Time Series Approaches

Cliff, *et al.* (1993, pp. 360–410) have tested a variety of time series models on Icelandic measles data. The models used, including *SIR* for comparison, and the advantages and disadvantages of each are summarised in **Table 6.5**. As Figure 6.32 shows, the time series of Icelandic measles epidemics comprises two main states: epidemic and no epidemic. A persistent difficulty from a modelling viewpoint with such two-state series, even with different models for each state, is devising a rule to switch models from the no epidemic to the epidemic state in the correct time period. And modelling the epidemic state is made problematic by the non-stationarity of the build up and fade out phases of an epidemic. The impact of these issues is seen in Table 6.5. Forecasts produced by different models often miss the start of epidemics by a month and then echo the shape of the epidemic curve one month in arrears – the so-called one month lag effect in Table 6.5. Then the non-stationarity of the build up and fade out phases can cause models to over-estimate epidemic size when the reported cases decline sharply after the epidemic peak.

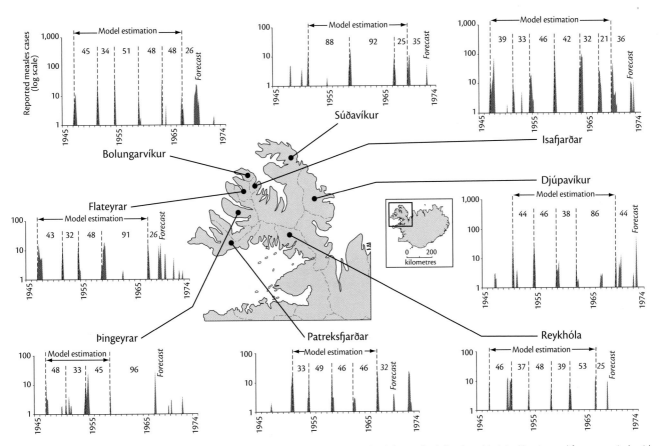

Figure 6.32 Iceland, northwest fjords, 1945–74: time series of reported measles cases in eight medical districts. Model calibration and forecast periods with inter-epidemic intervals in months are given. *Source*: Cliff and Ord (1995, Figure 8.6, p. 155).

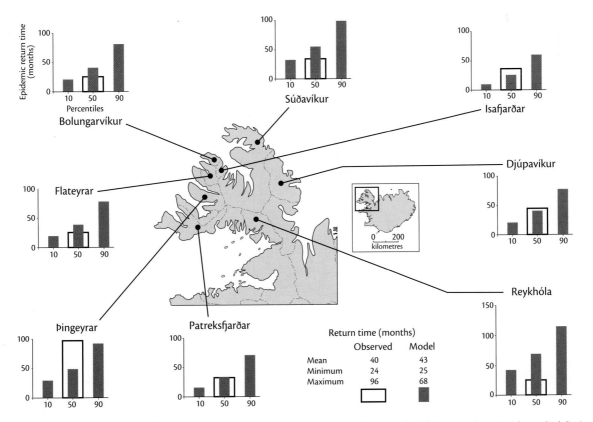

Figure 6.33 Iceland, northwest fjords, 1945–74: measles epidemic return times. Observed and projected epidemic return times in eight medical districts. Median, 10th and 90th percentiles for 50 simulations are plotted. *Source*: Cliff and Ord (1995, Figure 8.7, p. 157).

A further modelling complication with communicable diseases is the frequent non-congruence of data recording intervals and the *serial interval* of the disease; the serial interval is defined as the duration of time between the onset of symptoms of an index individual and the onset of symptoms in a second case directly infected by the first (Fine, 2003). A great deal of surveillance data for communicable diseases is reported for comparatively long discrete time intervals (e.g. weekly, monthly, quarterly), whereas the serial intervals for many communicable diseases of humans are often much shorter (e.g. a few days for influenza, about 14 days for measles). The spatial effect of this lack of congruence is that geographically widely separated cases, where the second is caused by the first, can appear as simultaneous events when they are in fact associated but separated temporally by a serial interval which is shorter than the data recording interval. Thus the spatial development of an epidemic on a monthly map series may appear as bursts of growth when there is in fact a causal chain between cases which would be observable if the data recording interval were of finer temporal granularity than the serial interval.

From the various time series models in Table 6.5, we have selected simultaneous equation models to illustrate how this issue may be tackled. **Figure 6.34** takes reported monthly cases of measles for seven Icelandic medical districts (Keflavíkur, Reykjavíkur, Akureyrar, Hofsós, Siglufjarðar, Ísafjarðar, Bolungarvíkur), 1945–70, and divides the data into a model calibration period (1945–57) and a forecast period (1958–70). The maps use vectors to show the measles diffusion chains modelled, reflecting the internal pathways identified in Figure 6.29A. Both time lags and spatial disease impulses between medical districts are incorporated. Mathematical details are given in Cliff, *et al.* (1993, pp. 383–88). The graphs show that the probability estimates of the likelihood of an epidemic are a better indication of observed epidemics than are the estimated number of cases. In addition, the size of epidemics as measured by number of reported cases is better modelled in larger than in smaller communities. This is unsurprising. As implied by Figure 1.18, the initiation of an epidemic in a small community is as likely to depend upon the chance arrival of an infective (e.g. a tourist; not allowed for in the model) as the systematic arrival of infection through the population size hierarchy of settlements.

Table 6.4 Iceland: inter-epidemic waiting times for measles, 1945–74. Observed and *ex-post* forecasts for groups of settlements

| Settlement group (n) | Parameter | Inter-epidemic interval (months) | | | |
| | | Observed | Model percentile | | |
			50	10	90
Group 1 (9)	Median	36	29.9	13.5	65.3
	Mean	62.9	34.9	17.4	71.6
	Minimum	34.0	20.2	6.7	52.3
	Maximum	167.0	57.4	34.4	100.6
	Corr (obs, 50th percentile)	0.76			
Group 2 (29)	Median	46	41.4	20.1	85.7
	Mean	58	43.9	22.3	88.7
	Minimum	24	24.4	8.1	63.1
	Maximum	168	89.1	57.7	146.0
	Corr (obs, 50th percentile)	0.26			
Group 3 (6)	Median	44	39.5	18.2	85.4
	Mean	52	38.6	17.6	83.8
	Minimum	26	32.5	13.2	75.8
	Maximum	92	42.6	20.4	89.0
	Corr (obs, 50th percentile)	0.03			

Table 6.5 Time series forecasting models. Characteristics with Icelandic measles data, 1945–70

| Model | Application format | | Main data inputs | | Temporal parameter structure | | Comments |
	Single region	Multiple region	S	I	Fixed	Variable	
SIR	×		×	×	×		Good at forecasting epidemic recurrence years ahead; average to poor at estimating epidemic size.
Autoregressive	Reykjavík			×		×	Initial one-month lag effect; adapts to changing phase characteristics; overestimates epidemic size.
GLIM (Generalised linear integrated model)		Northwest Iceland	×	×	×		Use of main town as epidemic lead indicator produces good estimates of epidemic starts in other medical districts; poor estimates of epidemic size.
Kalman filter	Reykjavík			×		×	Initial lag effect; locks on to epidemic course but overestimates epidemic size.
Bayesian entropy	Reykjavík		×	×		×	Separate models for epidemic and no epidemic states. One-month lag effect in predicting epidemic curve; probability forecasts of epidemic/no epidemic good; model switches states in correct month.
Simultaneous equation		Multi-region chains		×	×		Areas studied as causal chains; phase characteristics guaranteed by model formulation.
Logit		Multi-region chains		×	×		Good probability forecasts of epidemic/no epidemic states; slow state switching.

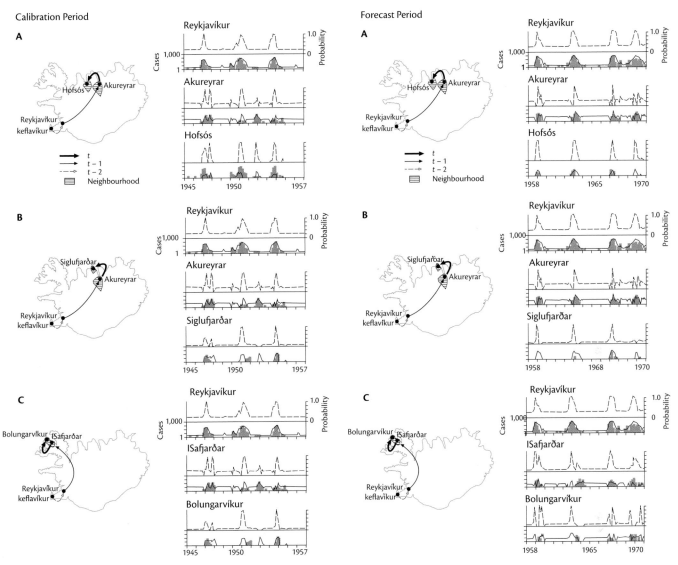

Figure 6.34 Icelandic measles diffusion chains: simultaneous equation models. The maps show (A) spread from Keflavíkur to Reykjavíkur, on to Akureyrar, and finally from Akureyrar into the local medical districts of Hofsós and (B) Siglufjarðar. (C) Spread from Keflavíkur to Reykjavíkur across to Ísafjarðar, with local spread (neighbourhood) from thence to Bolungarvíkur. The identifiers, t, $t-1$ and $t-2$, reflect the monthly time steps in the causal chains. Arrows run from impulse districts to the response districts. The graphs plot the district monthly reported cases of measles (grey bars) against simultaneous equation estimates of cases (solid black lines) and epidemic probabilities (pecked lines). The model calibration period is 1945–57 and the forecast period is 1958–70. *Source*: Cliff, *et al.* (1993, parts of Figure 14.12, p. 384 and Figure 15.6, p. 404).

Model Assessment

Forecasting the return times and sizes of epidemics of communicable diseases is still an art form and much remains to be done. In this, epidemic forecasting is no different from forecasting in other fields like economics, public health, or indeed the weather in the UK. Our broad conclusions after experimenting with many models over a spectrum of diseases and geographical areas are as follows:

(i)   We have yet to find the Rosetta stone of a model which produces accurate projections of both epidemic recurrence times and epidemic size. All too often, if a model is devised which will forecast recurrence acceptably, epidemic size is over-estimated. To forecast inter-epidemic times accurately, it is generally necessary to tune the model to be sensitive to

changes signalling the approach of an epidemic, with the result that it overshoots when the epidemic is in progress.

(ii)   Models which are based only on the size of the infective population in previous time periods consistently fail to detect the approach of an epidemic. Instead, they provide reasonable estimates of cases reported, but lagged in time.

(iii) Models with parameters fixed through time have a tendency to smooth through epidemic highs and lows because they are unable to adapt to the changes between the build-up and fade-out phases. Time-varying parameter models are better at avoiding this problem.

(iv)   Epidemic recurrences can be reasonably anticipated only by incorporating information on the size of the susceptible population and/or properly identifying the lead–lag structure for disease transmission among geographical areas. Addition of spatial interaction information markedly improves our ability to forecast recurrences in lagging areas. Information on susceptible population levels also serves to prime a model to the possibility of a recurrence. Models based on susceptible populations, but which are single- rather than multi-region, tend to miss the start of epidemics but rapidly lock on to the course of an epidemic thereafter. Models which are dominated by spatial transmission information, at the expense of information on the level of the susceptible population in the study region, produce estimates of epidemic size which reflect the course of the epidemic in the triggering regions rather than in the study region.

(v) Stochastic process models enhance our understanding of disease transmission across geographical space and increase the chances of devising time series models appropriate to the task of forecasting.

These conclusions highlight the fact that naïve models produce poor results. However, Table 6.5 also indicates the gains to be made for each extra element of complexity added to our models, namely:

(i) time-varying parameters to handle the non-stationary nature of within-epidemic structure, particularly the fundamentally different character of the build-up and fade-out phases;

(ii) separate models for epidemic and inter-epidemic episodes to recognise the different character of these periods;

(iii) spatial lead–lag information to improve our ability to forecast epidemic recurrences and to understand the transmission of disease between areas;

(iv) incorporation of data upon the susceptible population level to improve estimates both of epidemic size and likely recurrence intervals.

And it is important to be able to identify the gains obtained by increasing model complexity, since it is all too easy to specify sophisticated models which are either insoluble or contain multiplicative structures that magnify errors when applied to data of variable quality.

6.5 Intervention, Value-for-Money and Demography

All health interventions cost money, and the associated opportunity costs of the other uses to which the money used for health interventions could be put. Against the costs must be weighed the gains in lives saved and extended, the improvements in the quality of life which interventions can yield, and potential economic and social benefits in the labour market from a healthier population. In the end, resolution of the tensions between costs and benefits are resolved by societal debate and political choices. Sometimes the politicians buffer themselves from the difficult choices. In the United Kingdom, for example, the independent National Institute for Health and Clinical Excellence (NICE) was set up in 1999 to reduce variation in the geographical availability and quality of the UK's National Health Service (NHS) treatments and care. NICE's evidence-based guidance is designed to assist in resolving

uncertainty about which medicines, treatments, procedures and devices represent the best quality care and which offer the best value for money for the NHS. Inevitably, NICE's value-for-money guidance leads to making uncomfortable decisions to restrict or deny certain drugs on cost grounds to the NHS as opposed to the benefits gained (e.g. prolonging life for terminally-ill patients by a few months). No-one enjoys making these choices but they are the reality of the current world (cf. Figure 6.1).

In this section, we look at ways of assessing the impact of interventions to prevent the geographical spread of communicable diseases, costs, benefits and demographic outcomes. We begin by examining ways of measuring intervention impacts.

Measuring Intervention Impacts

Substantial resources are devoted to reducing the incidence, duration and severity of major diseases that cause morbidity and mortality, and to reducing their impact on people's lives. It is important to capture both fatal and non-fatal health outcomes in summary measures of average levels of population health. For mortality, one of the earliest and still most commonly used ways of measuring intervention impact is to assess the extension of life produced by intervention as compared with no-intervention scenarios.

Years of Potential Life Lost (YPLL)

Agencies such as the World Health Organization and the US Centers for Disease Control and Prevention have been experimenting with statistics which measure *years of potential life lost* (YPLL). This takes into account the year at which a death occurs as compared with their life expectancy at, say, birth, as given in the life tables published by most national population agencies. If an individual dies before their normal life expectancy, the difference between date of death and life expectancy in years represents one measure of YPLL. More complicated versions of this simple model exist because life expectancy itself changes with age. Thus, in England in 2000, a 20-year-old male could expect on average to live for another 55 years (60 for a female) whereas an 80-year-old male could expect to live on average for another seven years. So under YPLL, the two deaths would be weighted differently, the younger death having a weight much higher than the older.

The effect of measures of this kind is to change the order of some leading causes of death, as compared with the list order based on death rates alone, all tending to give greater weight to the infectious diseases (which especially affect children) and to injuries (which especially affect young people); where these conditions cause mortality, it is most commonly in the first two decades of life. YPLL also reduces the relative importance of heart disease and cancers (which tend to affect the old).

Disability-Adjusted Life Years (DALYs) and Healthy Life Expectancy (HALE)

With illness and disability, rather than mortality, similar arguments may be used, giving special weight to diseases which cause a lifetime of disability (so-called *disability-adjusted life years*, DALYs) rather than a brief illness. The World Health Organization makes frequent use of *healthy life expectancy* or HALE. HALE at birth sums expectation of life for different health states, adjusted for severity distribution, making it sensitive to changes over time or differences between countries in the severity distribution of health states. It gives the average number of years that a person can expect to live in 'full health' by taking into account years lived in less than full health due to disease and/or injury. A full account of the many different measures which have been proposed to quantify what is meant by 'full health' is given in Murray, *et al.* (2002). Yet other weighting systems attempt to weight morbidity data by quality of life measures. But the difficulty with all these approaches is defining unambiguous and generally accepted sets of weights.

Figure 6.35 shows the YPLL, DALY and HALE maps for the countries of the European Union for infectious and parasitic diseases in the first decade of the new millennium. All show essentially the same pattern of higher loss of life and poorer health primarily in southern Europe and the new republics of Eastern Europe which were originally part of the former USSR. The YPLL map focuses on death before age 65, so the figures give an indication of the premature loss of economically productive life. In the EU-27, the average YPLL is 116 per 100,000 men, as compared with 47 YPLL per 100,000 women. The increased resilience of women against infectious and parasitic diseases is a well known biological fact. The highest losses of potential life due to infectious diseases among men were found in Portugal (538 YPLL per 100,000 men) and in Romania (444 per 100,000 men). The variance is high in the highest quintile, showing the patchy nature of local epidemics in people under 65: in Lisboa the number of YPLL increased to over 1,000 among men. The lowest figures were found in the Czech Republic (23.1 YPLL). The same geographical pattern is found among women, with the highest YPLL again found in Romania (190) and Portugal (157, with 300 in Lisboa). The lowest figures were returned by Malta (only 1.5 years, which may be an artefact of Malta's small population) and the Czech Republic (10.3 YPLL).

Global Immunization Vision and Strategy: Intervention Costs and Benefits

As discussed in Section 4.4, the Expanded Programme on Immunization (EPI) was established in 1974 through a World Health Assembly resolution (WHA27.57) to build on the success of the global smallpox eradication programme and to ensure that all children in all countries benefited from life-saving vaccines. The operations of the EPI are currently set within the framework of the Global Immunization Vision and Strategy (GIVS), launched as a joint initiative of the WHO and the United Nations Children's Fund (UNICEF) in 2006.

GIVS was developed in the context of increasing resources for immunisation. As described in Section 4.4 and in Wolfson, *et al.* (2008), in 2000 a public–private partnership, the Global Alliance for Vaccines and Immunisation (GAVI) was initiated to provide financial support for immunisation in the world's poorest countries. By the end of 2005, government and private sources had pledged a total of US$3.3 billion to the GAVI Alliance, enabling it to provide support to 73 of 75 eligible countries. Between 2000 and 2005, total GAVI Alliance disbursements were US$760.5 million. GAVI Alliance's resource outlook over the next decade has improved with the launch of two innovative funding mechanisms: the International Finance Facility for Immunisation (IFFIm), which could provide up to US$4 billion over the next 10 years, and the Pneumo Advance Market Commitment (AMC), which will provide US$1.5 billion to support low-income countries for the purchase of new vaccines against *Streptococcus pneumoniae*, a leading cause of childhood meningitis and pneumonia mortality.

In 2005, WHO and UNICEF undertook, as a companion to the GIVS document, to estimate the costs to reach immunisation goals which had been established, and Wolfson, *et al.* (2008) report on the methods and results of that exercise. A model was developed to estimate the total cost of reaching GIVS goals by 2015 in 117 low- and lower-middle-income countries. Current spending was estimated by analysing data from country planning documents, and scale-up costs were estimated using a bottom-up, ingredients-based approach. Financial costs were estimated by country and year for reaching 90% coverage with all existing vaccines; introducing a discrete set of new vaccines (rotavirus, conjugate pneumococcal, conjugate meningococcal A and Japanese encephalitis); and conducting immunisation campaigns to protect at-risk populations against poliomyelitis, tetanus, measles, yellow fever and meningococcal meningitis (**Figure 6.36**).

The 72 poorest countries of the world spent US$2.5 (range: US$1.8–4.2) billion on immunisation in 2005, an increase from US$1.1 (range: US$0.9–1.6) billion in 2000. By 2015 annual immunisation costs will on average increase to about US$4.0 (range US$2.9–6.7) billion. Total immunisation costs for 2006–2015 are estimated at US$35 (range US$13–40) billion; of this, US$16.2 billion are incremental costs, comprising US$5.6 billion for system scale-up and US$8.7 billion for vaccines; US$19.3 billion is required to maintain immunisation programmes at 2005 levels. In all 117 low- and lower-middle-income countries, total costs for 2006–2015 are estimated at US$76 (range: US$23–110) billion, with US$49 billion for maintaining current systems and $27 billion for scaling-up. These projected costs are staggeringly large, particularly in the context of the state of the global debt and sovereign debt crises existing at the end of the first decade of the new millennium. In the 72 poorest countries, US$11–15 billion (30%–40%) of the overall resource needs are unmet if the GIVS goals are to be reached. While the authors acknowledge that the methods they used are approximate estimates with limitations, they do provide some idea of the financing gaps that need to be filled to scale up immunisation by 2015 if the world's communicable disease control aspirations are to be converted into practical reality.

What are the benefits? If the immunisation goals are realised, Wolfson, *et al.* (2008, pp. 35–6) estimate that, by 2015, more than 70 million children in the world's 72 poorest countries can be protected annually against 14 major childhood diseases if an additional US$1 billion per year can be invested towards immunisation, saving some 10 million more lives in the decade, 2006–15. The cost equates to an additional US$0.5 per capita per year above current levels (< US$1 per capita) of investment in immunisation. Wolfson and colleagues argue that, at such modest per capita costs and high benefits, immunisation continues to be one of the best values for public health investment today. They see other benefits too over and above saving lives: (i) in impoverished countries, lives saved boost economies, potentially yielding a rate of return of up to 18%; (ii) immunisation can serve as a platform to strengthen health systems and deliver other life-saving interventions such as those against non-communicable conditions like malnutrition, as well as other communicable infections like malaria and intestinal worms.

Failure to control the spread of communicable diseases has consequences other than demographic; it also throws sudden burdens upon healthcare systems, potentially leading to degradation of other services. For example, **Figure 6.37** shows the country by country impact of the 2009 swine flu scare upon healthcare services

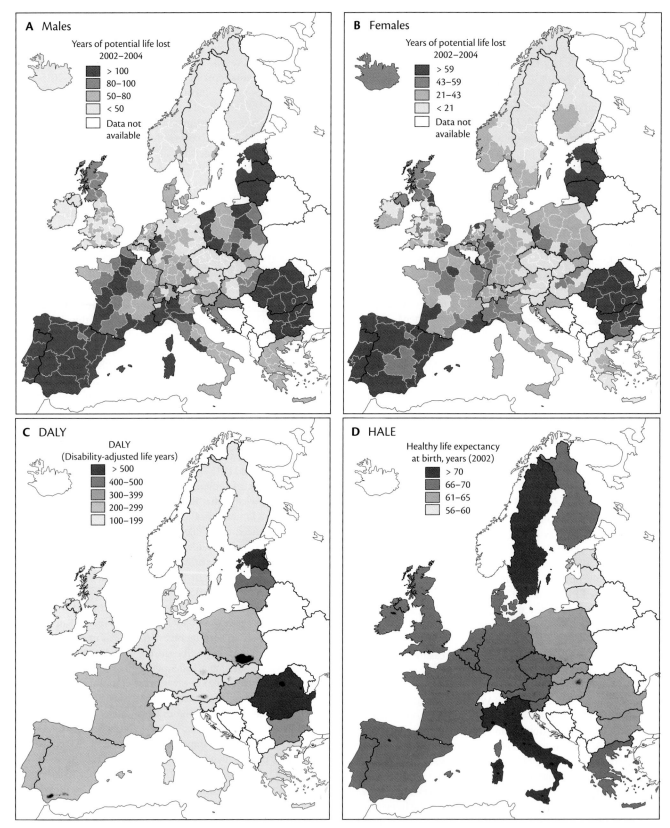

Figure 6.35 YPLL, DALY and HALE maps for the countries of the European Union. (A) Male YPLL. (B) Female YPLL. The YPLL is estimated against an age of death of 65. (C) Age-standardised DALYs per 100,000 population. (D) HALE. The YPLL and DALY maps are for infectious and parasitic diseases at the beginning of the new millennium. The HALE map gives the estimated healthy life expectancy for all persons at birth. In the British Isles, although the total burden of deaths from infectious and parasitic diseases was small at the millennium, the map shows that the greatest YPLL and lowest expectations of good health were in Scotland and the London area. The conurbations in South and West Yorkshire, Greater Manchester, and in the West Midlands also experienced comparatively high risks of premature mortality from infectious and parasitic diseases as did the Welsh Marches. *Sources*: (A) and (B) redrawn from Eurostat Statistical Books (2009, Figures 6.3 and 6.4, pp. 46–47). (C) WHO Global Burden of Disease data by member countries, 2004. (D) Data from World Health Organization (2004f, pp. 132–35).

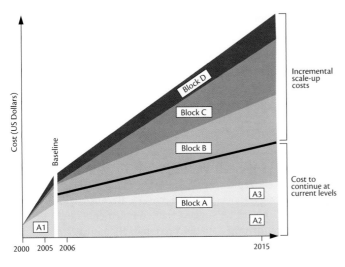

Figure 6.36 GIVS costing blocks.

Block A: maintenance of current routine system (baseline cost)
Current levels of investment in immunisation were estimated using available data from 40 Financial Sustainability Plans (Block A1), and extrapolated for the period 2006–2015 by accounting for the impact of inflation and population increases (Block A3). They assume no change in vaccination schedules and no improvement in immunisation coverage levels (Block A2). This does not include campaigns or vaccine costs.

Block B: vaccine costs
Vaccine costs were estimated by using coverage targets, population projections and applying the most recent available data on unit prices of different vaccine presentations. The estimates account for wastage rates and the need for buffer stock. The cost of safe injection equipment is bundled in the vaccine cost estimates. The element *below the line* represents the vaccine costs to continue immunisation at 2005 levels, and *above the line* is the vaccine portion of scaling-up.

Block C: scaling-up of routine system
This is estimated using an ingredients-based approach.

Block D: campaigns
A schedule of needed campaigns was generated based on a combination of the projections of vaccine coverage and the epidemiological coverage required to reduce rapidly the burden of disease. Campaign costs include both operational costs and vaccine costs.
Source: Wolfson, *et al.* (2008, Figure 1, p. 31).

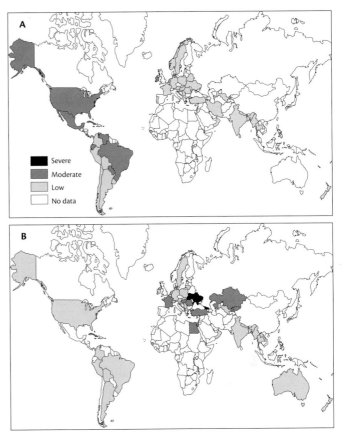

Figure 6.37 Pandemic (A/Swine/H1N1) influenza, 2009: global impact upon healthcare services. Impact refers to the degree of disruption of healthcare services from increased levels of acute respiratory diseases attributed to the pandemic, and is mapped at four levels of intensity for WHO member countries. (A) Early October 2009; (B) mid December 2009. *Source*: World Health Organization Map Production: Public Health Information and Geographic Information System (GIS).

for two months of the pandemic: the first week of November and the third week of December, 2009. Note the shift from an Americas focus of high impact to Europe as the pandemic spread from its hearth continent to another geographical region.

6.6 Conclusion

This chapter concludes our analysis of the control of the geographical spread of human infectious diseases. We have tried to show the ways in which modelling approaches, linked to real-time surveillance, can be used to guide intervention strategies using quarantine, isolation and vaccination to interrupt spatial spread. These interventions all have the capacity to reduce the global burden of transmissible infectious diseases which ruin lives, increase mortality rates, and drain public health resources. There is little sign that, in the foreseeable future, the spread of re-emerging old infections and the emergence of new infections will cease. As we noted in the Preface to this book, if pestilence, prayer and appeals to saints to control the spatial spread of communicable diseases are thought of solely as quaint relics of medieval life, the late twentieth century

came as a nasty shock. Since 1981, 25 millions have died from the AIDS pandemic, and Africa alone has 12 million AIDS orphans. The worldwide toll of HIV infection today has reached 35 million and in some African countries, one-quarter of the adult population is infected. Worries over new H5N1 and H1N1 strains of human influenza rekindle memories of the devastating Spanish influenza pandemic of 1918–19. The brief outbreak of SARS in 2003 showed how rapidly viruses can now race through the global urban network. Indeed, as this conclusion is being written, China has just reported (31 December 2011) its first death from H5N1 bird flu for over a year in the southern city of Shenzhen.

Study of the temporal history of human disease shows that 'new' or 'renewed' infectious diseases are a constant theme rather than a recent episode. Very old diseases such as measles or cholera undergo periodic eruptions and invasions which share many of the features now associated with emerging diseases. This longer-run perspective helps to set the context within which current events are viewed. It enables the exceptional conditions which are forcing the present rapid pace of disease change to be more readily isolated. In the twenty-first century, the world is still working at control, eradication and elimination of the spatial spread of infectious diseases, just as the Italian states and principalities, along with their saints, did seven centuries ago when confronted by plague epidemics. And it reinforces our need to intervene to control the spread of communicable diseases in timely and cost-effective ways.

Appendix 6.1: Swash–Backwash Model Equations

Let the first month of an influenza season (July, say) be coded as $t = 1$. The subsequent months of the season are then coded serially as $t = 2$, $t = 3$, ... , $t = T$, where T is the number of monthly periods from the beginning to the end of the season (i.e. $T = 12$ in our yearly cycle). We call the month in which an influenza case is first recorded in a given geographical unit the *leading edge* (LE) of the outbreak in that unit, and the last month of record as the following edge (FE). As described in Cliff and Haggett (2006), standard statistical analysis of the distribution of the two edges enables us to define a time-weighted arithmetic mean, $\bar{t}_{LE}$ and $\bar{t}_{FE}$ for each edge. For the leading edge, the equation is

$$\bar{t}_{LE} = \frac{1}{N}\sum_{t=1}^{T} tn_t \tag{A1}$$

where n_t is the number of units whose leading edge occurred in month t and $N = \sum n_t$. The time-weighted mean is a useful measure of the velocity of the wave in terms of average time to unit infection. A similar equation can be written for FE, and higher order moments can also be specified. To allow comparison between diseases with different wave characteristics, we convert these time-weighted means to a velocity ratio, $V, (0 \leq V \leq 1)$,

$$V_{LE} = 1 - \frac{\bar{t}_{LE}}{D} \tag{A2}$$

where D is the duration of the wave. A similar equation can be written for V_{FE}.

The conventional *basic reproduction number* (or *rate* or *ratio*), R_0, is defined as the ratio between an infection rate (β) and a recovery rate (μ):

$$R_0 = \frac{\beta}{\mu}. \tag{A3}$$

In the spatial domain, A, the spatial reproduction number, R_{0A}, is the average number of secondary infected geographical units produced from one infected unit in a virgin area. In a given study area, the integral S_A (the proportion of the study area at risk of infection) is given by:

$$S_A = \frac{(\bar{t}_{LE} - 1)}{T} \tag{A4}$$

while the proportion of the area which is infected (the infected area integral) is

$$I_A = \frac{\bar{t}_{FE}}{T} - S_A. \tag{A5}$$

The recovered area integral, R_A, is

$$R_A = 1 - (S_A + I_A). \tag{A6}$$

All three integrals are dimensionless numbers with values in the range [0, 1]. S parallels the reciprocal of β; a small value of S_A indicates a very rapid spread. The integral R_A parallels μ in that a large value suggests very rapid recovery. Because S_A is inversely related to its power we suggest that complements might be substituted in estimating a spatial version of R_0, namely

$$R_{0A} = \frac{1 - S_A}{1 - R_A}. \tag{A7}$$

Other formulations of R_{0A} are possible. For example, Smallman-Raynor and Cliff (2013) have used $R_{0A} = (1 - S_A)/R_A$ equally successfully.

Such a spatial basic reproduction number would measure the propensity of an infected geographical unit to spawn other infected units in later time periods. In effect it provides an indicator of the tendency of an infected unit to produce secondaries. Values of R_{0A} calibrate the velocity of such spread (the larger the value, the greater the rate of spread). It is important not to over-stretch the analogy between R_0 and R_{0A}. R_0 is defined for the hypothetical situation when a new case is introduced into a *wholly susceptible population*. While R_{0A} is defined for a virgin region, it is calculated using spatial data for the entire span of the outbreak. As a result, it is contaminated with data from the later phases of the outbreak when many spatial sub-areas are no longer virgin. This may account for the frequent small calculated values. Normal R_0 is useful because it distinguishes between situations where an epidemic can take off ($R_0 > 1$) and those where it cannot ($R_0 < 1$), and this is arguably the most important attribute of R_0 as a summary parameter in epidemiology. R_0's spatial cousin, R_{0A}, does not share this property – for example in Tables 6.1–6.3 there are analyses of real epidemics that had sustained spread from one district to another in which $R_{0A} < 1$. But it does allow large numbers of spatial settings to be examined and the relative velocity at different stages of outbreaks to be assessed and compared. Finally, it should be noted that the parameters R_{0A}, LE and FE are correlated, but each gives slightly different insights into the progress of an outbreak through a geographical area.

References and Author Index

Note: numbers in square brackets after references indicate the sections in the text where the item is cited. Where a section is denoted by a single digit, the cited work appears in the caption to the first figure of the corresponding chapter.

Ahmad, A., Andraghetti, R. (2007). *SARS Control: Effective and Acceptable Strategies for the Control of SARS and New Emerging Infections in China and Europe. Control Measures Implemented by the Non-European SARS Affected Countries.* Work Package 8. WHO EURO CSR Department. [3.4]

Alderson, M. (1981). *International Mortality Statistics.* London: Macmillan. [2.2]

Alward, R.B., Bilous, J., Tangermann, R.H., Sanders, R., Maher, C., Sato, Y., Omi, S. (1997). 'Strengthening routine immunization services in the Western Pacific through the eradication of poliomyelitis.' *Journal of Infectious Diseases*, 175 (suppl. 1), S268–71. [4.4]

Anderson, R.M. (2009). 'How well are we managing the influenza A/H1N1 pandemic in the UK?' *British Medical Journal*, 339, b2897, 15 July. [6.2]

Anderson, R.M., Fraser, C., Ghani, A.C., Donnelly, C.A., Riley, S., Ferguson, N.M., Leung, G.M., Lam, T.H., Hedley, A.J. (2004). 'Epidemiology, transmission dynamics and control of SARS: the 2002–2003 epidemic.' *Philosophical Transactions of the Royal Society London*, B359, 1091–1105. [3.4]

Anderson, R.M., May, R. (1991). *Infectious Disease of Humans: Dynamics and Control.* Oxford: Oxford University Press. [1.4, 6.1]

Andrus, J.K., de Quadros, C.A., Solórzano, C.S., Periago, M.R., Henderson, D.A. (2011). 'Measles and rubella eradication in the Americas.' *Vaccine* (http://dx.doi.org/10.1016/j.vaccine.2011.04.059; last viewed 27 February 2012). [5.5]

Anonymous (1942a). 'The outbreak of jaundice in the army.' *Journal of the American Medical Association*, 120, 51–3. [4.6]

Anonymous (1942b). 'Jaundice following yellow fever vaccination.' *Journal of the American Medical Association*, 119, 1110. [4.6]

Anonymous (1947a). 'Epidemiological notes.' *The Medical Officer*, LXXVII, 260. [6.3]

Anonymous (1947b). 'Acute poliomyelitis: memorandum by Medical Officers of the Ministry of Health.' *Lancet*, II, 155–6. [6.3]

Anonymous (1947c). 'Topical and local incidence of poliomyelitis.' *The Medical Officer*, LXXVIII, 23. [6.3]

Anonymous (2009). 'Communicable disease and health protection quarterly review: January to March 2009.' *Journal of Public Health Medicine*, 31, 298–9. [4.6]

Asaria, P., MacMahon, E. (2006). 'Measles in the United Kingdom: can we eradicate it by 2010?' *British Medical Journal*, 333, 890–5. [4.6]

Aylward, B., Hennessey, K.A., Zagaria, N., Olivé, J.-M., Cochi, S. (2000). 'When is a disease eradicable? 100 years of lessons learned.' *American Journal of Public Health*, 90, 1515–20. [5.1, 5.4]

Bailey, N.T.J. (1975). *The Mathematical Theory of Infectious Diseases.* London: Griffin. [1.4, 6.1]

Baker, J.P. (2003). 'The pertussis vaccine controversy in Great Britain, 1974–1986.' *Vaccine*, 21, 4003–10. [4.6]

Barbera, J., Macintyre, A., Gostin, L., Inglesby, T., O'Toole, T., DeAtley, C., Tonat, K., Layton, M. (2001). 'Large-scale quarantine following biological terrorism in the United States: scientific examination, logistic and legal limits, and possible consequences.' *The Journal of the American Medical Association*, 286, 2711–18. [3.4]

Baroyan, O.V., Genchikov, L.A., Rvachev, L.A., Shashkov, V.A. (1969). 'An attempt at large-scale influenza epidemic modelling by means of a computer.' *Bulletin of the International Epidemiology Association*, 18, 22–31. [6.4]

Baroyan, O.V., Rvachev, L.A., Basilevsky, U.V., Ermakov, V.V., Frank, K.D., Rvachev, M.A., Shashkov, V.A. (1971). 'Computer modelling of influenza epidemics for the whole country (USSR).' *Advances in Applied Probability*, 3, 224–6. [6.4]

Baroyan, O.V., Rvachev, L.A., Ivannikov, Y.G. (1977). *Modelling and Prediction of Influenza Epidemics in the USSR* (in Russian). Moscow: N.F. Gamaleia Institute of Epidemiology and Microbiology. [6.4]

Bart, K.J., Foulds, J., Patriarca, P. (1996). 'Global eradication of poliomyelitis: benefit-cost analysis.' *Bulletin of the World Health Organization*, 74, 35–45. [5.3]

Bartlett, M.S. (1957). 'Measles periodicity and community size.' *Journal of the Royal Statistical Society A*, 120, 48–70. [1.4]

Basu, R.N., Jezek, Z., Ward, N.A. (1979). *The Eradication of Smallpox from India.* New Delhi: WHO South-East Asia Regional Office. [2.7]

Bellhouse, D.R. (2011). 'A new look at Halley's life table.' *Journal of the Royal Statistical Society A*, 174, 823–32. [2.3]

Bellini, W.J., Rota, P.A. (2011). 'Biological feasibility of measles eradication.' *Virus Research*, 162, 72–9. [5.5]

Beltrami, L. (1882). 'Il lazzaretto di Milano.' *Archivio Storico Lombardo*, 9, 403–41. [1.2]

Benenson, A.S. (ed.) (1990). *Control of Communicable Diseases in Man (15th Edition).* Washington, D.C.: American Public Health Association. [3.1]

Bienia, R.A., Stein, E., Bienia, B.H. (1983). 'United States Public Health Service hospitals (1798–1981) – the end of an era.' *New England Journal of Medicine*, 308, 166–8. [3.2]

Biraben, J.N. (1975–76). *Les Hommes et la Peste en France et dans les Pays Européens et Méditerranéens.* Paris: Mouton. [1.2]

Black, F.L. (1966). 'Measles endemicity in insular populations: critical community size and its evolutionary implication.' *Journal of Theoretical Biology*, 11, 207–11. [1.4]

Bland, J., Clements, J. (1998). 'Protecting the world's children: the story of WHO's immunization programme.' *World Health Forum*, 19, 162–73. [4.4]

Blume, S., Geesink, I. (2000). 'A brief history of polio vaccines.' *Science*, 288, 1593–4. [4.6]

Böckh, R. (1886). *Statistisches Jahrbuch der Stadt Berlin, Zwölfter Jahrgang. Statistik des Jahres 1884*. Berlin: P. Stankiewicz. [6.2]

Boëlle, P.Y., Bernillon, P., Desenclos, J.C. (2009). 'A preliminary estimation of the reproduction ratio for new influenza A(H1N1) from the outbreak in Mexico, March–April 2009.' *Eurosurveillance*, 14, issue 19, 14 May, 10–13. [6.2]

Bordley, J., Harvey, A.Mc. (1976). *Two Centuries of American Medicine 1776–1976*. Philadelphia: W.B. Saunders Co. [3.2]

Bottero, A. (1942). 'La peste in Milano nel 1399–1400 e l'opera di Giangaleazzo Visconti.' *Atti e Memorie dell'Academia di Storia del Arte Sanitaria*, ser. 2, no. 8. [1.2]

Boulton, J., Schwarz, L. (2010). 'Yet another inquiry into the trustworthiness of eighteenth-century London's *Bills of Mortality*.' *Local Population Studies*, 85, 28–45. [2.3]

Brauer, F., Van den Driessche, P., Wu, J., Allen, L.J.S. (eds.) (2008). *Mathematical Epidemiology*. Berlin: Springer-Verlag. [3.3]

Brown, T.M. (2006). 'International public health before the World Health Organization.' *Global Forum for Health Research*, Forum 10, Cairo, Egypt, 29 October–2 November 2006. Geneva: Global Forum for Health Research. [2.3]

Bruce-Chwatt, L.J. (1987). 'Malaria and its control: present situation and future prospects.' *Annual Review of Public Health*, 8, 75–110. [5.4]

Bryder, L. (1984). 'Papworth Village Settlement – a unique experiment in the treatment and care of the tuberculous?' *Medical History*, 28, 372–90. [3.3]

Burton, A., Monasch, R., Lautenbach, B., Gacic-Dobo, M., Neill, M., Karimov, R., Wolfson, L., Jones, G., Birmingham, M. (2009). 'WHO and UNICEF estimates of infant immunization coverage: methods and processes.' *Bulletin of the World Health Organization*, 87, 535–41. [4.4]

Bush, K. (2000). 'Polio, war and peace.' *Bulletin of the World Health Organization*, 78, 281–2. [5.3]

Butler, A.G. (1943). *The Australian Army Medical Services in the War of 1914–1918, Volume III*. Melbourne: Australian War Memorial. [6.2]

Butler, D. (2011). 'WHO to decide fate of smallpox stocks.' *Nature*. doi:10.1038/news.2011.288. [5.7]

Carmichael, A.G. (1986). *Plague and the Poor in Renaissance Florence*. Cambridge: Cambridge University Press. [1.2]

Carmichael, A.G. (1991). 'Contagion theory and contagion practice in fifteenth-century Milan.' *Renaissance Quarterly*, 44, 213–56. [1.2]

Carmichael, A.G. (1993). 'Leprosy.' In: K.F. Kiple (ed.), *The Cambridge World History of Human Disease*. Cambridge: Cambridge University Press, 834–9. [3.3]

Carmichael, A.G. (1997). 'Leprosy: larger than life.' In: K.F. Kiple (ed.), *Plague, Pox and Pestilence: Disease in History*. London: Weidenfeld and Nicolson, 50–7. [3.3]

Castillo-Salgado, C. (2010). 'Trends and directions of global public health surveillance.' *Epidemiologic Reviews*, 32, 93–109. [2.7, 2.8]

Castillo-Solórzano, C.C., Matuz, C.R., Tambini, G. (2009). *Images that Inspire: The Mobilization of the Americas to Eliminate Measles and Rubella*. Washington, D.C.: Pan American Health Organization. [4.4, 5.5]

Cello, J., Paul, A.V., Wimmer, E. (2002). 'Chemical synthesis of poliovirus cdna: generation of infectious virus in the absence of natural template.' *Science*, 297, 1016–18. [5.6]

Centers for Disease Control (1974). *Neurotropic Diseases Surveillance: Poliomyelitis*. Atlanta: Centers for Disease Control. [4.5]

Centers for Disease Control (1981). *Poliomyelitis Surveillance: Summary, 1979*. Atlanta: Centers for Disease Control. [4.5]

Centers for Disease Control (1982). *Poliomyelitis Surveillance: Summary, 1980–81*. Atlanta: Centers for Disease Control. [4.5]

Centers for Disease Control (1988). 'Guidelines for evaluating surveillance systems.' *Morbidity and Mortality Weekly Report*, 37 (suppl. S–5), 1S–10S. [2.1]

Centers for Disease Control and Prevention (1993a). 'Summary of notifiable diseases, United States 1993.' *MMWR Summary of Notifiable Diseases*, 42, 1–91. [4.5]

Centers for Disease Control and Prevention (1993b). 'Recommendations of the International Task Force for Disease Eradication.' *MMWR Recommendations and Reports*, 42 (RR-16), 1–38. [5.1, 5.5, 5.8]

Centers for Disease Control and Prevention (1994a). 'Human plague – India, 1994.' *Morbidity and Mortality Weekly Report*, 43, 689–91. [3.4]

Centers for Disease Control and Prevention (1994b). 'Update: human plague – India, 1994.' *Morbidity and Mortality Weekly Report*, 43, 722–3. [3.4]

Centers for Disease Control and Prevention (1995). 'Lack of evidence for wild poliovirus circulation – United States, 1993.' *Morbidity and Mortality Weekly Report*, 43, 957–9. [4.5]

Centers for Disease Control and Prevention (1996). 'History of CDC.' *Morbidity and Mortality Weekly Report*, 45, 526–30. [2.4]

Centers for Disease Control and Prevention (1997a). 'Paralytic poliomyelitis – United States, 1980–1994.' *Morbidity and Mortality Weekly Report*, 46, 79–83. [4.5]

Centers for Disease Control and Prevention (1997b). 'Follow-up on poliomyelitis – United States, Canada, Netherlands.' *Morbidity and Mortality Weekly Report*, 46, 1195–9. [4.5]

Centers for Disease Control and Prevention (2005). *Epidemic Intelligence Service*. Atlanta: CDC. [2.4]

Centers for Disease Control and Prevention (2008). *Bioterrorism Agents/Diseases*. Atlanta: CDC. [5.6]

Centers for Disease Control and Prevention (2011a). 'Measles – United States, January–May 20, 2011.' *Morbidity and Mortality Weekly Report*, 60, 666–8. [4.5]

Centers for Disease Control and Prevention (2011b). 'Update on vaccine-derived polioviruses – worldwide, July 2009–March 2011.' *Morbidity and Mortality Weekly Report*, 60, 846–50. [5.3]

Centers for Disease Control and Prevention (2011c). 'State Electronic Disease Surveillance Systems – United States, 2007 and 2010.' *Morbidity and Mortality Weekly Report*, 60, 1421–23. [2.4]

Centers for Disease Control and Prevention (2011d). 'Progress toward poliomyelitis eradication – Afghanistan and Pakistan, January 2010–September 2011.' *Morbidity and Mortality Weekly Report*, 60, 1523–7. [5.3]

Centers for Disease Control and Prevention (2012a). *CDC Wonder*. Atlanta: CDC (available at http://wonder.cdc.gov; last viewed 27 February 2012). [2.4]

Centers for Disease Control and Prevention (2012b). *Epi-X: The Epidemic Information Exchange*. Atlanta: CDC (available at http://www.cdc.gov/epix; last viewed 27 February 2012). [2.4]

Centers for Disease Control and Prevention (2012c). *Epi Info*™. Atlanta: CDC (available at http://wwwn.cdc.gov/epiinfo; last viewed 27 February 2012). [2.4]

Centers for Disease Control and Prevention (2012d). *National Notifiable Diseases Surveillance System*. Atlanta: CDC (available at http://www.cdc.gov/osels/ph_surveillance/nndss/nndsshis.htm; last viewed 27 February 2012). [2.4]

Chapin, G., Wasserstrom, R. (1983). 'Pesticide use and malaria resurgence in Central America and India.' *Social Science and Medicine*, 17, 273–90. [5.4]

Choi, B.C.K., Pak, A.W.P. (2003). 'A simple approximate mathematical model to predict the number of severe acute respiratory syndrome cases and deaths.' *Journal of Epidemiology and Community Health*, 57, 831–35. [6.2]

Choi, B.C.K., Pak, A.W.P., Ottoson, J.M. (2002). 'Understanding the basic concepts of public health surveillance.' *Journal of Epidemiology and Community Health*, 56, 402–11. [2.9]

Chowell, G., Ammon, C.E., Hengartner, N.W., Hyman, J.M. (2006). 'Estimation of the reproductive number of the Spanish flu epidemic in Geneva, Switzerland.' *Vaccine*, 24, 6747–50. [6.2]

Chowell, G., Hengartner, N.W., Castillo-Chavez, C., Fenimore, P.W., Hyman, J.M. (2004). 'The basic reproductive ratio number of Ebola and the effects of public health measures: the cases of Congo and Uganda.' *Journal of Theoretical Biology*, 229, 119–26. [6.2]

Ciofi, M.B. (1984). 'La peste del 1630 a Firenze con particolare riferimento ai provvedimenti igienico-sanitari e sociali.' *Archivio Storico Italiano*, 142, 47–75. [1.2]

Cipolla, C.M. (1973). *Christofano and the Plague: A Study in the History of Public Health in the Age of Galileo*. London: Collins. [1.2, 1.3]

Cipolla, C.M. (1976). *Public Health and the Medical Profession in the Renaissance*. Cambridge: Cambridge University Press. [Preface]

Cipolla, C.M. (1978). 'The 'Bills of Mortality' of Florence.' *Population Studies*, 32, 543–8. [2.3]

Cipolla, C.M. (1981a). *Fighting the Plague in Seventeenth-Century Italy*. Madison: University of Wisconsin Press. [1.2]

Cipolla, C.M. (1981b). *Faith, Reason, and the Plague in Seventeenth-Century Tuscany*. New York: Norton. [1.2]

Clements, C.J., Baopong, Y., Crouch, A., Hipgrave, D., Mansoor, O., Nelson, C.B., Treleaven, S., van Konkolenberg, R., Wiersma, S. (2006). 'Progress in the control of hepatitis B infection in the Western Pacific Region.' *Vaccine*, 24, 1975–82. [4.4]

Cliff, A.D., Haggett, P. (1981). 'Methods for the measurement of epidemic velocity from time-series data.' *International Journal of Epidemiology*, 11, 82–9. [6.3]

Cliff, A.D., Haggett, P. (1985). *The Spread of Measles in Fiji and the Pacific: Spatial Components in the Transmission of Epidemic Waves through Island Communities*. Department of Human Geography publication number HG/18. Canberra: Research School of Pacific Studies, Australian National University. [3.2]

Cliff, A.D., Haggett, P. (1988). *Atlas of Disease Distributions: Analytic Approaches to Epidemiological Data*. Oxford: Blackwell Reference. [4.5]

Cliff, A.D., Haggett, P. (1989). 'Spatial aspects of epidemic control.' *Progress in Human Geography*, 13, 315–47. [4.3, 5.1]

Cliff, A.D., Haggett, P. (1990). 'Epidemic control and critical community size: spatial aspects of eliminating communicable diseases in human populations' In: R.W. Thomas (ed.), *Spatial Epidemiology*. London Papers in Regional Science 21. London: Pion, 93–110. [4.3]

Cliff, A.D., Haggett, P. (2004). 'Time, travel and infection.' *British Medical Bulletin*, 69, 87–99. [3.4]

Cliff, A.D., Haggett, P. (2006). 'A swash–backwash model of the single epidemic wave.' *Journal of Geographical Systems*, 8, 227–52. [6.3, Appendix 6.1]

Cliff, A.D., Haggett, P., Ord, J.K. (1986). *Spatial Aspects of Influenza Epidemics*. London: Pion. [4.3, 6.3]

Cliff, A.D., Haggett, P., Ord, J.K., Versey, G.R. (1981). *Spatial Diffusion: An Historical Geography of Epidemics in an Island Community*. Cambridge: Cambridge University Press. [6.4]

Cliff, A.D., Haggett, P., Smallman-Raynor, M. (1993). *Measles: An Historical Geography of a Major Human Viral Disease from Global Expansion to Local Retreat, 1840–1990*. Oxford: Blackwell. [1.4, 2.2, 4.5, 4.6, 5.2, 5.3, 6.4]

Cliff, A.D., Haggett, P., Smallman-Raynor, M. (1998). *Deciphering Global Epidemics: Analytical Approaches to the Disease Records of World Cities, 1888–1912*. Cambridge: Cambridge University Press. [2.2, 2.6, 3.2, 5.5]

Cliff, A.D., Haggett, P., Smallman-Raynor, M. (2000). *Island Epidemics*. Oxford: Oxford University Press. [3.2, 3.4, 4.3, 6.2, 6.4]

Cliff, A.D., Haggett, P., Smallman-Raynor, M. (2004). *World Atlas of Epidemic Diseases*. London: Arnold. [2.2, 3.3, 6.3]

Cliff, A.D., Ord, J.K. (1995). 'Estimating epidemic return times.' In: A.D. Cliff, P.R. Gould, A.G. Hoare & N.J. Thrift (eds.), *Diffusing Geography*. Institute of British Geographers Special Publications Series, 31. Oxford: Blackwell, 135–67. [6.4]

Cliff, A.D., Smallman-Raynor, M.R., Stevens, P.M. (2009). 'Controlling the geographical spread of infectious disease: plague in Italy, 1347–1851.' *Acta Medico-Historica Adriatica*, 7, 197–236. [1.2]

Cliff, A.D., Smallman-Raynor, M.R., Haggett, P., Stroup, D.F., Thacker, S.B. (2009). *Infectious Diseases. Emergence and Re-Emergence: A Geographical Analysis*. Oxford: Oxford University Press. [2.2, 2.3, 2.4, 2.7, 2.8, Appendix 2.1, 3.2, 3.4, 4.3, 5.4, 6.2, 6.3]

Clifford, J. (1995). *Eyam Plague 1665–1666*. Cromford, Derbyshire: Scarthin Books. [3.3]

Clifford, J.G., Clifford, F. (1993). *Eyam Parish Register, 1630–1700*. Chesterfield: Derbyshire Record Society. [3.3]

Coan, P.M. (1997). *Ellis Island Interviews: In Their Own Words*. New York: Facts on File, Inc. [3.2]

Cochi, S.L., Hull, H.F., Sutter, R.W., Wilfert, C.M., Katz, S.L. (1997). 'Commentary: the unfolding story of global poliomyelitis eradication.' *Journal of Infectious Diseases*, 175 (suppl. 1), S1–3. [2.7]

Commission Centrale Suisse pour la Lutte Antituberculeuse (Schweizerische Zentralkommission zur Bekämpfung der Tuberkulose) (1917). *Die Tuberkulose und ihre Bekämpfung in der Schweiz*. Bern: Francke. [3.3]

Communicable Disease Center (1964). *Poliomyelitis Surveillance: Report No. 283*. Atlanta: Communicable Disease Center. [4.5]

Cooper, B.S., Pitman, R.J., Edmunds, W.J., Gay, N.J. (2006). 'Delaying the international spread of pandemic influenza.' *PLoS Medicine*, 3(6): e212. doi:10.1371/journal.pmed.0030212. [3.4]

Corradi, A. (1865–94). *Annali delle Epidemie Occorse in Italia dalle Prime Memorie Fino al 1850*. Bologna: Gamberini e Parmeggiani. [1.2]

Creighton, C. (1891–94). *A History of Epidemics in Britain. From A.D. 664 to the Great Plague (Vol. I). From the Extinction of the Plague to the Present Time (Vol. II)*. Cambridge: Cambridge University Press. [2.3]

Cumpston, J.H.L. (1919). *Influenza and Maritime Quarantine in Australia*. Melbourne: Service Publication No. 18, Quarantine Service, Commonwealth of Australia. [6.2]

Cumpston, J.H.L., Lewis, M.J. (1989). *Health and Disease in Australia: A History*. Canberra: Australian Government Publishing Service. [6.2]

Cutts, F.T. (1990). *Measles Control in the 1990s: Principles for the Next Decade*. Geneva: WHO Expanded Programme on Immunization. [4.3]

Daley, D.J., Gani, J. (1999). *Epidemic Modelling*. Cambridge: Cambridge University Press. [6.1]

Davey, V.J., Glass, R.I. (2008). 'Rescinding community mitigation strategies in an influenza pandemic.' *Emerging Infectious Diseases*, 14, 365–72. [3.4]

Davies, R.E.G. (1964). *A History of the World's Airlines*. London: Oxford University Press. [3.4]

de Koeijer, A., Heesterbeek, H., Schreuder, B., Oberthür, R., Wilesmith, J., van Roermund, H., de Jong, M. (2004). 'Quantifying BSE control by calculating the basic reproduction ratio R_0 for the infection among cattle.' *Journal of Mathematical Biology*, 48, 1–22. [6.2]

Decio, C. (1900). *La Peste in Milano nell'Anno 1451 e il Primo Lazzaretto a Cusago: Appunti Storici e Note Inedite Tratte degli Archive Milanese*. Milan: Cogliati. [1.2]

Declich, S., Carter, A.O. (1994). 'Public health surveillance: historical origins, methods and evaluation.' *Bulletin of the World Health Organization*, 72, 285–304. [2.2, 2.3]

del Fiumi, A. (1981). 'Medici, medicine, e peste nel veneto durante il secolo XVI.' *Archivio Veneto*, ser. 5, 116. [1.2]

Department of Health (2003). *Guidelines for Smallpox Response and Management in the Post-Eradication Era [Version 2]*. London: Department of Health. [5.6]

Diekmann, O., Heesterbeek, J.A.P. (2000). *Mathematical Epidemiology of Infectious Diseases: Model Building, Analysis and Interpretation*. New York: Wiley. [6.1]

Dietz, K. (1975). 'Transmission and control of arbovirus diseases.' In: D. Ludwig & K.L. Cooke (eds.), *Epidemiology*. Philadelphia: Society for Industrial and Applied Mathematics, 104–21. [6.2]

Dietz, K. (1993). 'The estimation of the basic reproduction number for infectious diseases.' *Statistical Methods in Medical Research*, 2, 23–41. [6.2]

Dixon, C.W. (1962). *Smallpox*. London: Churchill Livingstone. [3.3]

Dowdle, W.R. (1998). 'The principles of disease elimination and eradication.' *Bulletin of the World Health Organization*, 76 (suppl. 2), 22–5. [5.1]

Dowdle, W.R. (1999). 'Influenza A virus recycling revisited.' *Bulletin of the World Health Organization*, 77, 820–8. [6.3]

Dowdle, W.R., Birmingham, M.E. (1997). 'The biologic principles of poliovirus eradication.' *Journal of Infectious Diseases*, 175 (suppl. 1), S286–92. [5.3]

Dublin, L.I., Lotka, A.J. (1925). 'On the true rate of natural increase of a population.' *Journal of the American Statistical Association*, 20, 305–39. [6.2]

Duintjer Tebbens, R.L., Pallansch, M.A., Cochi, S.L., Wassilak, S.G.F., Linkins, J., Sutter, R.W., Aylward, R.B., Thompson, K.M. (2011). 'Economic analysis of the global polio eradication initiative.' *Vaccine*, 29, 334–43. [5.3]

Dutt, A.K, Akhtar, R., McVeigh, M. (2006). 'Surat plague of 1994 re-examined.' *Southeast Asian Journal of Tropical Medicine and Public Health*, 37, 755–8. [3.4]

Eastern Bureau of the League of Nations Health Organisation (1926a). *Half-Yearly Bulletin of the Eastern Bureau, January–June 1926*. Singapore: League of Nations Health Organisation Eastern Bureau. [2.6]

Eastern Bureau of the League of Nations Health Organisation (1926b). *League of Nations, Health Organisation Eastern Bureau. Annual Report for 1925 and Minutes of the Advisory Council Meeting held in Singapore, January, 4th to 6th 1926*. Singapore: Eastern Bureau of the League of Nations Health Organisation. [2.6]

Eastern Bureau of the League of Nations Health Organisation (1927). *League of Nations, Health Organisation Eastern Bureau. Annual Report for 1926 and Minutes of the Advisory Council Meeting held in Singapore, January, 6th to 10th 1927*. Singapore: Eastern Bureau of the League of Nations Health Organisation. [2.6]

Eastern Bureau of the League of Nations Health Organisation (1928). *League of Nations, Health Organisation Eastern Bureau. Annual Report for 1927 and Minutes of the Third Session of the Advisory Council held in New Delhi, December, 26th to 29th 1927*. Singapore: Eastern Bureau of the League of Nations Health Organisation. [2.6]

Eastern Bureau of the League of Nations Health Organisation (1939). *Annual Report for 1939*. Singapore: Eastern Bureau of the League of Nations Health Organisation. [2.6]

Eichner, M., Hadeler, K., Dietz, K. (1994). 'Stochastic models for the eradication of poliomyelitis: minimum population size for polio virus persistence.' In: V. Isham & G. Medley (eds.), *Models for Infectious Human Diseases: Their Structure and Relation to Data*. Cambridge: Cambridge University Press, 315–27. [4.5]

Ell, S.R. (1989). 'Three days in October of 1630: detailed examination of mortality during an early modern plague epidemic in Venice.' *Reviews of Infectious Diseases*, 11, 128–41. [1.2]

Ellis, A.E. (1958). *The Rack*. London: Heinemann. [3.3]

Epstein, J.M., Goedecke, D.M., Yu, F., Morris, R.J., Wagener, D.K., Bobashev, G.V. (2007). 'Controlling pandemic flu: the value of international travel restrictions.' *PloS ONE*, 2(5): e401. doi:10.1371/journal.pone.0000401. [3.4]

Etheridge, E.W. (1992). *Sentinel for Health: A History of the Centers for Disease Control*. Berkeley: University of California Press. [2.4]

European Centre for Disease Prevention and Control (2010). *Annual Threat Report 2009*. Stockholm: ECDC. [2.8]

Eurostat Statistical Books (2009). *Health Statistics – Atlas on Mortality in the European Union*. Luxembourg: Office for Official Publications of the European Communities. [6.5]

Ewert, D.P., Thomas, J.C., Chun, L.Y., Enguidanos, R.C., Waterman, S.H. (1991). 'Measles vaccination coverage among Latino children aged 12 to 59 months in Los Angeles County: a household survey.' *American Journal of Public Health*, 81, 1057–9. [4.6]

Fee, E., Cueto, M., Brown, T.M. (2008). 'WHO at 60: snapshots from its first six decades.' *American Journal of Public Health*, 98, 630–3. [2]

Fenner, F. (1986). 'The eradication of infectious diseases.' *South African Medical Journal*, 66 (suppl.), 35–9. [5.1, 5.2, 5.3]

Fenner, F., Henderson, D.A., Arita, I., Jesek, Z., Ladnyi, I.D. (1988). *Smallpox and its Eradication*. Geneva: World Health Organization. [2.7, 3.3, 4.2, 5.2]

Ferguson, N.M., Donnelly, C.A., Anderson, R.M. (2001). 'The foot-and-mouth epidemic in Great Britain: pattern of spread and impact of interventions.' *Science*, 292, 1155–60. [6.2]

Ferguson, N.M., Donnelly, C.A., Woolhouse, M.E.J., Anderson, R.M. (1999). 'Estimation of the basic reproduction number of BSE: the intensity of transmission in British cattle.' *Proceedings of the Royal Society B*, 266, 23–32. [6.2]

Fiji Legislative Council (1903). *Annual Report on Indian Immigration, etc., 1902*. Levuka, Fiji: Legislative Council Paper No. 20, 1903. [3.2]

Fine, P.E.M. (1993). 'Herd immunity: history, theory, practice.' *Epidemiologic Reviews*, 15, 265–302. [6.2]

Fine, P.E.M. (2003). 'The interval between successive cases of an infectious disease.' *American Journal of Epidemiology*, 158, 1039–47. [6.4]

Finlay, R. (1981). *Population and Metropolis: The Demography of London 1580-1650*. Cambridge: Cambridge University Press. [2.3]

Fracastoro, G. (1546). *De Contagione et Contagiosis Morbis et Eorum Curatione (On Contagion, Contagious Diseases and Their Cure)*. Venice: Junta, 1546. English translation by Wilmer Cave Wright (New York/London: G. P. Putnam, 1930). [3.3]

Fraser, C., Donnelly, C.A., Cauchemez, S., Hanage, W.P., van Kerkhove, M.D., Hollingsworth, T.D., Griffin, J., Baggaley, R.F., Jenkins, H.E., Lyons, E.J., Jombart, T., Hinsley, W.R., Grassly, N.C., Balloux, F., Ghani, A.C., Ferguson, N.M., Rambaut, A., Pybus, O.G., Lopez-Gatell, H., Alpuche-Aranda, C.M., Chapela, I.B., Zavala, E.P., Guevara, D.M.E., Checchi, F., Garcia, E., Hugonnet, S., Roth, C. (2009). 'Pandemic potential of a strain of influenza A (H1N1): early findings.' *Science*, 324, 1557–61. [6.2]

Fraser, S.M.F. (1980). 'Leicester and smallpox: the Leicester Method.' *Medical History*, 24, 315–32. [3.3]

Frati, P. (2000). 'Quarantine, trade and health policies in Ragusa-Dubrovnik until the age of George Armmenius-Baglivi.' *Medicina nei Secoli*, 12, 103–27. [1.2]

Freifeld, C.C., Mandl, K.D., Reis, B.Y., Brownstein, J.S. (2008). 'HealthMap: global infectious disease monitoring through automated classification and visualization of Internet media reports.' *Journal of the American Medical Association*, 15, 150–7. [2.8]

Fritz, C.L., Dennis, D.T., Tipple, M.A., Campbell, G.L., McCance, C.R., Gubler, D.J. (1996). 'Surveillance for pneumonic plague in the United States during an international emergency: a model for control of imported emerging diseases.' *Emerging Infectious Diseases*, 2, 30–6. [3.4]

Furesz, J. (1979). 'Poliomyelitis outbreaks in the Netherlands and Canada.' *Canadian Medical Association Journal*, 120, 905–6. [4.5]

Furman, B. (1973). *A Profile of the United States Public Health Service, 1798-1948*. Washington, D.C.: US Government Printing Office. [3.2]

Gale, A.H. (1948). 'Poliomyelitis in England and Wales in 1947.' *Monthly Bulletin of the Ministry of Health and the Public Health Laboratory Service*, 7, 127–32. [6.3]

Gale, A.H. (1959). *Epidemic Diseases*. Harmondsworth: Pelican Books. [2.3]

Gay, N.J. (2004). 'The theory of measles elimination: implications for the design of elimination strategies.' *Journal of Infectious Diseases*, 189 (suppl. 1), S27–35. [4.3]

Gensini, G.F., Yacoub, M.H., Conti, A.A. (2004). 'The concept of quarantine in history: from plague to SARS.' *Journal of Infection*, 49, 257–61. [1.2, 3.4]

Gillion, K.L. (1962). *Fiji's Indian Migrants: A History to the End of Indenture in 1920*. Melbourne: Oxford University Press. [3.2]

Global Polio Eradication Initiative (2010). *Global Polio Eradication Initiative Strategic Plan 2010-2012*. Geneva: World Health Organization. [5.3]

Goodman, N.M. (1952). *International Health Organizations and Their Work*. London: J. & A. Churchill, Ltd. [2.5, 2.6, 2.7]

Goodman, R.A., Bauman, C.F., Gregg, M.B., Videtto, J.F., Stroup, D.F., Chalmers, N.P. (1990). 'Epidemiologic field investigations by the Centers for Disease Control and Epidemic Intelligence Service, 1946–87.' *Public Health Reports*, 105, 604–10. [2.4]

Gould, P.R. (1970). 'Is *Statistix Inferens* the geographical name for a wild goose?' *Economic Geography*, 46 (supplement), 439–48. [6.3]

Grassly, N.C., Fraser, C. (2008). 'Mathematical models of infectious disease transmission.' *Nature Reviews Microbiology*, 6, 477–87. [6.1]

Graunt, J. (1662). *Natural and Political Observations Mentioned in a Following Index, and Made Upon the Bills of Mortality*. London: Printed by Tho. Roycroft for John Martin, James Allestry, and Tho. Dicas. [2.3]

Gravenor, M.B., Papasozomenos, P., McLean, A.R., Neophytou, G. (2004). 'A scrapie epidemic in Cyprus.' *Epidemiology and Infection*, 132, 751–60. [6.2]

Greene, J.C. (1977). 'The United States Public Health Service: A bicentennial report.' *Military Medicine*, 142, 511–13. [3.2]

Greenhalgh, D. (1986). 'Optimal control of an epidemic by ring vaccination.' *Stochastic Models*, 2, 339–63. [4.3]

Greenwood, B., Salisbury, D., Hill, A.V.S. (2011). 'Vaccines and global health.' *Philosophical Transactions of the Royal Society B*, 366, 2733–42. [4.7]

Griffiths, D.A. (1973). 'The effect of measles vaccination on the incidence of measles in the community.' *Journal of the Royal Statistical Society A*, 136, 441–9. [4.3, 4.5]

Haber, M.J., Shay, D.K., Davis, X.M., Patel, R., Jin, X., Weintraub, E., Orenstein, E., Thompson, W.W. (2007). 'Effectiveness of interventions to reduce contact rates during a simulated influenza pandemic.' *Emerging Infectious Diseases*, 13, 581–9. [3.4]

Haggett, P. (2000). *The Geographical Structure of Epidemics*. Oxford: Oxford University Press. [4.3]

Hagmann, R., Charlwood, J.D., Gil, V., Ferreira, C., do Rosário, V., Smith, T.A. (2003). 'Malaria and its possible control on the island of Principe.' *Malaria Journal*, 2, 15. [6.2]

Hall, C.E., Cooney, M.K., Fox, J.P. (1970). 'The Seattle virus watch program. I. Infection and illness experience of virus watch families during a community wide epidemic of echovirus type 30 aseptic meningitis.' *American Journal of Public Health and the Nation's Health*, 60, 1456–65. [2.8]

Halley, E. (1693). 'An estimate of the degrees of mortality of mankind, drawn from curious tables of the births and funerals at the City of Breslaw; with an attempt to ascertain the price of annuities upon lives.' *Philosophical Transactions*, 17, 596–610. [2.3]

Hardy, A. (1983). 'Smallpox in London: factors in the decline of the disease in the nineteenth century.' *Medical History*, 27, 111–38. [2.3]

Health Protection Agency (2006). *Communicable Disease in London 2002–05. A Review by the Health Protection Agency in London*. London: HPA. [4.6]

Health Protection Agency (2008). 'Confirmed measles cases in England and Wales: an update to end-May 2008.' *Health Protection Report*, 2:25 (available at: http://www.hpa.org.uk/hpr/archives/back_issues.htm; last viewed 27 February 2012). [4.6]

Heesterbeek, J.A.P. (2002). 'A brief history of R_0 and a recipe for its calculation.' *Acta Biotheoretica*, 50, 189–204. [6.2]

Heesterbeek, J.A.P., Dietz, K. (1996). 'The concept of R_0 in epidemic theory.' *Statistica Neerlandica*, 50, 89–110. [6.2]

Heffernan, J.M., Smith, R.J., Wahl, L.M. (2005). 'Perspectives on the basic reproductive ratio.' *Journal of the Royal Society. Interface*, 2, 281–93. [6.2]

Henderson, J. (1994). *Piety and Charity in Late Medieval Florence*. Oxford: The Clarendon Press. [3.3]

Hethcote, H.W. (1975). 'Mathematical models for the spread of infectious diseases.' In: D. Ludwig & K.L. Cooke (eds.), *Epidemiology*. Philadelphia: Society for Industrial and Applied Mathematics, 122–31. [6.2]

Hethcote, H., Zhien, M., Shengbing, L. (2002). 'Effects of quarantine in six endemic models for infectious diseases.' *Mathematical Biosciences*, 180, 141–60. [3.4]

Heymann, D.L., Rodier, G.R., and the WHO Operational Support Team of the Global Outbreak Alert and Response Network (2001). 'Hot spots in a wired world: WHO surveillance of emerging and re-emerging infectious diseases.' *Lancet Infectious Diseases*, 1, 345–53. [2.7]

Hilleman, M.R. (1992). 'Past, present, and future of measles, mumps, and rubella virus vaccines.' *Pediatrics*, 90, 149–53. [Appendix 4.1]

Hinman, A.R., Orenstein, W.A., Papania, M.J. (2004). 'Evolution of measles elimination strategies in the United States.' *Journal of Infectious Diseases*, 189 (suppl. 1), S17–22. [4.5]

Hirsch, A. (1883). *Handbook of Geographical and Historical Pathology. Vol. I. – Acute Infective Diseases*. Translated from the second German edition by C. Creighton. London: The New Sydenham Society. [1.2]

Hirst, L.B. (1953). *The Conquest of Plague: A Study of the Evolution of Epidemiology*. Oxford: Clarendon Press. [1.2]

Hong Choi, Y., Gay, N., Fraser, G., Ramsay, M. (2008). 'The potential for measles transmission in England.' *BMC Public Health*, 8:338 (available at: http://www.biomedcentral.com/1471-2458/8/338; last viewed 27 February 2012). [4.6]

Hopkins, D.R., Ruiz-Tiben, E. (1991). 'Strategies for dracunculiasis eradication.' *Bulletin of the World Health Organization*, 69, 533–40. [5.4]

Hopkins, D.R., Ruiz-Tiben, E., Eberhard, M.L., Roy, S.L. (2011). 'Progress toward global eradication of dracunculiasis, January 2010–June 2011.' *Morbidity and Mortality Weekly Report*, 60, 1450–3. [5.4]

Howard, J. (1791). *An Account of the Principal Lazarettos in Europe; with Various Papers Relative to the Plague: Together with Further Observations on some Foreign Prisons and Hospitals; and Additional Remarks on the Present State of Those in Great Britain and Ireland*. London: J. Johnson. [1.2, 3.3]

Howard-Jones, N. (1981). *The Pan American Health Organization: Origins and Evolution*. History of International Public Health, No. 5. Geneva: World Health Organization. [2.5]

Huber, V. (2006). 'The unification of the globe by disease? The International Sanitary Conferences on Cholera, 1851–94.' *The Historical Journal*, 49, 453–76. [1.2]

Hull, H.F., Birmingham, M.E., Melgaard, B., Lee, J.W. (1997). 'Progress toward global polio eradication.' *Journal of Infectious Diseases*, 175 (suppl. 1), S4–9. [2.7, 5.3]

Jarcho, S. (1983). 'Some early Italian epidemiological maps.' *Imago Mundi*, 35, 9–19. [1.2]

John, T.J., Plotkin, S.A., Orenstein, W.A. (2011). 'Building on the success of the Expanded Programme on Immunization: enhancing the focus on disease prevention and control.' *Vaccine*, 29, 8835–7. [4.4]

Johnston, W.D. (1993). 'Tuberculosis.' In: K.F. Kiple (ed.), *The Cambridge World History of Human Disease*. Cambridge: Cambridge University Press, 1059–68. [3.3]

Johnstone, R.W. (1910). 'Report to the Local Government Board on occurrences of enteric fever in the Folkestone Urban District.' *Reports to the Local Government Board on Public Health and Medical Subjects, New Series*, No. 41. London: HMSO, 1–14. [3.3]

Kaplan, E.H., Craft, D.L., Wein, L.M. (2002). 'Emergency response to a smallpox attack: the case for mass vaccination.' *Proceedings of the National Academy of Sciences, USA*, 99, 10935–40. [6.2]

Katz, S.L., Hinman, A.R. (2004). 'Summary and conclusions: measles elimination meeting, 16–17 March 2000.' *Journal of Infectious Diseases*, 189 (suppl. 1), S43–7. [4.5]

Keegan, R., Dabbagh, A., Strebel, P.M., Cochi, S.L. (2011). 'Comparing measles with previous eradication programs: enabling and constraining factors.' *Journal of Infectious Diseases*, 204 (suppl. 1), S54–61. [5.5]

Keeling, M.J., Grenfell, B.T. (1997). 'Disease extinction and community size: modeling the persistence of measles.' *Science*, 275, 65–7. [1.4]

Keja, J., Henderson, R. (1984). 'The Expanded Programme on Immunization: global overview.' *World Health Organization Second Conference on Immunization Policies*, Karlovy Vary, 10–12 December. [4.4]

Kermack, W.O., McKendrick, A.G. (1927). 'A contribution to the mathematical theory of epidemics.' *Proceedings of the Royal Society*, 115, 700–21. [6.2]

Kew, O.M., Wright, P.F., Agol, V.I., Delpeyroux, F., Shimizu, H., Nathanson, N., Pallansch, M.A. (2004). 'Circulating vaccine-derived polioviruses: current state of knowledge.' *Bulletin of the World Health Organization*, 82, 16–21. [5.3]

Khan, M.M., Ehreth, J. (2003). 'Costs and benefits of polio eradication: a long-run perspective.' *Vaccine*, 21, 702–5. [5.3]

Kilwein, J.H. (1995a). 'Some historical comments on quarantine: Part one.' *Journal of Clinical Pharmacy and Therapeutics*, 20, 185–7. [3.4]

Kilwein, J.H. (1995b). 'Some historical comments on quarantine: Part two.' *Journal of Clinical Pharmacy and Therapeutics*, 20, 249–52. [3.4]

Kiple, K.F. (ed.) (1993). *The Cambridge World History of Human Disease*. Cambridge: Cambridge University Press. [1.2, 4.2]

Konstantinidou, K., Mantadakis, E., Falagas, M.E., Sardi, T., Samonis, G. (2009). 'Venetian rule and control of plague epidemics on the Ionian Islands during 17th and 18th centuries.' *Emerging Infectious Diseases*, 15, 39–43. [1.2]

Koplan, J.P., Thacker, S.B. (2001). 'Fifty years of epidemiology at the Centers for Disease Control and Prevention: significant and consequential.' *American Journal of Epidemiology*, 154, 982–4. [2.4]

Kretzschmar, M., van den Hof, S., Wallinga, J., van Wijngaarden, J. (2004). 'Ring vaccination and smallpox control.' *Emerging Infectious Diseases*, 10, 832–41. [4.3]

Kuczynski, R.R. (1928). *The Balance of Births and Deaths*, vol. 1. New York: Macmillan. [6.2]

Lancaster, H.O. (1990). *Expectations of Life: A Study in the Demography, Statistics and History of World Mortality*. Berlin: Springer-Verlag. [4.2]

Landers, J. (1993). *Death and the Metropolis: Studies in the Demographic History of London 1670–1830*. Cambridge: Cambridge University Press. [2.3]

Lane, J.M., Poland, G.A. (2011). 'Why not destroy the remaining smallpox virus stocks?' *Vaccine*, 29, 2823–4. [5.7]

Langmuir, A.D. (1963). 'The surveillance of communicable diseases of national importance.' *New England Journal of Medicine*, 268, 183–92. [2.1, 2.9]

Langmuir, A.D. (1976). 'William Farr: founder of modern concepts of surveillance.' *International Journal of Epidemiology*, 5, 13–18. [2.1]

Langmuir, A.D. (1980). 'The Epidemic Intelligence Service of the Centers for Disease Control.' *Public Health Reports*, 95, 470–7. [2.4]

Langmuir, A.D., Nathanson, N., Hall, W.J. (1956). 'Surveillance of poliomyelitis in the United States in 1955.' *American Journal of Public Health*, 46, 75–88. [4.6]

Lau, C.Y., Wahl, B., Foo, W.K. (2005). 'Ring vaccination versus mass vaccination in event of a smallpox attack.' *Hawaii Medical Journal*, 64, 34–6, 53. [4.3]

League of Nations Health Organisation (1931). *Health*. Geneva: Information Section, League of Nations. [2.6]

League of Nations Health Organisation (1932). 'Notifiable diseases in various countries in 1930.' *Statistics of Notifiable Diseases for the Year 1930*, E.I.15, 54–64. [2.7]

League of Nations Health Section (1922a). *Rapport Épidémiologique*, 19, 7 July 1922. [3.4]

League of Nations Health Section (1922b). *Rapport Épidémiologique*, 21, 17 July 1922. [3.4]

League of Nations Health Section (1922c). *Epidemiological Intelligence*, 4, September 1922. [3.4]

League of Nations Health Section (1922d). 'Introductory note.' *Epidemiological Intelligence: Eastern Europe in 1921*, E.I.1, 3. [2.6]

League of Nations Health Section (1938). 'Eastern Bureau Health Organisation at Singapore.' *Weekly Epidemiological Record*, 13, 583. [2.6]

Learmonth, A. (1988). *Disease Ecology: An Introduction*. Oxford: Basil Blackwell. [5.4]

Leavitt, J.W. (1996). *Typhoid Mary: Captive to the Public's Health*. Boston: Beacon Press. [3.3]

Lemon, S.M., Hamburg, M.A., Sparling, P.F., Choffnes, E.R., Mack, A. (2007). *Global Infectious Disease Surveillance and Detection: Assessing the Challenges – Finding Solutions, Workshop Summary*. Washington, D.C.: The National Academies Press. [2.7]

Lipsitch, M., Cohen, T., Cooper, B., Robins, J.M., Ma, S., James, L., Gopalakrishna, G., Chew, S.K., Tan, C.C., Samore, M.H., Fisman, D.,

Murray, M. (2003). 'Transmission dynamics and control of severe acute respiratory syndrome.' *Science*, 300, 1966–70. [6.2]

Lloyd-Smith, J.O., Galvani, A.P., Getz, W.M. (2003). 'Curtailing transmission of severe acute respiratory syndrome within a community and its hospital.' *Proceedings of the Royal Society B*, 270, 1979–89. [6.2]

Local Government Board (1882). *Tenth Annual Report of the Local Government Board, 1880–81. Supplement in Continuation of the Report of the Medical Officer of the Board for 1880–81, Containing a Report on the Use and Influence of Hospitals for Infectious Diseases by Sir Richard Thorne, F.R.S., with an Introduction by the Medical Officer of the Board*. London: His Majesty's Stationery Office, C. 3290. [3.3]

Local Government Board (1912). *Fortieth Annual Report of the Local Government Board, 1910–11. Supplement in Continuation of the Report of the Medical Officer of the Board for 1910–11, Containing a Report on Isolation Hospitals by H. Franklin Parsons, M.D., with an Introduction by the Medical Officer of the Board*. London: His Majesty's Stationery Office, Cd. 6342. [3.3]

Longini, I.M., Jr, Halloran, M.E., Nizam, A., Yang, Y. (2004). 'Containing pandemic influenza with antiviral agents.' *American Journal of Epidemiology*, 159, 623–33. [6.2]

Longmore, C. (1929). *The Old Sixteenth: Being a Record of the 16th Battalion, AIF [Australian Imperial Force], during the Great War 1914–1918*. Perth: History Committee of the 16th Battalion Association. [6.2]

Lothian, N.V. (1924). 'The Service of Epidemiological Intelligence and Public Health Statistics.' *American Journal of Public Health*, 14, 287–90. [2.6]

Lucas, A.O. (1968). 'The surveillance of communicable diseases.' *WHO Chronicle*, 22, 439–44. [2.1]

Luz, P.M., Codeco, C.T., Massad, E., Struchiner, C.J. (2003). 'Uncertainties regarding dengue modeling in Rio de Janeiro, Brazil.' *Memórias do Instituto Oswaldo Cruz*, 98, 871–78. [6.2]

MacDonald, G. (1952). 'The analysis of equilibrium in malaria.' *Tropical Diseases Bulletin*, 49, 813–29. [6.2]

Madan, T.N. (1995). 'The plague in India, 1994.' *Social Science and Medicine*, 40, 1167–8. [3.4]

Mafart, B., Perret, J.-L. (1998). 'Histoire du concept de quarantaine.' *Médecine Tropicale*, 58, 14S–20S. [3.4]

Magistrato della Sanità, Venice (1752). *An Authentick Account of the Measures and Precautions used at Venice by the Magistrate of the Office of Health for the Preservation of the Publick Health*. London: Edward Owen. [1.2]

Malthus, T.R. (1798). *An Essay on the Principle of Population, as it Affects the Future Improvement of Society*. London: J. Johnson. [3.3]

Manderson, L. (1995). 'Wireless wars in the Eastern Arena: epidemiological surveillance, disease prevention and the work of the Eastern Bureau of the League of Nations Health Organisation, 1925–1942.' In: P. Weindling (ed.), *International Health Organisations and Movements, 1918–1939*. Cambridge: Cambridge University Press. [2.6]

Mann, T. (1932). *The Magic Mountain*. New York: The Modern Library. [3.3]

Markel, H., Lipman, H.B., Navarro, J.A., Sloan, A., Michalsen, J.R., Stern, A., Cetron, M.S. (2007). 'Nonpharmaceutical interventions implemented by US cities during the 1918–1919 influenza pandemic.' *Journal of the American Medical Association*, 298, 644–54. [3.4]

Marshall, J. (1832). *Mortality of the Metropolis: A Statistical View of the Number of Persons Reported to have Died of Each of More than 100 Kinds of Disease, and Casualties within the Bills of Mortality in Each of the Two Hundred and Four Years, 1629–1831*. London: Treuttel, Würtz and Richter. [2.3]

Massad, E., Coutino, F.B.B., Burattini, M.N., Lopez, L.F. (2004). 'The Eyam plague revisited: did the village isolation change transmission from fleas to pulmonary?' *Medical Hypotheses*, 63, 911–15. [3.3]

Massey, A. (1933). *Epidemiology in Relation to Air Travel*. London: H.K. Lewis and Co. Ltd. [3.4]

Matossian, M.K. (1985). 'Death in London, 1750–1909.' *Journal of Interdisciplinary History*, 16, 183–97. [2.3]

Matthews, L., Haydon, D.T., Shaw, D.J., Chase-Topping, M.E., Keeling, M.J., Woolhouse, M.E.J. (2003). 'Neighbourhood control policies and the spread of infectious diseases.' *Proceedings of the Royal Society B*, 270, 1659–66. [6.2]

Mattox, H.E. (1989). *The Twilight of Amateur Diplomacy: The American Foreign Service and its Senior Officers in the 1890s*. Kent, Ohio: The Kent State University Press. [3.2]

McArthur, N. (1967). *Island Populations of the Pacific*. Canberra: Australian National University. [3.2]

McKhann, C.F., Chu, F.T. (1933). 'Use of placental extract in prevention and modification of measles.' *American Journal of Diseases of Children*, 45, 475–9. [Appendix 4.1]

McKinley, R.A. (ed.) (1958). *Victoria County History. A History of the County of Leicester, Volume 4: The City of Leicester*. London: Institute of Historical Research/Oxford University Press. [3.3]

McNabb, S.J.N., Chungong, S., Ryan, M., Wuhib, T., Nsubuga, P., Alemu, W., Carande-Kulis, V., Rodier, G. (2002). 'Conceptual framework of public health surveillance and action and its application in health sector reform.' *BMC Public Health*, 2:2. doi:10.1186/1471-2458-2-2. [2.9]

McQueen, H. (1975). '"Spanish flu" 1919: political, medical and social aspects.' *Medical Journal of Australia*, 1, 565–70. [6.2]

Melnick, J.L. (1978). 'Advantages and disadvantages of killed and live polio-myelitis vaccines.' *Bulletin of the World Health Organization*, 46, 21–38. [Appendix 4.1]

Melnick, J.L. (1997). 'Poliovirus and other enteroviruses.' In: A.S. Evans & R.A. Kaslow (eds.), *Viral Infections of Humans: Epidemiology and Control* (fourth edition). London: Plenum Medical Book Company, 583–663. [Appendix 4.1]

Meltzer, M.I. (2008). 'Pandemic influenza, reopening schools, and returning to work.' *Emerging Infectious Diseases*, 14, 507–8. [3.4]

Millard, C.K. (1914). *The Vaccination Question in the Light of Modern Experience*. London: Lewis. [3.3]

Miller, M., Roche, P., Spencer, J., Deeble, M. (2004). 'Evaluation of Australia's National Notifiable Disease Surveillance System.' *Communicable Diseases Intelligence*, 28, 311–23. [2.9]

Miller, M.A., Hinman, A.R. (2008). 'Economic analyses of vaccine policies.' In: S.A. Plotkin, W.A. Orenstein & P.A. Offit (eds.), *Vaccines* (fifth edition). Philadelphia: Saunders Elsevier, 1593–1609. [4.5]

Mills, C.E., Robins, J.M., Lipsitch, M. (2004). 'Transmissibility of 1918 pandemic influenza.' *Nature*, 432, 904–6. [6.2]

Mollison, D. (1977). 'Spatial contact models for ecological and epidemic spread.' *Journal of the Royal Statistical Society B*, 39, 283–326. [6.4]

Mollison, D. (1991). 'Dependence of epidemic and population velocities on basic parameters.' *Mathematical Biosciences*, 107, 255–87. [6.4]

Montague, A. (1922). *Annual Medical Report, 1921*. Levuka, Fiji: Legislative Council Paper No. 51. [3.2]

Morens, D.M., Folkers, G.K., Fauci, A.S. (2004). 'The challenge of emerging and re-emerging infectious diseases.' *Nature*, 430, 242–9. [5.6]

Morrison, A.S., Kirshner, J., Molho, A. (1985). 'Epidemics in Renaissance Florence.' *American Journal of Public Health*, 75, 528–35. [1.2]

Moss, W.J., Strebel, P. (2011). 'Biological feasibility of measles eradication.' *Journal of Infectious Diseases*, 204 (suppl. 1), S47–53. [5.5]

Murray, C.J.L., Salomon, J.A., Mathers, C.D., Lopez, A.D. (2002). *Summary Measures of Population Health: Concepts, Ethics, Measurement and Applications*. Geneva: World Health Organization. [6.5]

Mykhalovskiy, E., Weir, L. (2006). 'The Global Public Health Intelligence Network and early warning outbreak detection: a Canadian contribution to global public health.' *Canadian Journal of Public Health*, 97, 42–4. [2.8]

Nathanson, N., Langmuir, A.D. (1963a). 'The Cutter incident: poliomyelitis following formaldehyde-inactivated poliovirus vaccination in the United States during the spring of 1955. I. Background.' *American Journal of Hygiene*, 78, 16–28. [4.6]

Nathanson, N., Langmuir, A.D. (1963b). 'The Cutter incident: poliomyelitis following formaldehyde-inactivated poliovirus vaccination in the United States during the spring of 1955. II. Relationship of poliomyelitis to Cutter vaccine.' *American Journal of Hygiene*, 78, 29–60. [4.6]

Nettleton, C. (2002). *From Emergence to Extinction. The Geography of Poliomyelitis, 1850–2000*. Unpublished PhD Dissertation. Department of Geography, University of Cambridge. [4.5]

Office International d'Hygiène Publique (1909). 'Choléra en Russie en 1907 et 1908.' *Bulletin de l'Office International d'Hygiène Publique*, 1, 274–5. [3.4]

Offit, P.A., Davis, R.L., Gust, D. (2008). 'Vaccine safety.' In: S.A. Plotkin, W.A. Orenstein & P.A. Offit (eds.), *Vaccines* (fifth edition). Philadelphia: Saunders Elsevier, 1629–50. [4.6]

Olsen, S.J., Chang, H.L., Cheung, T.Y., Tang, A.F., Fisk, T.L., Ooi, S.P., Kuo, H.W., Jiang, D.D., Chen, K.T., Lando, J., Hsu, K.H., Chen, T.J., Dowell, S.F. (2003). 'Transmission of the severe acute respiratory syndrome on aircraft.' *New England Journal of Medicine*, 349, 2416–22. [3.4]

Omran, A.R. (1971). 'The epidemiologic transition: a theory of the epide-miology of population change.' *Milbank Memorial Fund Quarterly*, 49, 509–38. [2.3]

Orenstein, W.A., Papania, M.J., Wharton, M.E. (2004). 'Measles elimination in the United States.' *Journal of Infectious Diseases*, 189 (suppl. 1), S1–3. [4.5, 4.7]

Orenstein, W.A., Rodewald, L.E., Hinman, A.R., Schuchat, A. (2008). 'Immunization in the United States.' In: S.A. Plotkin, W.A. Orenstein & P.A. Offit (eds.), *Vaccines* (fifth edition). Philadelphia: Saunders Elsevier, 1479–510. [4.5]

Palmer, R.J. (1978). *The Control of Plague in Venice and Northern Italy, 1348–1600*. Doctoral dissertation, University of Kent at Canterbury, UK. [1.2]

Parish, H.J. (1965). *A History of Immunization*. Edinburgh and London: E. & S. Livingstone. [4.2]

Parish, H.J. (1968). *Victory with Vaccines: The Story of Immunization*. Edinburgh and London: E. &. S. Livingstone. [4.1, 4.2, Appendix 4.1]

Patterson, K.D., Pyle, G.F. (1991). 'The geography and mortality of the 1918 influenza pandemic.' *Bulletin of the History of Medicine*, 65, 4–21. [6.2, 6.3]

Paul, J.R. (1971). *The History of Poliomyelitis*. New Haven: Yale University Press. [4.6, Appendix 4.1]

Perkins, N.R., Webster, W.R., Wright, T., Denney, I., Links, I. (2011). 'Vaccination program in response to the 2007 equine influenza out-break in Australia.' *Australian Veterinary Journal*, 89 (suppl. 1), 126–34. [4.3]

Petitti, P. (1852). *Repertorio Administrativo ossia collezione di leggi, decreti, reali rescritti, ministeriali di massima regolamenti, ed istruzioni sull'amministrazione civile de Regno delle Due Sicilie*. Volume 3 (fifth edition). Naples: Tipografia di Gaetano Sautto. [1.4]

Plotkin, S.A., Orenstein, W.A., Offit, P.A. (eds.) (2008). *Vaccines* (fifth edition). Philadelphia: Saunders Elsevier. [4.4, Appendix 4.1]

Plotkin, S.L., Plotkin, S.A. (2008). 'A short history of vaccination.' In: S.A. Plotkin, W.A. Orenstein & P.A. Offit (eds.), *Vaccines* (fifth edition). Philadelphia: Saunders Elsevier, 1–16. [4.1, 4.2]

Pollitzer, R. (1954). *Plague*. Geneva: World Health Organization. [1.2]

Preto, P. (1978). *Peste e Società a Venezia nel 1576*. Venice: Neri Pozza. [1.2]

Pridie, E.D. (1936). 'Faits récents concernant la fièvre jaune dans le Soudan Anglo-Égyptien, en particulier la lutte contre les moustiques.' *Bulletin de l'Office International d'Hygiène Publique*, 28, 1292–1308. [3.4]

Prinzing, F. (1916). *Epidemics Resulting from Wars*. Oxford: Clarendon Press. [3.3]

Race, P. (1995). 'Some further consideration of the plague in Eyam, 1665–6.' *Local Population Studies*, 54, 56–65. [3.3]

Raggett, G.F. (1982a). 'A stochastic model of the Eyam plague.' *Journal of Applied Statistics*, 9, 212–25. [3.3]

Raggett, G.F. (1982b). 'Modeling the Eyam plague.' *IMA Journal*, 18, 221–6. [3.3]

Ramsay, A.M., Emond, R.T.D. (1978). *Infectious Diseases*. London: William Heineman. [4.3]

Ramsay, M.E., Jin, L., White, J., Litton, P., Cohen, B., Brown, D. (2003). 'The elimination of indigenous measles transmission in England and Wales.' *Journal of Infectious Diseases*, 187 (suppl. 1), S198–207. [4.6]

Regidor, E., de la Fuente, L., Gutiérrez-Fisac, J.L., de Mateo, S., Pascual, C., Sánchez-Payá, J., Ronda, E. (2007). 'The role of the public health official in communicating public health information.' *American Journal of Public Health*, 97, S93–7. [2.9]

Registry Department, Boston (1893). *Bills of Mortality, 1810–1849, City of Boston: With an Essay on the Vital Statistics of Boston, from 1810–1841*. Boston: Registry Department. [2.3]

Riley, S., Ferguson, N.M. (2006). 'Smallpox transmission and control: spatial dynamics in England and Wales.' *Proceedings of the National Academy of Sciences, USA*, 103, 12637–42. [5.6]

Riley, S., Fraser, C., Donnelly, C.A., Ghani, A.C., Abu-Raddad, L.J., Hedley, A.J., Leung, G.M., Ho, L.-M., Lam, T.-H., Thach, T.Q., Chau, P., Chan, K.-P., Lo, S.-V., Leung, P.-Y., Tsang, T., Ho, W., Lee, K.-H., Lau, E.M.C., Ferguson, N.M., Anderson, R.M. (2003). 'Transmission dynamics of the etiological agent of SARS in Hong Kong: impact of public health interventions.' *Science*, 300, 1961–6. [6.2]

Roeder, P.L. (2011). 'Rinderpest: the end of cattle plague.' *Preventive Veterinary Medicine*, 102, 98–106. [5.1]

Ross, R. (1911). *The Prevention of Malaria*. London: John Murray. [6.2]

Rothenberg, G. (1973). 'The Austrian sanitary cordon and the control of the bubonic plague: 1710–1871.' *Journal of the History of Medicine and Allied Sciences*, 28, 15–23. [1.2]

Rothstein, M.A., Alcalde, M.G., Majumder, M.A., Palmer, L.I., Stone, T.H., Hoffman, R.E. (2003). *Quarantine and Isolation: Lessons Learned from SARS*. Louisville, Kentucky: University of Louisville School of Medicine, Institute for Bioethics, Health Policy and Law. Report to the Centers for Disease Control and Prevention, Atlanta. [3.4]

Rudnick, S.N., Milton, D.K. (2003). 'Risk of indoor airborne infection transmission estimated from carbon dioxide concentration.' *Indoor Air*, 13, 237–45. [6.2]

Salierno, V. (2010). *Il Mediterraneo nella Cartografia Ottomana (Coste, Porti, Isole Negli Atlanti di Piri Reis)*. Lecce: Capone Editore. [1.4]

Salk, D., Salk, J. (1984). 'Vaccinology of poliomyelitis: a review.' *Vaccine*, 2, 59–74. [Appendix 4.1]

Sattenspiel, L., Herring, D.A. (2003). 'Simulating the effect of quarantine on the spread of the 1918–19 flu in central Canada.' *Bulletin of Mathematical Biology*, 65, 1–26. [3.4]

Savage, E., Ramsay, M., White, J., Beard, S., Lawson, H., Hunjan, R., Brown, D. (2005). 'Mumps outbreaks across England and Wales in 2004: observational study.' *British Medical Journal*, 330, 1119–20. [4.6]

Savage, E., White, J.M., Brown, D.E.W., Ramsay, M.E. (2006). 'Mumps epidemic – United Kingdom, 2004–2005.' *Morbidity and Mortality Weekly Report*, 55, 173–5. [4.6]

Schleisner, P.A. (1851). 'Vital statistics of Iceland.' *Quarterly Journal of the Statistical Society of London*, 14, 1–10. [6.3]

Schonberger, L.B., Kaplan, J., Kim-Farley, R., Moore, M., Eddins, D.L., Hatch, M. (1984). 'Control of paralytic poliomyelitis in the United States.' *Reviews of Infectious Diseases*, 6 (suppl. 2), S424–6. [4.5]

Scott, S., Duncan, C.J. (2001). *Biology of Plagues: Evidence from Historical Populations*. Cambridge: Cambridge University Press. [1.2]

Sehdev, P.S. (2002). 'The origin of quarantine.' *Clinical Infectious Diseases*, 35, 1071–2. [1.2]

Sharma, V.P. (1996). 'Re-emergence of malaria in India.' *Indian Journal of Medical Research*, 103, 26–45. [5.4]

Sharp, F.R., Lotka, A.J. (1911). 'A problem in age distribution.' *Philosophical Magazine*, 6, 435–8. [6.2]

Simpson, J.Y. (1868). 'Proposal to stamp out smallpox etc.' *Medical Times and Gazette*, 5–6, 32–3. [3.3]

Simpson, W.J. (1905). *A Treatise on Plague, Dealing with the Historical, Epidemiological, Clinical, Therapeutic and Preventive Aspects of the Disease*. Cambridge: Cambridge University Press. [1.2]

Slack, P. (1985). *The Impact of Plague in Tudor and Stuart England*. London: Routledge and Kegan Paul. [3.3]

Smallman-Raynor, M., Cliff, A.D., Trevelyan, B., Nettleton, C., Sneddon, S. (2006). *Poliomyelitis. A World Geography: Emergence to Eradication*. Oxford: Oxford University Press. [4.5, 4.6, 5.3, 6.3]

Smallman-Raynor, M.R., Cliff, A.D. (2004). *War Epidemics: An Historical Geography of Infectious Diseases in Military Conflict and Civil Strife*. Oxford: Oxford University Press. [3.3, 5.6, 6.2, 6.3]

Smallman-Raynor, M.R., Cliff, A.D. (2012). *Atlas of Epidemic Britain: A Twentieth Century Picture*. Oxford: Oxford University Press. [1.4, 3.2, 3.3, 4.6, 5.6]

Smallman-Raynor, M.R., Cliff, A.D. (2013). 'Abrupt transition to heightened poliomyelitis epidemicity in England and Wales, 1947–57, associated with a profound shift in the geographical rate of disease propagation'. In review. [Appendix 6.1]

Smallman-Raynor, M.R., Johnson, N., Cliff, A.D. (2002). 'The spatial anatomy of an epidemic: influenza in London and the county boroughs of England and Wales, 1918–19.' *Transactions of the Institute of British Geographers, New Series*, 27, 452–70. [6.2]

Soper, G. (1907). 'The work of a chronic typhoid germ distributor.' *Journal of the American Medical Association*, 48, 2019–22. [3.3]

Soper, G. (1919). 'Typhoid Mary.' *The Military Surgeon*, 45, 1–15. [3.3]

Soper, G. (1939). 'The curious career of Typhoid Mary.' *Bulletin of the New York Academy of Medicine*, 15, 698–712. [3.3]

Sprengell, C. (1727). 'A farther account of the Bills of Mortality, &c. of several considerable towns in Europe, for the years 1722 and 1723, extracted from the *Acta Breslaviensia*.' *Philosophical Transactions*, 35, 365–74. [2.3]

Stanwell-Smith, R. (1996). 'Immunization: celebrating the past and injecting the future.' *Journal of the Royal Society of Medicine*, 80, 509–13. [5.1]

Stegeman, A., Bouma, A., Elbers, A.R., de Jong, M.C., Nodelijk, G., de Klerk, F., Koch, G., van Boven, M. (2004). 'Avian influenza A virus (H7N7) epidemic in The Netherlands in 2003: course of the epidemic and effectiveness of control measures.' *Journal of Infectious Diseases*, 190, 2088–95. [6.2]

Strebel, P.M., Sutter, R.W., Cochi, S.L., Biellik, R.J., Brink, E.W., Kew, O.M., Pallansch, M.A., Orenstein, W.A., Hinman, A.R. (1992). 'Epidemiology of poliomyelitis in the United States one decade after the last reported case of indigenous wild virus-associated disease.' *Clinical Infectious Diseases*, 14, 568–79. [4.5]

Stroup, D.F., Brookmeyer, R., Kalsbeek, W.D. (2003). 'Public health surveillance in action: a framework.' In: R. Brookmeyer & D.F. Stroup (eds.), *Monitoring the Health of Populations: Statistical Principles and Methods for Public Health Surveillance*. New York: Oxford University Press, 1–36. [2.9]

Stroup, D.F., Thacker, S.B. (2007). 'Epidemic Aid investigations (Epi-Aids), the teenage years: 1956–1965.' *EIS Bulletin*, Special Conference Issue. Atlanta: CDC, 12–18. [2.4]

Stuard, S.M. (1973). 'A communal program of medical care: medieval Ragusa/Dubrovnik.' *Journal of the History of Medicine and Allied Sciences*, 28, 126–42. [1.2]

Sutter, R.W., Cáceres, V.M., Lago, P.M. (2004). 'The role of routine polio immunization in the post-certification era.' *Bulletin of the World Health Organization*, 82, 31–9. [5.6]

Sutter, R.W., Markowitz, S.E., Bennetch, J.M., Morris, W., Zell, E.R., Preblud, S.R. (1991). 'Measles among the Amish: a comparative study in primary and secondary cases in households.' *Journal of Infectious Diseases*, 163, 12–16. [4.6]

Szucs, T. (2000). 'Cost-benefits of vaccination programmes.' *Vaccine*, 18 (suppl. 1), S49–51. [4.5]

Tangermann, R.H., Hull, H.F., Jafari, H., Nkowane, B., Everts, H., Aylward, R.B. (2000). 'Eradication of poliomyelitis in countries affected by conflict.' *Bulletin of the World Health Organization*, 78, 330–8. [5.3]

Tatham, J. (1888). 'On extension of the system of notification of infectious disease, with especial reference to a proposed national system of disease registration.' *British Medical Journal*, 2, 402–4. [1.1]

Thacker, S.B. (2010). 'Historical development.' In: L.M. Lee, S.M. Teutsch, S.B. Thacker & M.E. St. Louis (eds.), *Principles and Practice of Public Health Surveillance* (third edition). New York: Oxford University Press, 1–17. [2.3]

Thacker, S.B., Berkelman, R.L. (1988). 'Public health surveillance in the United States.' *Epidemiologic Reviews*, 10, 164–90. [2.4]

Thacker, S.B., Dannenberg, A.L., Hamilton, D.H. (2001). 'Epidemic Intelligence Service of the Centers for Disease Control and Prevention: 50 years of training and service in applied epidemiology.' *American Journal of Epidemiology*, 154, 985–92. [2.4]

Thacker, S.B., Stroup, D.F. (2007a). 'Epidemic Aid investigations, 1946–1955.' *EIS Bulletin*, March issue. Atlanta: CDC, 34–44. [2.4]

Thacker, S.B., Stroup, D.F. (2007b). 'Epidemic Aid investigations, the third decade: 1966–1975.' *EIS e-Bulletin*, Vol. e2, Issue e3 (June). Atlanta: CDC. [2.4]

Thacker, S.B., Stroup, D.F. (2008). 'Epidemic Aid investigations, the fourth decade: 1976–1985.' *EIS e-Bulletin*, Vol. e3, Issue e1 (March). Atlanta: CDC. [2.4]

Thacker, S.B., Stroup, D.F., Sencer, D.J. (2011). 'Epidemic assistance by the Centers for Disease Control and Prevention: role of the Epidemic Intelligence Service, 1946–2005.' *American Journal of Epidemiology*, 174 (suppl.), S4–15. [2.4]

Thompson, K.M., Duintjer Tebbens, R.J. (2006). 'Retrospective cost-effectiveness analyses for polio vaccination in the United States.' *Risk Analysis*, 26, 1423–40. [4.5]

Tinline, R.R. (1972). *A Simulation Study of the 1967–68 Foot-and-Mouth Epizootic in Great Britain*. Unpublished D.Phil dissertation. Department of Geography, University of Bristol, UK. [4.3]

Tobler, W.R. (1970). 'A computer movie simulating urban growth in the Detroit region.' *Economic Geography*, 46 (supplement), 234–40. [6.3]

Trail, R.R. (1961). 'Papworth and Enham-Alamein Village Settlements.' *Diseases of theChest*, 40, 381–5. [3.3]

Trevelyan, B., Smallman-Raynor, M.R., Cliff, A.D. (2005). 'The spatial dynamics of poliomyelitis in the United States: emergence to vaccine-induced retreat, 1910–1971.' *Annals of the Association of American Geographers*, 95, 269–93. [6.3]

Trigg, P.I., Kondrachine, A.V. (1998). 'Malaria control in the 1990s.' *Bulletin of the World Health Organization*, 76, 11–16. [5.4]

Uemura, K. (1988). 'World health situation and trend assessment from 1948 to 1988.' *Bulletin of the World Health Organization*, 66, 679–87. [2.7]

US Department of Health and Human Services (2005). *Pandemic Influenza Plan*. Washington, D.C.: Department of Health and Human Services (available at: http://www.hhs.gov/pandemicflu/plan; last viewed: 27 February 2012). [3.4]

US Department of Health and Human Services (2007). *Interim Pre-pandemic Planning Guidance: Community Strategy for Pandemic Influenza Mitigation in the United States – Early, Targeted, Layered Use of Non-pharmaceutical Intervention*. Washington, D.C.: Department of Health and Human Services. [3.4]

US Department of State (1889). *Register of the Department of State Corrected to December 1, 1888*. Washington, D.C.: Government Printing Office. [3.2]

US Department of the Treasury (1875). *Cholera Epidemic of 1873 in the United States*. Washington, D.C.: Government Printing Office. [3.2]

van den Bosch, F., Metz, J.A.J., Diekmann, O. (1990). 'The velocity of spatial population expansion.' *Journal of Mathematical Biology*, 28, 529–65. [6.4]

Varrier-Jones, P. (1935). 'Papworth Village Settlement: its history and aims.' *Chest*, 1, 8–21. [3.3]

Viboud, C., Grais, R.F., Lafont, B.A., Miller, M.A., Simonsen, L. (2005). 'Multinational impact of the 1968 Hong Kong influenza pandemic: evidence for a smoldering pandemic.' *Journal of Infectious Diseases*, 192, 233–48. [6.3]

Vynnycky, E., Trindall, A., Mangtani, P. (2007). 'Estimates of the reproduction numbers of Spanish influenza using morbidity data.' *International Journal of Epidemiology*, 36, 881–9. [6.2]

Walford, C. (1878). 'Early bills of mortality.' *Transactions of the Royal History Society*, 7, 212–48. [2.3]

Weinberger, D.M., Krause, T.G., Mølbak, K., Cliff, A., Briem, H., Viboud, C., Gottfredsson, M. (2012). 'Influenza epidemics in Iceland over nine decades: changes in timing and synchrony with the United States and Europe.' *Emerging Infectious Diseases* (forthcoming). [6.4]

Whaley, F. (2006). 'Flight CA112: facing the spectre of in-flight transmission.' In: S. Omi (ed.), *SARS: How a Global Epidemic was Stopped*. Manila: WHO Western Pacific Region, 149–54. [3.4]

WHO Vaccines, Immunization and Biologicals (2005). *Statistics and Graphs*. Geneva: World Health Organization. [4.6]

WHO Western Pacific Region (2008). *Western Pacific Regional Strategy for Increasing Access to and Utilization of New and Underutilized Vaccines*. Manila: WHO Regional Office for the Western Pacific. [4.4]

Williams, R.C. (1951). *The United States Public Health Service, 1798–1950*. Washington, D.C.: Commissioned Officers of the United States Public Health Service. [3.2]

Winslow, O.E. (1974). *A Destroying Angel: The Conquest of Smallpox in Colonial Boston*. Boston: Houghton-Mifflin. [4.2]

Wolfson, L.J., Gasse, F., Lee-Martin, S.-P., Lydon, P., Magan, A., Tibouti, A., Johns, B., Hutubessy, R., Salama, P., Okwo-Beled, J.-M. (2008). 'Estimating the costs of achieving the WHO–UNICEF Global Immunization Vision and Strategy, 2006–2015.' *Bulletin of the World Health Organization*, 86, 27–39. [6.5]

Wonham, M.J., de-Camino-Beek, T., Lewis, M.A. (2004). 'An epidemiological model for West Nile virus: invasion analysis and control applications.' *Proceedings of the Royal Society B*, 271, 501–7. [6.2]

Wood, W. (1865). *The History and Antiquities of Eyam; with a Minute Account of the Great Plague, which Desolated that Village in the Year 1666* (fourth edition). London: Bell and Daldy. Reprinted 2006, Little Longstone: Country Books/Ashridge Press. [3.3]

Woolhouse, M.E.J., Anderson, R.M. (1997). 'Understanding the epidemiology of BSE.' *Trends in Microbiology*, 5, 421–4. [6.2]

World Health Organization (1958). *The First Ten Years of the World Health Organization*. Geneva: World Health Organization. [2.5, 2.6, 2.7, 3.2]

World Health Organization (1968). *The Second Ten Years of the World Health Organization, 1958–1967*. Geneva: World Health Organization. [2.7]

World Health Organization (1978). 'Poliomyelitis surveillance – Canada.' *Weekly Epidemiological Record*, 53, 259. [4.5]

World Health Organization (1988). *41st World Health Assembly. WA41/1988/REC/1: Resolutions and Decisions. Annexes*. Geneva: World Health Organization. [5.3]

World Health Organization (1997). *Polio: The Beginning of the End*. Geneva: World Health Organization. [5.3]

World Health Organization (1998a). 'Expanded Programme on Immunization (EPI): progress towards poliomyelitis eradication in Africa, 1997.' *Weekly Epidemiological Record*, 73, 97–101. [4.6]

World Health Organization (1998b). 'Acute flaccid paralysis (AFP) surveillance: the surveillance strategy for poliomyelitis eradication.' *Weekly Epidemiological Record*, 73, 113–17. [2.7]

World Health Organization (2000a). 'Global laboratory network for poliomyelitis eradication 1997–1999: development and expanding contributions.' *Weekly Epidemiological Record*, 75, 70–5. [2.7]

World Health Organization (2000b). 'Ebola strikes Uganda.' *Action Against Infection*, 3, 3. [3.3]

World Health Organization (2003). *Report of the Eighth Meeting of the Technical Consultative Group (TCG) on the Global Eradication of Poliomyelitis, Geneva, 24–25 April 2003* (WHO/V&B/03.13). Geneva: World Health Organization. [5.3]

World Health Organization (2004a). 'Progress towards poliomyelitis eradication in Nigeria, January 2003–March 2004.' *Weekly Epidemiological Record*, 79, 162–7. [4.6]

World Health Organization (2004b). 'Wild poliovirus importations in west and central Africa, January 2003–March 2004.' *Weekly Epidemiological Record*, 79, 206–10. [4.6]

World Health Organization (2004c). 'Progress towards global eradication of poliomyelitis, 2003 and January–April 2004.' *Weekly Epidemiological Record*, 79, 229–34. [4.6]

World Health Organization (2004d). 'Global Polio Eradication Initiative – recent developments in polio eradication in Nigeria.' *Weekly Epidemiological Record*, 79, 289. [4.6]

World Health Organization (2004e). *Public Health Response to Biological and Chemical Weapons: WHO Guidance*. Geneva: World Health Organization. [5.6]

World Health Organization (2004f). *World Health Report*. Geneva: World Health Organization. [6.5]

World Health Organization (2005a). *GIVS: Global Immunization Vision and Strategy 2006–2015*. Geneva: World Health Organization. [4.4]

World Health Organization (2005b). 'Poliomyelitis outbreak escalates in the Sudan: case from Sudan reported in Saudi Arabia.' *Weekly Epidemiological Record*, 80, 2–3. [4.6]

World Health Organization (2005c). 'Progress towards poliomyelitis eradication – poliomyelitis outbreak in Sudan, 2004.' *Weekly Epidemiological Record*, 80, 42–6. [4.6]

World Health Organization (2005d). 'Poliomyelitis outbreak spreads across Yemen; case confirmed in Indonesia.' *Weekly Epidemiological Record*, 80, 157–8. [4.6]

World Health Organization (2005e). *Global Outbreak Alert and Response Network: Worldwide Distribution of GOARN Partner Institutions and Networks*. Geneva: World Health Organization. [2.7]

World Health Organization (2005f). *Summary of Probable SARS Cases with Onset of Illness from 1 November 2002 to 31 July 2003*. Geneva: World Health Organization. [3.4]

World Health Organization (2006). *Constitution of the World Health Organization*. Geneva: World Health Organization. [2.7]

World Health Organization (2007). *Putting People and Health Needs on the Map*. Geneva: World Health Organization. [2.8]

World Health Organization (2008a). *The Third Ten Years of the World Health Organization, 1968–1977*. Geneva: World Health Organization. [2.7]

World Health Organization (2008b). *International Health Regulations (2005)* (second edition). Geneva: World Health Organization. [3.2]

World Health Organization (2010a). *WHO Vaccine-Preventable Diseases: Monitoring System. 2010 Global Summary*. Geneva: WHO Immunization, Vaccines and Biologicals. [4.4]

World Health Organization (2010b). *Global Eradication of Measles: Report by the Secretariat*. Sixty-Third World Health Assembly, A63/18. Geneva: World Health Organization. [5.1, 5.5]

World Health Organization (2011a). *History of the Development of the ICD*. Geneva: World Health Organization. [2.2]

World Health Organization (2011b). 'Second meeting of the GPEI Independent Monitoring Board.' *Weekly Epidemiological Record*, 86, 177–9. [5.3]

World Health Organization (2011c). 'Progress towards eradicating poliomyelitis – Nigeria, January 2010–June 2011.' *Weekly Epidemiological Record*, 86, 356–63. [4.6]

World Health Organization (2011d). 'Fourth meeting of the Global Polio Eradication Initiative's Independent Monitoring Board.' *Weekly Epidemiological Record*, 86, 557–8. [5.3]

World Health Organization (2011e). *World Malaria Report 2011*. Geneva: World Health Organization. [5.4]

World Health Organization (2012). *Accelerating Work to Overcome the Global Impact of Neglected Tropical Diseases: A Roadmap for Implementation. Executive Summary*. Geneva: World Health Organization. [Preface]

Wright, J.W., Fritz, R.F., Haworth, J. (1972). 'Changing concepts of vector control in malaria eradication.' *Annual Review of Entomology*, 17, 75–102. [5.4]

Wrigley, E.A., Schofield, R.S. (1981). *The Population History of England, 1541–1871: A Reconstruction*. London: Edward Arnold. [3.3]

Yach, D. (1998). 'Telecommunications for health – new opportunities for action.' *Health Promotion International*, 13, 339–47. [2.6]

Yorke, J.A., Nathanson, N., Pianigiani, G., Martin, J. (1979). 'Seasonality and the requirements for perpetuation and eradication of viruses in populations.' *American Journal of Epidemiology*, 109, 103–22. [4.3]

Zanetti, D.E. (1976). 'La morte a Milano nei secoli XVI-XVII. Apunti per una ricerca.' *Revista Storica Italiana*, 87, 803–51. [1.2]

Zhou, F., Reef, S., Massoudi, M., Papania, M.J., Yusuf, H.R., Bardenheier, B., Zimmerman, L., McCauley, M.M. (2004). 'An economic analysis of the current universal 2-dose measles-mumps-rubella vaccination program in the United States.' *Journal of Infectious Diseases*, 189 (suppl. 1), S131–45. [4.5]

Zinsser, H. (1935). *Rats, Lice and History*. London: Routledge. [3.3]

Index

Note: Figure numbers in italics refer to colour plates in the colour section.